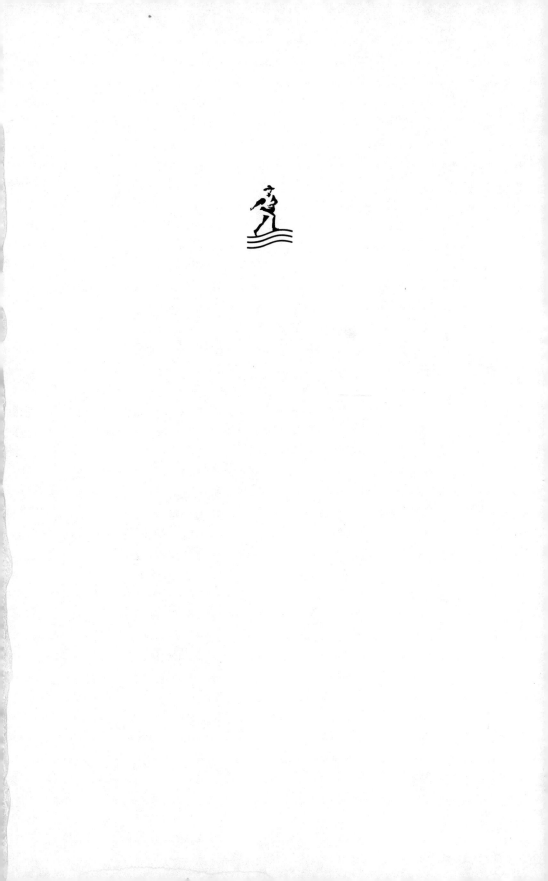

Immortal Bird

A Family Memoir

DORON WEBER

Simon & Schuster

NEW YORK LONDON TORONTO SYDNEY NEW DELHI

Simon & Schuster
1230 Avenue of the Americas
New York, NY 10020

First Simon & Schuster hardcover edition February 2012

SIMON & SCHUSTER and colophon are
registered trademarks of Simon & Schuster, Inc.

For information about special discounts for bulk purchases,
please contact Simon & Schuster Special Sales at 1-866-506-1949
or business@simonandschuster.com.

The Simon & Schuster Speakers Bureau can bring authors to your live event.
For more information or to book an event
contact the Simon & Schuster Speakers Bureau at 1-866-248-3049
or visit our website at www.simonspeakers.com.

Designed by Ruth Lee-Mui

Manufactured in the United States of America

1   3   5   7   9   10   8   6   4   2

Library of Congress Cataloging-in-Publication Data
Weber, Doron.
Immortal bird : a family memoir / Doron Weber. — 1st Simon & Schuster hardcover ed.
p. cm.
1. Weber, Damon, 1988–2005 — Health. 2. Congenital heart disease in children — Patients —
New York (State) — Biography. 3. Heart — Transplantation — Patients — New York (State) —
Biography. 4. Heart — Transplantation — Complications — New York (State) I. Title.
RJ426.C64W43 2012
362.198'921280092 — dc22
[B]   2011011481

ISBN 978-1-4516-1806-8
ISBN 978-1-4516-1808-2 (ebook)

For Sam and Miranda, two ineffably brave, beautiful beings whose appearance in these pages is perforce brief but whose blessed presence in my life—all days past, present, and future—is a source of perpetual joy, infinite pride, and the profoundest gratitude and love.

For Shealagh Alison Macleod De Beurges Rosenthal Weber, my co-creator and full partner in the miracle of Damon, Sam, and Miranda and for a quarter century the love of my life.

For Robert and Helga, beloved parents, dear friends and fellow travelers, and true keepers of the faith, who always have been, and always will be, with me.

Thou wast not born for death, Immortal Bird!
No hungry generations tread thee down;
The voice I hear this passing night was heard
In ancient days by emperor and clown:
Perhaps the self-same song that found a path
Through the sad heart of Ruth, when, sick for home,
She stood in tears amid the alien corn;
The same that ofttimes hath
Charm'd magic casements, opening on the foam
Of perilous seas, in faery lands forlorn.

—From "Ode to a Nightingale"
by John Keats (1795–1821)

Part I

Part 1

Chapter 1

I am walking up Prospect Avenue with my twelve-year-old son, striding side by side along the mottled sidewalk, when it strikes me he has not grown for a while. I look across at him. Damon's head—that flame-red, leonine head—still falls below my shoulders, roughly where it had reached the previous year. He is so vital and engaging one easily forgets his size. But now his clipped stature feels like a withholding of fruition, as if his legs were young shoots held back by a clinging, invisible vine. I want to reach down and cut him loose so he can sprout. I don't want a big change but I feel he needs a little nudge, one more click to get him over the next hump of development.

"So how was school?" I ask. Damon wears baggy jeans, a gray hooded sweatshirt, and Adidas sneakers, with a Walkman round his neck and a cell phone on his belt loop.

"Good. I got picked to read my essay for Kick Butts day." He speeds up as we talk, swinging his arms to keep up with me, and explains that Hillary Clinton, now running for a Senate seat, is part of the visiting delegation for this stop-smoking educational campaign.

"Congrats." I salute him. "Need any help with the essay?"

"I'll do a draft and show you," Damon says. We stop at Venus Video and select a musical for his audition. "Can Jon sleep over Saturday?" he asks.

"If you get your work done, I don't see why not." I pay for the rental.

"Yes! Thanks, Dad!" Damon smiles as we exit, his cerulean eyes dancing with open vistas. But as we continue strolling up the avenue, I again ponder his unsprung height.

He is due for a growth spurt—he is overdue—and I don't need a tape measure or a doctor to verify my judgment. I can always gauge the slightest change in his body, to a hair's breadth, and I have a built-in monitor of his progress embedded deep inside me, like a microchip—or is it a mirror? If we are not exactly joined at the hip, we have more than the usual father-son bond connecting us.

Damon is the oldest of our three children. Born on 8/8/88—a date so fortuitous that in China they performed premature Caesarians to snag this birthday—he was an only child for nearly five years before his brother, Sam, arrived. For most of this time, he also was a sick child who required, and received, extraordinary love and attention from his mother, Shealagh, and from me. Even after his sister, Miranda, appeared in 1995, a healthier Damon remained the focus of our family, the pacesetter.

He was born with a malformed heart, for no known reason.

Most notably, Damon lacks a second ventricle like you and I have. His good ventricle, the left, pumps red, oxygen-rich blood throughout his body. But when the blood returns from his body to the lower right chamber of his heart—blue blood now because it has given up its oxygen—there is no second ventricle to pump it back into the lungs, where it can pick up fresh oxygen and expel carbon dioxide. So Damon was a "blue baby" whose organs and tissues did not get enough oxygen. He was smaller and weaker than other infants and his gross motor skills developed more slowly. But his brain, his manual and verbal dexterity, and his imagination never lagged.

By age four, Damon had undergone two open-heart surgeries, and the second operation, known as a modified Fontan, alleviated his problem. A "passive flow" system, it bypasses his right side altogether and shunts the returning blue blood directly to his lungs, where it can take on vital oxygen and discharge carbon dioxide.

After the modified Fontan, Damon's body received sufficient oxygen-rich blood, and he flourished.

He grew and scrambled back onto the growth charts for height and weight, even catching up to some of his friends. His color improved, his energy increased, and he became physically more active. He is a tortoise, not a hare, but he is intrepid and takes delight in activity of all kinds, from karate and kayaking to soccer and skiing.

Damon is in seventh grade now, attending the Salk School of Science in Manhattan, where he excels academically. He also is an actor who performs in every school play and then in more advanced theater workshops outside school. And he's become increasingly popular in middle school, more of a star than he's ever been. When he spiffs up his unruly red hair and dons a dress shirt for the school dance, cruising the room like a confident young blade, he makes an impression. He outshines the taller boys because he actually dances and *talks* to the girls.

Damon is never going to be the biggest kid in the class or run a four-minute mile, but otherwise he's in great shape. He's been healthy for the eight years since his last operation and free of all medications. He sees his cardiologist every six months and she marvels at his progress.

I am keenly aware of all this as we walk together this afternoon. We have lived through a protracted nightmare and survived to talk about it as a page from history, a backstory. I know all about patience and keeping your eye on the fundamentals. Shealagh and I have our own set of milestones for Damon, outside the standard configuration, and we feel inordinately proud of his advancement and the kind of person he's become.

So on this early fall day of the first year of the new millennium, with the soft yellow leaves raining down from the sky and starting to blur the margins of the pavement, I dismiss my concerns as exaggerated, a common defensive ploy to contemplate the worst, just so you can say it ain't so.

We turn into the wide embrace of Terrace Place, with the great park at one end, and walk up the front porch into our two-story brick house with its long driveway and small backyard that boasts a bona fide peach tree and a fig tree, our own patch of Eden.

Chapter 2

A perfect spring evening at Yankee Stadium. The air is warm, with the slightest breeze ruffling the flag. The baselines and foul lines are stamped in fresh white chalk.

I have taken Damon and two of his closest friends, Kyle and Keith, to a night game against the Boston Red Sox. The stadium is packed, the fight songs blaring and the beer flowing, as befits these longtime archrivals. But the three teens don't really care. They enjoy the aesthetics and ambience of the game as much as the competition.

"Check out the body-paint dudes!" Keith points at the bleachers, where seven rowdy males spell "Go Yanks!" in bold lettering across bare torsos.

"I think they're drunk." Kyle wrinkles her nose at the beefy, soft-bellied roisterers.

"Man with crazy chef's hat, six o'clock!" Damon gestures three rows ahead, where a fan sits in a billowing, brimless white hat. "The Mad Hatter is blocking the view—"

"It's called a toque." Kyle corrects Damon with her sweet Natalie Portman smile.

"Duh, I think it's a mascot for Sheffield—he's 'the Chef,'" Keith interjects, correcting Kyle.

"Really? Whatever . . ." Kyle giggles as she takes in the information.

"Hey, Dad, can we get Cracker Jacks? Kyle needs brain food."

Kyle is Damon's oldest and closest friend, a girl he rescued in kindergarten when the school bus dropped her off at the wrong stop. They are the same age but Damon is a grade ahead, which makes him the sage elder. Now almost thirteen, Kyle changes her hair color every week—today it's purple with blond streaks—and she wears bangles and bracelets and layers of colorful clothing. She is bright, vital, and quite beautiful, but her identity shifts like a kaleidoscope, with a propensity toward the darker hues.

The Cracker Jacks arrive in a giant box and Kyle and Keith dive in looking for the prize. "If it's a ring, it's mine!" Keith smiles.

Keith is a tall, wiry African American, wry, sensitive, and hyperarticulate. He and Damon attend Salk together. Handsome and fine-featured, like a model, Keith lives alone with his young single mother in Harlem and spends weekends with his grandmother in Queens.

"Okay, guys, we need to root for the Yankees," Damon announces late in the game. "I think they're losing"—he checks the scoreboard—"and we don't want my dad to go home unhappy."

And indeed, after eight lackluster innings, the Yanks rally and pull out the game with two home runs in the bottom of the ninth. The stadium erupts. Damon and I exchange excited high fives, connecting in the moment's primitive ecstasy. Although not a committed fan, Damon appreciates raw emotion and the thrill of the come-from-behind. And he is impressed by my militant cheerleading for someone other than him. As he embraces Kyle in the pandemonium, I note he looks a little hamstrung, as if nursing an injury.

I wonder if it's the aftereffects of his "fight." Five weeks earlier, Damon came home from school with deep cuts and a grapefruit-sized swelling across his forehead. He'd gotten into an altercation with the school bully, a humongous lout twice his size.

"This kid kept shoving me and trying to get in my face," Damon explained. "He bumped me with his chest: 'Come on, little guy, fight me!'" I told him I wasn't afraid of him but I didn't want to fight, so I started to walk away when he rushed me from behind and smashed my head against the cafeteria table. I never saw him coming."

Damon sustained contusions, a hematoma, and a concussion. Head injuries even in healthy people are notoriously complex, as both Shealagh and I know: Shealagh did research on war veterans with head wounds at the Radcliffe Infirmary Neuropsychology Unit at Oxford, where we met, and I boxed for Oxford University and learned about concussions firsthand. We kept Damon at home while I initiated disciplinary action against his attacker, a notorious troublemaker, and made sure this could never happen again.

Damon appeared physically traumatized yet stubbornly proud, incised with fresh, deep wounds he's worn since like a badge of honor. He recovered, and his standing up to the class bully only enhanced his status in school as a leader. But the incident forced me to confront his vulnerability, and my own possible complicity in it. I had always taught Damon to stand up for himself and to hold his ground. But now I felt torn between a father's pride at his son's courage and concern that Damon not follow my example too closely, because he lacks the physical resources to defend himself. I quickly realized, however, that any cautionary advice at this stage was futile because Damon's character had long been formed. All I could do was hug my brave-hearted bantamweight while privately resolving to watch him like a hawk.

We return from Yankee Stadium in high spirits, dropping Keith off in Harlem and Kyle in Ditmas Park. Shealagh, waiting up, gets a full report from her beaming son as we sit in the downstairs kitchen. Damon even eats his mother's rhubarb pie as he fills her in on the triumphant game.

It's been a good day. But now it's late and there's school tomorrow, so Damon moseys up to the middle floor, where he and Sam have adjacent bedrooms. Shealagh goes to talk to him and get a little private time—mother and son have their own very special bond—before she kisses him good night and leaves.

As I pass through on my way to the top floor, Damon cracks the bathroom door and calls to me from the doorway. "Hey, Dad, can you come here a minute?"

I can sense something amiss as I head to the bathroom. Normally Damon asks his mother about routine matters and saves me for the big stuff.

As I walk inside, Damon closes the bathroom door with mysterious urgency. I feel the burden of a pending revelation and brace myself.

"I wanted to show you this, Dad . . ."

Damon pulls down his pants and lowers his boxers under the overhead bulb.

"Oh man!" I shake my head. "What happened?" His testicles hang down, hugely swollen. They look four times their normal size. He's a young kid and I am all for his sexual development, but this is alarming. "When did . . . ?"

"I noticed it Friday but thought I should wait a day. But it hasn't gotten better."

"Poor guy . . . Does it hurt, D-man?"

He hesitates. "It's uncomfortable." Damon has experienced real pain and never exaggerates about such matters. "And it's kinda awkward, you know—"

"Sure. Okay, this isn't right and we're going to take care of it. Pronto!"

I talk to Shealagh, then call a few doctor friends. Two scenarios emerge. A hernia, the most likely, or a twisted testicle, rarer and more urgent. And given Damon's history, there's always an extra element of uncertainty and fear.

We decide not to risk waiting until morning and call my parents to come over and babysit Sam and Miranda before we speed off to Columbia Presbyterian Hospital, which has treated Damon since shortly after his birth. It's a long drive, but Columbia knows his complex case and we trust them. It's past midnight when we reach the sprawling medical complex in Washington Heights.

Eons ago, we did hard time in this hospital and feared we'd never escape. Once, when he weighed only eleven pounds, Damon spent thirty days in the ICU, trying to come off the respirator. Now as we arrive, the dread memories rise up.

We walk past ambulances, EMT personnel, and two burly cops and enter into the perpetual twilight zone of the emergency room, a cacophony of coughing, moaning, shouting, and crying. We pick our way through the tumult and despair and request immediate care for our son. Damon's cardiologist, Dr. Hayes, has called ahead and told them to expect us.

The admissions clerk nods, unimpressed, and gives us forms to fill out.

A well-organized unit, we establish ourselves on three plastic chairs. Shealagh distributes juice and snacks and fills out forms, I call home to check on the kids and gather intel from the staff, and Damon, after sweeping the room, disappears into his copy of *The Subtle Knife* by Philip Pullman.

Eventually an intake nurse admits us and we enter a more orderly if still-hectic space. Someone takes Damon's vitals and he gets a bed with a flimsy half curtain. We wait until a young resident pops by. He checks Damon's groin and instantly declares he has a hernia. A bona fide inguinal hernia, the gross rupture will need to be surgically repaired, but he finds no twisted testicle or undue cause for alarm.

I feel a measure of relief but continue talking to the doctor as he examines Damon. Because he is unfamiliar with my son's anatomy—Damon's heart is on the right side and several other organs are reversed—I fill him in while he asks questions and offers observations. I've long grasped that medicine is an imperfect art, fifty to a hundred years from being an exact science, so I gather information from every possible source. I've also learned that good doctors are not necessarily the senior people with fancy reputations—often quite the opposite—and a young resident, if he observes thoroughly and with an open mind, can tell me as much as anyone.

This resident—he has the gift; you can tell in the first thirty seconds—palpates Damon's abdomen and casually mentions his liver is enlarged, which I've never heard before. When I inquire further, he lets me feel how the liver presses against the abdomen, its margins extending beyond the normal range. Damon watches us with quiet, alert eyes, always the model patient, and I wonder if this enlarged liver could explain why his belly protrudes, giving him a slouching appearance. Even in karate class, with his *gi* neatly belted and his back erect, his stomach seems to slump forward, and zipped into a black wet suit for swimming, he looks paunchy despite his leanness.

Shealagh and I have questioned his cardiologist about this anomaly and we once dragged Damon to a chiropractor to try to sort it out. We exhort our son to stand up straight and pull his shoulders back. Now it strikes us a protruding liver could explain his posture more than any deficiency of spine or will. We feel a stab of guilt that we held Damon even partially responsible. Later, when we pursue the oversized liver with the chief of surgery, he says it is completely normal for children with Damon's heart condition and he sees it frequently. We wonder why no one ever told us this before.

We schedule the surgery promptly but try to minimize the disruption to Damon's life. He hates to miss school and has started rehearsal for *Charlie and the Chocolate Factory*.

Chapter 3

When the morning of his hernia operation dawns, we tell ourselves it is a routine procedure, but with Damon's medical history, nothing is routine. We envy all our friends who freak out over their kids' colds.

On the ride in, Damon and I discuss a new play I'm supporting with Alan Alda playing the Nobel Prize–winning physicist Richard Feynman. I work for a well-established philanthropic foundation and one of my roles is to help develop plays, films, and television shows with science and technology themes.

We arrive at the hospital, sign in, and go to the fourth-floor pediatrics ward.

The secretary makes several copies of our insurance and asks us to fill out the same form about Damon's medical history, several pages long, for the umpteenth time.

A nurse takes Damon's blood pressure and temperature, weighs and measures him, and exchanges his familiar jeans and T-shirt for a hospital gown that ties loosely at the back. A hearty, decent sort, she means well but her idea of small talk is to ask him three times if he's nervous. "A little," Damon says to mollify her.

Another nurse comes in to start an IV. Damon has pale, spidery veins and sticking him requires precision. After an initial adjustment, she gets the line in.

Then a young doctor, bright-eyed with self-importance, saunters in and beams at Damon. "Hi, I'm the resident. Have you ever had any serious medical conditions?"

At first, we think he's kidding, but he's not. Damon turns away, too polite to sneer, and Shealagh groans in disbelief. I fire off a rapid, testy medical summary. "Next time do your homework and read the chart!" I say. He slinks out of the room, red-faced.

We wait with other tense parents and their sick children until they send us to the preoperative holding area. A fountain of gurgling water, pink-lit, is meant to soothe our nerves. A tall doctor with a Hungarian accent walks in and mumbles that they want to put Damon under general anesthesia because a local injection could lower his blood pressure, and his pressure is already low. The anesthesiologist tries to rush our consent but we won't give it until he answers each of our questions and reviews all the options. General anesthesia carries a known risk of mortality, compounded, like everything else, in Damon's case, and we have learned not to take anything for granted.

The surgeon arrives in his scrubs and quickly runs through the procedure. An affable, highly competent man, he does not anticipate problems and wants to get started. We each ask questions, including Damon—"When can I go back to my karate class?"—before signaling that we are ready. The nurse releases the brakes on the gurney and the anesthesiologist, turning to follow the rolling bed, suggests we say our good-byes now.

"No," I tell him. "We always go into the operating room with our son. It's part of our routine." Damon watches us from the gurney, upset—we touch his arm to calm him—before the surgeon tells the anesthesiologist it's okay for us to accompany our son.

We quickly throw yellow moon suits over our clothes and don protective face masks before plodding down the corridor beside Damon's gurney like a team of sterilized astronauts. We turn and push through sealed doors into the operating theater.

It's a large, cool, brilliantly lit room with state-of-the-art medical equipment surrounded by a tinted observation booth. A lone bed rises in the center, with a giant stainless steel arm arcing above it. A modern setting for sacrifice and, hopefully, healing—a place for testing one's faith.

I tell myself it's not as dire this time—this is standard procedure for a hernia—but still, I can't believe we're going through this ordeal *again*.

I keep up a running banter with Damon as they wheel him into position and Shealagh chimes in with reassuring comments. Damon remains stoic and game throughout but he likes having us nearby. I want Mom and Dad to be the last thing he sees when he closes his eyes and the first when he opens them again.

Damon climbs onto the narrow steel bed and they immediately place a mask over his head and tell him to inhale. A team of nurses, doctors, and assistants attaches lines and sensors to Damon. They prick his finger with a needle and he says "ouch" through the mask, but then the nitrous oxide reaches his central nervous system and he begins to laugh. We watch his lips pull back over his large front teeth all the way to the gums as he giggles uncontrollably. His big face with the bright red hair and pale skin fills with induced mirth. Then he is out cold. An array of monitors reads live data input from his unconscious body. We kiss him one last time and leave the operating theater.

We sit in a common room with gray lockers and a coffeepot. We make our calls, try to read the paper, stare into space.

The wait that lasts an eternity.

At some point, the surgeon emerges and walks toward us. We scour his face and body language for clues to our son's fate. He reaches us and immediately says, "Everything's okay." So time begins again, and now we can listen to what he says.

It was a surprisingly big hernia that demanded more surgery than anticipated—"The hernia of the week," the surgeon confides with a trace of professional pride—but all is well now. We should see improvement within seventy-two hours. Damon will be sore for a few days but the rupture is repaired and the problem solved.

We thank the surgeon profusely, then go to the recovery room to see Damon.

"Hi, sweetie." Shealagh hugs Damon, who's groggy from the anesthesia.

"You did great, D-man." I kiss his brow and congratulate him. He smiles weakly.

We sit by the bedside, each of us holding one of his pale, slender hands. We feed him ice chips until he's permitted to drink.

The next morning we leave the hospital and take Damon home.

Everything seems to have gone well. Damon had a hernia, which any healthy person can get, and now it's fixed. There is no apparent connection to his underlying heart disease, nor any long-term ramification. He'll be back at school within a week and right as rain. We had a spot of bad luck but it's behind us now.

We try to reassure ourselves with this official prognosis but sense in our depths that something has changed, some seismic but as yet undetectable shift.

Something *has* changed, but we do not understand it yet.

Chapter 4

"Help, help me!"

I am jolted awake. It is early on a Saturday morning and somewhere in the house, Shealagh is screaming.

I leap out of bed and follow the trail of cries down the long staircase.

My wife hovers on the middle steps, bent over in agony.

Her back has seized up and she cannot move.

Shealagh has experienced back trouble for the past few years. A tall, robust young woman and a competitive athlete when we met—swimming, rowing, riding—she no longer competes but maintains a physically active life, so the worsening condition takes its toll.

She works three twelve-hour days a week as a therapist for the New York City Health and Hospitals Corporation, shuttling to a clinic in East New York, where she ministers to an underprivileged minority clientele. Meanwhile, she chauffeurs her three kids everywhere; kneels down with them over class projects; helps design and build sets and costumes, especially for Damon's theatricals; and cleans, cooks, shops, and gardens.

Now she's beginning to slow down, and it's not just from passing forty. She gets out of breath and uses an inhaler. Her afflicted back makes sitting at a desk for long periods untenable. Often, she must lie down in the middle of the day. She is less mobile and energetic and needs assistance with routine chores.

I pick up some slack and also get outside help. But I fret about this atypical lassitude in such a strong, vigorous person, and I worry about my wife.

One friend suggests it is partly psychological, a delayed result of Damon's illness and the stress surrounding those early years. Now that Damon is better and we have three wonderful kids, none of which came easily, now that our lives and careers are flourishing, the suppressed trauma of that period is returning for a full accounting.

I fear the worst when I find Shealagh frozen on the stairs this Saturday morning. She hangs on to the banister like a lifeline, paralyzed and sobbing in pain.

"I can't move!" she cries.

Slowly, with excruciating care, I maneuver Shealagh down the steps and into our car. We drive straight to the emergency room—the nearest one, in Brooklyn, this time.

Several long days, intrusive MRIs, and expert consults later, the consensus is that Shealagh requires back surgery. She has extrusion and disc herniation, with severe compression of the nerve root. She has lost some sensation and mobility in her left leg—she has minor "neurological deficit"—and the doctors don't want to risk more damage.

It is late July and we have planned our big August vacation on the Isle of Skye, our traditional retreat in the Scottish Hebrides. Shealagh will need four to six weeks of rest and rehab following the surgery, so Skye is out of the question for her. I'm beginning to feel like a professional caretaker and I'm ready to cancel all our plans so I can focus on Shealagh. My tenderhearted wife, the devoted mother of my three children and my dearest friend and confidante, she also is my secret sharer in the special project that is Damon. Our union has deep roots. On a more mundane level, Shealagh is Super Mom, whereas Dad, useful for schoolwork, sports, and outdoor adventure, mostly writes in the summer, so it's unclear how the kids would eat, dress, or sleep on clean sheets with *him* in charge.

But Shealagh does not want her children deprived of their big summer holiday and wonders if we can go on vacation without her. Maybe, too, she needs a break from us so she can concentrate on her rehabilitation and get some personal time. Her biggest concern is whether we four can survive with Dad as the sole parent, especially since I planned to do my summer writing in Skye. I assure her I'm up to the task and will defer the writing if I must. She should stop worrying about anything but her recovery.

Shealagh's spine surgery is considered elective but proves more harrowing than we expected, especially after our recent experience with Damon.

My wife lies sprawled on her side as they lift the back muscles off her spine and expose the nerve root, forcing aside the protective membrane so they can remove any obstructive disc matter. I sit alone in the hospital's designated waiting area and call my best friend, David, who lives in Seattle, to get my mind off the unthinkable.

Damon is very concerned about his mother's well-being but helps to divert Sam and Miranda, who stay with him at my parents' house. I phone him to provide updates. He talks to me from the room I slept in when I was his age and I feel like I'm talking to my younger self, only an improved version.

"So when will the surgery be over?" Damon asks pointedly. Responsibility comes naturally to him.

"Another hour or so. It's always longer than they say. This is routine, D-man."

"I know. Sam wanted to talk to Mom but I said she was sleeping."

"That's true, well done," I praise him. "So the little ones are okay?"

"Yeah. They're watching *Jungle Book* on the VCR and eating ice cream with Grandma and Granddad. Miranda's already asleep but Sam is being stubborn."

"He'll drop off soon . . . I'll call you when Mom's out of the OR. Okay?"

"Don't worry about me, Dad. Just watch over Mom's doctors like you watch over mine."

Shealagh's flashy, expensive surgeon shows up in the waiting room after the surgery wearing a tux. He says the patient is fine, he did his job, and now we must wait to see if they got all the disc material out—because of course you can never tell.

After the surgery, Shealagh invites her best friend, Sonja, who is single and mobile and also happens to be a doctor, to stay in our house through August. My wife wants us to go on holiday with a clear conscience. Sonja is a very kind, loyal, and super-efficient friend, so we couldn't leave Shealagh in better hands. Still, the kids and I all feel a pang, and not a few gnawing doubts, when, loaded with suitcases, backpacks, and wet suits, we set off for our summer vacation in Scotland without Mom.

Chapter 5

Damon assists me from the start of our motherless Hebridean sojourn, even before we've landed. He supervises Sam and Miranda on the airplane, escorting them to the toilet, refereeing card games, and showing them how to work the in-flight remote.

At Glasgow airport, he insists on pushing the second luggage cart, even when it proves unwieldy and spins around on him. On the winding drive through northwest Scotland, he entertains his younger siblings with stories. When they get cranky and fight, he adroitly applies the carrot and stick—"You want to hear what happened next? Then stop bickering!"—until they beg him to continue, promising peace treaties until the end of time.

My own exhortations to look out the window at the lochs, mountains, and medieval castles dotting the Scottish Highlands fall on deaf, jet-lagged ears. Nevertheless, the Isle of Skye casts its misty magic the instant we make landfall, and we are transported as we drive through the magnificent twisting Black Cuillin. Snowcaps gleam while lush vegetation flourishes—purple heather, yellow gorse, and red rowans dazzle our bleary eyes—and torpid sheep blithely cross the highway.

We drive toward Portree harbor, then veer off the highway, singing "Donald, Where's Your Troosers?" as we skirt the moors along a serpentine valley road. Across from us rises a broad, heather-clad mountain, Ben Tianavaig, which overlooks the cold blue bay that reputedly welcomed Bonnie Prince Charlie ashore in the eighteenth century.

We descend sharply into the tiny loch-lapped village of Camastianavaig and head for the White Cottage, a compact stone croft house with a slate roof. The somnolent village consists of about twenty houses with small plots and open grazing land dotted about a paved circle that loops the picturesque bay at the base of Ben Tianavaig. Government subsidies keep this rural crofting community afloat and support the few die-hards who still tend the ubiquitous, black-faced sheep, who outnumber the cars and the people and overrun the place at will.

"Sheep attack!" Damon grins at the familiar swarm of waddling, woolly frames, bleating faces, and clipping hooves that greets us.

Although we are outsiders, Shealagh is a maternal descendant of the island's ruling clan, the Macleods, and entitled by tradition to wear the tartan. Her ancestors cannot lay claim to Dunvegan Castle, the imposing twelfth-century Macleod seat that still draws tourists, but her great-grandfather Jack Macleod bottled Macleod whiskey and made his fortune bootlegging to the States during Prohibition. He built schools and hotels on the island and his offspring prospered, several becoming members of Parliament and one marrying the daughter of a billionaire media tycoon. My own link is far more tenuous but I spent a year living alone in the isolated family croft two decades earlier, without heating save for coal-banked fires and without a phone. We weren't married yet—I'd graduated Oxford and Shealagh still had a year to go—so I paid rent and wrote every day in near-perfect solitude, developing the daily discipline that's sustained me since and forming a deep attachment to this windswept Celtic aerie. I may also harbor a sweet spot for Scotland because my father grew up in Glasgow and still speaks with a faint brogue.

Now our kids have discovered the splendors of this rugged island. Our sheltered bay gives them the freedom to play outdoors and run wild with other parent-free children, and they fit right in with their bright hair and fair, freckled complexions.

Damon and Miranda—she's a vivid blonde, unlike her two redheaded brothers, but her general coloration matches—both have friends in the village from previous visits, while Sam, the middle child, tags along, buffeted between competing camps. Because the village has a limited pool of children, the kids are more adaptable and less finicky about age differences—seventeen-year-olds willingly play with seven-year-olds—but sibling rivalry and group exclusion appear immutable.

Damon is leader of the pack and chief organizer, ruling his siblings and negotiating between two main friends, Lachlann and Jamie. Lachlann, compact, agile, and mischievous, has a six-year-old sister, Kerry, who plays with Miranda, and an older brother, Alasdair, who sometimes joins the boys. Jamie, tall, handsome, and soft-spoken, lives down the hill with his parents and offers a quieter alternative.

We quickly develop a routine. I rise around five A.M., stroll down to the bay—examining tidal seaweed and occasionally spotting a seal or a heron— then pick up fresh eggs from Lachlann's house (his mother raises chickens) after depositing a brass one-pound coin in the squeaky metal honor box. I return to the croft and write for several hours before anyone wakes up.

Sam rises first and I give him writing assignments. His work is meticulous but spare, and I must coax him to explicitness.

"What you wrote is very good, but you need more than one paragraph!"

Sam at eight has curly red hair, lighter than Damon's; pale blue eyes; and a dusting of freckles across winsome features. He is lean and rubbery with a sweet disposition. Mostly quiet and self-contained, he also possesses a stubborn streak that can erupt into tantrums. We call him El Shrieko for his piercing cry. He is our wild card.

"Can you help me write a postcard to Marwan?" Sam asks today.

"Sure," I say, nodding. Marwan is a Palestinian boy from Lebanon who Sam met in first grade and with whom he formed a tight, biblical-style friendship. Marwan's family, lacking a green card, had to leave Brooklyn for the United Arab Emirates, but despite the distance and the passing years, the two boys call each other almost every week and stay in close touch.

After Sam, Miranda comes tumbling down the narrow stairs. I give her juice and a sheet of math problems, which she knocks off in a trice.

"All done!" Miranda beams. She is quick and clever, a loquacious six-year-old charmer dubbed "the blond bombshell" by her brothers. Sensitive but pragmatic, Miranda is always thinking two steps ahead.

I enjoy these private morning sessions with Sam and Miranda but when Damon gets up—I hear him prop open the skylight upstairs and can visualize him inhaling the pristine air and the dazzling bay in one luxurious gulp—I usually let him slide on the schoolwork. I want him to relax and recharge, and after years of working with him, I know he's absorbed my lessons and internalized my approach.

"Morning, D-man. How'd you sleep?" I smile at him in the low doorway.

"Good. I always have the deepest sleeps here." He yawns. "What time is it?"

While Damon washes up in the one tiny bathroom, I prepare a big communal breakfast. This first meal of the day becomes increasingly well attended, just like our lunches and dinners. The kids' friends drift in at mealtimes because they've discovered I'm a naïve profligate—I over-shop—and a soft touch, at least where food is concerned. I smile as they tear into Nutella sandwiches and stacks of funny-face ham and frosted wheat cereal that comes in sheets.

After breakfast, I stand on the metal grate by the door and make my restive offspring put on sun hats, sunscreen—it doubles as a midge repellent, so they don't complain so much—and Wellington boots. The high rubber boots prove practical not only for the marshy bogs and moors but as protection against the sheep shit that litters our front yard. The sheep have discovered a gap in our sagging wire fence.

Damon, the ringleader, claps on his blue canvas legionnaire's hat, which has side flaps and covers the back of his neck. He wears bottle-green wellies, scraggly shorts, and a *Save the Panda* T-shirt. I make sure he takes his EpiPen—an emergency shot of epinephrine against bee stings, to which he's allergic.

Once the kids have passed inspection, I unhook the big swinging front gate and let them all out with their friends. "See you for lunch," I say, waving, as they scamper off.

Damon, who dominates indoors with his force of personality, immediately falls behind as all the kids run up the hill to Lachlann's. He follows his own meandering path to obscure this fact, veering off to beat the roadside thistles with a stick and bending down to discover natural wonders en route.

When he can, Damon also deploys his younger siblings as cover. Sam, though gangly, benign, and worshipful of his older brother, is already too fast, but little Miranda happily lingers for Damon's attentions. Damon takes her by the hand and carries her off to the side of the road when a car comes by. He lifts her over a puddle or ditch, as if she were more helpless than she is.

"Don't worry, I got you, Mirandy," Damon says protectively.

Miranda plays along with her adored big brother until she gets bored and races off with the fleet Kerry—"Gonna beat you, Kerry!"—leaving Damon exposed again.

The others wait at the top as Damon slogs up the steep hill to join them. I watch him swing his hips and push his upper body forward while his striving legs lift and his feet drag and scrape the ground in their clunky rubber boots.

Damon struggles, but he always smiles and maintains his self-possession, and he always gets there. He's not even that far behind.

"Okay, guys, what are we doing?" He catches his breath at the crest and quickly reestablishes leadership. "I know. Let's go on a treasure hunt!"

Chapter 6

Due to his medical history, Damon has never learned to ride a bicycle. At home, I practice with him in the anonymity of Prospect Park, but it's a struggle because it's taken so long and now he's afraid to let go. I wait for the summer, when we'll have more time together. A few more falling-down sessions and I know we'll get there.

But it's trickier than I anticipated once we're in Skye. Damon is almost thirteen now; there's no privacy in this tiny village, and I don't want to embarrass him in front of his friends and his siblings. I watch Lachlann do amazing wheelies and other high-wire tricks on his bicycle and I decide to ask him to teach Damon. For a fee, of course. Lachlann loves commerce and jumps on the idea—I offer him a hundred dollars, which makes his eyes pop.

"Och aye, I'll teach him to bike up Ben Tianavaig for a hundred dollars!" Lachlann says, beaming.

Damon likes the idea too. It's a challenge and an adventure for two twelve-year-old boys. They spend the next few days practicing nonstop. I can hear fragments and catch glimpses of their budding collaboration from my study window. They come down the hill at a good clip, Lachlann running alongside Damon's bicycle with one hand on the handlebars.

"Good job, Damon . . . Och, but keep the damn thing straight, man!"

"I'm trying," Damon squeals, "but it has a mind of its own—oh no . . . !"

Damon takes several spills, gasping and giggling as he scrapes his leg or tumbles over Lachlann. I give the boys a stern safety lecture and make them practice on the flat parts, but I do not stop them. They're having a great time together. And I know, underneath the playfulness, how much this matters. I can see Damon's confidence and comfort level grow by the day.

One afternoon Damon calls to me from the road. "Hey, Dad, come out here for a minute, I have something to show you!" I step out of the croft. The sun pours gold over the entire valley, the granite peaks of the Red Cuillin glow, and the glassy blue bay shimmers.

"Come on, Dad!" Damon grins, beckoning me closer.

He perches over a black mountain bike at the top of the hill.

"You watching?" he asks excitedly. I nod. I have seen him perform onstage many times but this is a riskier kind of role for him. He straddles the metal frame and counts off, rehearsing in his head. "Ready?" he says, priming himself as much as me.

"Just do it, Damon!" Lachlann cries. "Before the bloody midges eat us alive."

Damon places one tentative foot on the upraised pedal. He takes a deep breath, then pushes off more authoritatively with his back leg.

The impelled bike immediately starts to zigzag in wide arcs.

"Whoa!" Damon tries to get a grip on the shaky handlebars but the bicycle careens toward a roadside gully, making straight for the gutter.

"No!" Damon yells, bracing for disaster. But with the bike rim on the verge of the ditch, he recovers and steers it back to the center of the road.

Still a tad off-kilter, Damon hunkers forward and to the left as the bike leans to the right. I've never seen anything like this, except maybe at the circus.

Damon and his bicycle tilt in *opposite* directions.

"Hang on, Damon!" Lachlann shouts, fearing the worst.

I hold my breath. Damon appears to be falling out of the saddle as he overcompensates on the left to offset the rightward drift of the bicycle. The bike sways and jitters as if it's about to spin away from him. But somehow Damon manages to keep it balanced and finds a strange new equilibrium.

A tightly focused Damon now pedals past me with set jaw. In the corners of his mouth, I spot the wisp of a proud smile forming. He grips the handlebars with tremulous intensity and turns right on a steep slope, speeding downhill. The bike wobbles but Damon confidently hangs on and stays astride all the way to the bay.

"Attaboy, D-man!" I holler and whoop, startling the sheep. Lachlann stands by a gorse bush, beaming at his student and avidly contemplating payday.

My son pushes his bike up the hill, breathless with excitement. "See that, Dad?"

I flash a thumbs-up as Damon remounts and pushes off again. He's got the hang of it now, and he's having fun. A panicked sheep runs out in front of him and Damon swerves expertly around it. "Naughty ewe!" he chides, grinning.

The look on his face as he makes the bicycle do his bidding is extraordinary to behold. I watch him grasp all the lost ground he's recovered and the new powers he's unleashed as he rejoins his cohort and celebrates a major rite of passage.

I call Shealagh in New York. "Guess what your son did today?" Delighted, she wants to congratulate Damon, so he trudges into the croft and indulges his mother with nonchalant teen pride—"Yeah, Mom, I know"—before running out again.

Shealagh is mending and Sonja is taking excellent care of her. She misses us all but is happy her kids are having a great summer in such a beautiful place. We discuss the progress of each child, then linger over Damon's latest accomplishment.

"This is huge," Shealagh says. "A few years late, but he did it. Our Damon!"

The Skye idyll continues, with a few minor setbacks. One day, a breathless Sam slips into the croft with a garbled tale that he and Damon had gone into the woods searching for a tree house, and now Damon is apparently injured and needs help!

Frantic, I race out the door and down the valley to the bay, then charge up the facing hill, searching through bushes and a thick copse of birch that Sam points me to.

"I don't see him, Sam! You sure this is the place? Think carefully!"

Sam is flustered and confused so I ask him to calm down and retrace their route.

We scour the area in a wide swath. I cup my hands and yell. Nothing.

Just when I'm wondering if this is a bad dream—the dense wooded hillside, though visible from the croft, would take me hours to comb through, and it's already growing dark—we stumble upon Damon lolling on a bed of bracken. He reclines on one elbow, enacting a battle scene on the peaty ground with twigs deployed as toy soldiers.

"Hey, Dad." He greets me as if I've just dropped by his room. It transpires my venturesome firstborn was swinging on a rotten tree branch when it collapsed under his weight. He tried to walk back but it became too painful so he sent Sam for help.

I hoist Damon onto my back and carry him down the hill and back up to the croft. Inside, I lay him on the couch and examine him carefully for injuries. Sam insists he was only a foot off the ground when he fell, and in truth, he does not appear seriously hurt. A couple of minor scrapes and bruises, a sore ankle. But he's had a scare, and so have I.

I'm struck by Damon's frailty as I carry him through the sinking twilight back to the croft, how small and fragile he feels in my arms and how tightly he clings to me. It takes so little to knock him off course. And I'm struck by my own powerlessness, how hard it is for me to safeguard my son if I also want him to have a normal life.

Back home, Damon explains how his little brother propped him up and carried him down the hill until it got too hard and Sam ran for help. We both agree eight-year-old Sam showed impressive maturity and presence of mind.

I cook Damon his favorite dishes and read to him on the couch while he mends. Sam and Miranda get bedtime stories but Damon needs more mature fare—all three kids bunk in the same room—so I select literary works for him, which we two discuss.

On request, I also give my recuperating son therapeutic massages. He has a stiff upper body with a thick neck and a relatively narrow back, solid and compact, except for two bony shoulder blades. You can see where his powerful underlying frame, the rugged core that is Damon's original blueprint, has been attenuated by cardiac insufficiency. I knead the tight, sensitive muscles around his scapula and gently work out the knots, praying that the young body at my fingertips reaches its full potential.

One day, when I return from a run with a bad cramp in my own back, Damon offers to give *me* a massage. I'm glad he's feeling better but I tell him it's not necessary. Besides, my back has defeated trained people twice his size. But Damon insists.

I sit on the edge of the couch bowed in grateful wonder, a hunched father in sopping T-shirt, as my diligent son bends over the knotted, sweaty terrain of my back and, asking for feedback, zeroes in on my cramp. "Wow, Dad, it's like a rock!"

I feel the fierce, loving, and focused determination as Damon pinpoints the area of tightness and exerts precise force with his elbows and thumbs. It's a sweet treat, and I enjoy the pleasant sense of bonding with my own flesh and blood.

As the summer wears on, I undertake more outings with the kids. We go to the Skye Highland Games in Portree and the sheepdog trials in Talisker Bay. When the sun's out, we slide down boulders and splash in the bone-cold Varragill River. Damon's lips turn purple but his smiling enthusiasm for our watering hole is undimmed.

We take riding lessons at the Portree stables. All the kids enjoy horseback riding and Damon proves surprisingly adept. During one exercise, I glance over my shoulder and catch him clearly outclassing me as he trots.

"Nice, D-man!" I yell, realizing with a start that this is how it's supposed to be.

I throw Damon a big thirteenth-birthday party with a big cake, inviting half the village to celebrate. "Make a Skye wish!" Miranda says as Damon blows out his candles. His vivid face glows before the moors, the lochs, and the mountains.

Per tradition, we drive down to visit Shealagh's uncle and aunt in their remote summer retreat, running into huge, gorgeous cattle lolling on the single-track road, until we reach the loch-edged house with its daunting view of the Black Cuillin.

Philip and Catriona are warm, genuine people, not what you'd necessarily assume from their upper-class English accents and manor house in Berkshire, England. They've long been like surrogate parents to Shealagh and very hospitable to me, and they embrace our kids and welcome them amid their visiting children and grandchildren.

We putter on a small motorboat and picnic on Coral Island before heading back to the house, where it's tea, juice, and gingerbread with lots of kids, including my children's lovely teenage cousins, flitting about. Damon seizes the moment, enthralling the coltish girls with his patter and mimicry. He stands on a stool and impersonates a cartoonish cigar-chomping American mogul. The girls applaud and ask for more, which Damon happily provides, but I can't help noticing how he shivered out on the water and looks puffier in the face now.

Chapter 7

We have been waiting for a clear day to climb Ben Tianavaig. The mountain behind our croft is only about fourteen hundred feet high, but the weather changes very fast on the Misty Isle, and we cannot risk getting fogged out. Every year, climbers on the Cuillin disappear due to inclement weather. Ben Tianavaig is tamer, a pleasant hour-and-a-half hike under the right conditions, but none of my kids has ever reached the top.

On a crystalline blue day, we set off on a path behind our house. I carry a backpack with food, water, and sweaters—it gets chilly at the top—and Lachlann, for whom the ascent is a dawdle, carries a second pack. He also annoys us all by blasting "Lucy in the Sky with Diamonds" on his tape player and screeching along nonstop.

We pass behind a neighboring croft, following a well-trod path through bracken and fern up the first steep slope. Damon and Lachlann lead while I bring up the rear, taking Miranda by the hand. Sam, the middle child, walks in the middle.

It's narrow during the initial climb, and we hike single file through dense overgrowth. Damon, in a broad khaki hat, marches proudly ahead while Lachlann flits on the margins beside him, ducking to avoid scratches. Damon beats the bushes with a stick, kicks obstacles from the path, and relishes being in front. I know it won't last but I enjoy watching Damon feel his oats. He's a natural-born leader who rarely gets to exercise physical command, but now he's unchallengeably in the lead.

"Wow, that's sharp!" Damon whacks a stinging nettle.

Sam, in a Buzz Lightyear T-shirt and a flap hat, eagerly follows behind the two older boys, nipping at Damon's heels. Sam has a high, darting gait, like a show horse, and he's bursting with raw energy. "Easy—no tailgating!" I warn Sam, recognizing his impulse to prove himself and pass his big brother. Part of me roots for Sam—I know about being the second child—while another part seeks to restrain Sam for Damon's sake. I want both my boys to succeed, but just now, it's Damon who needs my help.

As we advance up the mountain, the valley quickly drops away and recedes into a tiny, sun-drenched hollow of lines and colors—grass-green, peat-brown, and gorse-gold, with streaks of heath-purple—revealing other mountains and moors and cliffs, a vast geology of which it is only one small part.

I notice Damon straining and Miranda slowing. "Let's take a break," I announce.

We stretch out on a carpet of bell heather and pass around the water bottle. Lachlann discovers McVitie's chocolate cookies and devours them with yelps of pleasure. Damon pushes up his hat and scans the horizon like a veteran climber.

"It's nice up here. Everything looks so *small*." Damon eyes the neat cliffs and tidy bay at the mouth of our little valley, savoring the infinitesimal scale.

"Isn't that Lachlann's house?" Miranda points to a far-off tiny green roof.

"No way!" Sam dismisses both the idea and its proponent.

"Aye, that's our wee shed glinting through the trees," Lachlann replies.

"Good eye, Mirandy!" Damon pats his sister, and Miranda sticks her tongue out at Sam. The pesky midges swarm and I spray the kids with more insect repellent.

"Midges don't bother you above one thousand feet," I tell them.

We resume climbing and make slow but steady progress. Only there's a catch.

Ben Tianavaig rises out of the ocean like a rough volcanic pyramid, with its southern flank—the side that shelters our croft and village, the side we climb—sliced diagonally with a series of sweeping setbacks that can deceive the first-time climber, who experiences two "false" summits before reaching the third and final, or "true," apex.

So despite my admonitions, the kids believe they've reached the top long before we get there. Miranda rides on my back while the others struggle but won't admit it.

Damon propels himself through sheer will. He's like a car on empty, determined to squeeze every drop from the reserve tank and then push from behind if necessary. Sam too is exhausted but still intent on beating Damon. He stumbles about, complaining—"Are we there yet? How much farther?"—but then he shoots up the hillside in a sudden spurt to join Lachlann and smiles down at us. Damon glances up at his younger brother and his friend, frustrated and quietly seething.

I call several breaks but Damon insists it's not necessary.

"No, let's keep going," he says between clenched teeth. "I'm fine, Dad."

Finally I stop by a boulder. "I need a rest from carrying Miranda." I set my daughter down and make Damon sit too. I give them each juice, then pull him aside.

"Listen, D-man, you're doing great. With your oxygen level, you're carrying *three* Mirandas . . . So let's not overdo it. If we don't make it this time, we'll try another day."

Damon nods at what I'm saying but his mind, or rather his iron will, is set.

"I'm okay, Dad. I just needed to catch my breath." He glances up the mountain. "It's farther than it looks—and steeper!" He grins, then snaps his fingers. "Let's do it!"

He stands with his windblown lion's mane flapping and his hat flying behind him on a tie-string. He's got everything it takes, all the heart in the world, just not the heart function. I cheer silently and send him invisible boosts and rungs of support.

We march on. The scrub trees have long yielded to stubbly mountain grass. No more heather at this height. Not even thistles. It's hot, arduous, and unforgiving.

My kids look dazed and punch-drunk. But no one wants to give up.

I trail Damon with Miranda on my back, lending a hand when he starts to falter and taking a longer but more graduated path to help him pace the ascent.

"We're almost there now!" I say, wondering if he can hang on.

We pass the second false summit and see the true peak up ahead. Damon's eyes light up, his arms swing into action, and his stride quickens. He end-runs Sam, who's flagging again, and makes for the finish line. A violent wind suddenly rushes in from all sides and swirls about him, creating a turbulent barrier.

"Arrrgh!" Damon charges, locking on the column that marks the mountaintop.

Sam spots the column too, but he's been outflanked by his older brother, so he just makes a run for it. But Damon hits the target first. Lachlann swoops in beside Damon, landing like an eagle. Miranda scrambles off my back and agrees to walk the final stretch. She grabs my hand as we all reach the apex and converge at the column.

Ben Tianavaig lifts its high craggy shoulders, with a sheer drop over the ridge. We teeter on the naked, windswept summit, with cliffs and rocky precipices below.

"Awesome!" Damon's eyes glint at the harsh confluence of land, sea, and sky.

A lowering storm suddenly looms above our heads as fast-moving clouds scud across the peak. The clouds turn into chunks of mist and pelt us like hailstones, engulfing the summit and shrouding us in blinding swirls of fog. We get pummeled.

Just as quickly as they came, the storm clouds move past, and sunshine pours down again from a luminous blue vault, revealing a sparkling, vertiginous panorama.

No one speaks. Damon leans a proprietary arm against the summit column, catching his breath. His brow is damp, his cheeks flushed, but his chest swells proudly.

The Black Cuillin hover beyond our sunlit valley like a pale, jagged mirage.

"We're on top of the world!" Damon grins like a conquistador and hoists an unsuspecting Miranda onto the summit shaft, planting her there like a flag.

Miranda, frightened at first, relaxes and leans back, her legs extending from her torso like a ballerina's as her golden tresses fly in the wind. Damon guards his baby sister, slinging her legs across his shoulder, while Sam presses close, holding down his flap hat. Lachlann beams in the pure ether, a humble knight to my trio.

We're close to heaven, and everyone feels it.

A chill, bitter wind eventually forces us down to a lower spot. Lachlann inflates orange balloons and shows the others how to tie them into swords so they can fight and duel on the mountain. Swashbuckling Damon, who's reading *The Count of Monte Cristo,* corners the slippery Lachlann while Sam jabs him and Miranda jumps on his back. Their yodeling carries down the valley and in no time Lachlann's sister and mother, out on their own trek, clamber up to join our cavorting.

For the finale, inspired and cued by Damon, we set all the balloons free, watching as they catch the fierce wind and float over the valley like migrating orange swallows.

Chapter 8

A week before leaving Skye, after I've asked Damon to review for his high school entrance exams, he steps out of the croft to talk to me. I'm sitting in a white patio chair facing what's left of the sun, reading foundation proposals FedExed to me from New York, when he stands in the doorway and looks at me with a curious expression.

"I got this funny feeling in my side, Dad."

I put down my papers and walk over. "What kind of feeling?"

"I don't know. But it hurts in a weird way, like a shooting pain."

"That's not good." I put my hand on his shoulder. "When did this start?"

"Not sure. I had it Tuesday but then it went away. But just now I felt it again."

I lean over him, peering. "Where exactly is the pain?"

He points to a large area, running his hand from his rib cage to his hip.

"Could you have fallen down and gotten bruised without knowing it?" I ask.

"No, it's not like that . . ."

"Then what's it like, D-man?" I press because he's starting to worry me.

"I don't know . . ." He frowns. "It just went through me and it felt really weird."

Just then something weird goes through *me*—right through *my* side—and I do not like the feeling. If there's an innocent or logical explanation, why can't I think of one?

"It's not that bad, Dad," Damon finally says, reading my unquiet thoughts. "I just thought you should know."

I watch him closely over the next days but he insists the pain is gone. He believes it was a false alarm, maybe even growing pains, but I remain uneasy. I start seeing warning signs everywhere but maybe I'm looking for them.

The day before departing, I take the kids to the Portree stables. We plan to skip the lesson for a big farewell trek. Damon's regular horse, Bootise, is indisposed, so they give him a bigger horse, Jasper. We're about to roll out when I notice Damon is close to tears. He can't tell me what's wrong but it seems the immense horse, close to eighteen hands tall, has him rattled. Damon says he's too far off the ground and he wants to get down.

We dismount and he calms somewhat. But he's still too overwrought to try a different horse and I won't force him, even if it means canceling our last ride.

I've rarely seen Damon so distraught and I'm baffled by it. Until today, he's shown complete confidence and proficiency on a horse. Did I push him too fast? It's always a balancing act but he seemed to enjoy the riding as much as his siblings and he's even started to surpass us. Maybe the sudden chill has affected him? It's been raining and the temperature has dropped sharply, as it does at the end of August.

Or maybe he's upset we're leaving Skye and wants more time with his friends? Or he got into a fight and didn't tell us, as happened once before?

I can't figure it out but it's completely out of character. I tell a disappointed Sam and Miranda that the trek is off and take them for fish and chips by the harbor.

We sit by a railing overlooking the brackish quay and watch as swift hands fry each fresh fillet of cod, anoint glazed chips with salt and vinegar, and wrap it all up in thick white paper. Damon perks up with the hearty food and laughs when a big, cheeky seagull swoops onto our cramped table and steals a fry right out of my hand.

He seems to have recovered by evening and is up to his old tricks with his pals. They goof around and play hide and seek. They jump on the trampoline. When Harry's white van makes its weekly visit, Damon braves the midges to buy treats from the mobile grocery while Harry, the white-haired Wizard of Skye, tells me about Damon's island ancestors, who looked just like him.

That night I invite our village friends for farewell drinks and food. The kids play video games and have pillow fights choreographed by Damon with boisterous hilarity.

When we leave the Isle of Skye the following morning, everyone agrees it was a great summer. But as we drive over the bridge at Kyleakin, I cannot shake an inchoate sense of dread about Damon. I check for him in the rear-view mirror and watch him surreptitiously in the backseat, where he retreats with a Walkman and a book into his gray hooded sweatshirt, stares glumly out the window, and dozes off for long stretches.

Chapter 9

On the eve of September 11, 2001, ten days after returning from Skye, I sense, along with many people in the United States, that something nasty is brewing.

I read the papers and track news coverage from around the world. I'm aware of public threats made by al-Qaeda and other Islamic fundamentalist groups, and of U.S. government alerts responding to those threats. Although I have no security clearances, my job puts me in touch with a range of government officials—at State, Defense, the CIA—and I know many leading scientists and policymakers.

I also have less-mainstream connections and more offbeat sources. As a former taxi driver who regularly takes cabs, I talk to cabbies and listen to their chatter. I'm also writing a thriller set in the Middle East—I was born in Israel and spent the first seven years of my life in the Levant—and I've read widely about Jihadism and terrorism.

So I develop a palpable sense of impending attack, and I even think I know the occasion: a September 23 Salute to Israel parade, when Governor George Pataki will welcome Israeli prime minister Ariel Sharon to New York. My mistake is, I'm working off an outdated model—the 1980s assassination of President Bashir Gemayel in Beirut, Lebanon—and I do not just overshoot the date by twelve days, but I miscalculate the number of deaths and the level of destruction by several orders of magnitude.

There is something sickeningly familiar, as well as shocking and monstrous, about what happens on 9/11. I've seen it, in paler versions, before—as a child in Israel, whenever I revisit the Middle East, and even in Europe. But never *here*, not in America and in the quintessentially progressive, tolerant city where I live with my family. It belongs back there, in the feudalistic, tribal world I left behind.

Like most people, on the day itself my immediate concern is my family. Sam and Miranda attend PS 29, very near to the Brooklyn Heights clinic where Shealagh now works. I reach my wife on the phone—she can see the burning tower from her window on Montague Street—and we agree she should pick up the two younger children because she has the car, while I decide what to do about Damon, who's in Manhattan.

Shealagh leaves for the school on Henry Street. The wind blows east, from downtown Manhattan to Brooklyn. Out on the street, thick smoke fills the air and white ash floats down like dirty snowflakes on Shealagh's head. She hurries, worried about the white ash, which is asbestos from the towers, though officials will deny it for months.

Inside the school, hundreds of frightened children gather in the auditorium, where teachers in face masks organize the evacuation. Panicked parents rush in, clutch their kids, and sign them out. Some kids will wait all day because several PS 29 parents work in the World Trade Center and never will make it out alive.

While Shealagh collects Sam and Miranda, I ponder what to do about Damon. His school is near Gramercy Park, but the bridges and subways are closed. When my wife returns with the car, I'm ready to drive in anyway, but Shealagh's seen police stopping drivers on the bridge and doesn't want me to go. I suggest riding my bike past the roadblock but she worries I'll be arrested; even if I get across, my wife doesn't want me cycling back with Damon on the handlebars. She feels he's safe at school—we track the news nonstop—and doesn't want us to risk further family separation.

I call my sister, Anat, on a landline—cell phones still don't work. She lives near Damon's school and reports all is calm in the area. I ask her to check up on Damon for me. She walks to East Twentieth Street, upwind of the explosions, where everything appears normal. Classes remain in session and Damon wants to stay. My sister agrees to meet him after school and take him back to her apartment, where he can spend the night.

I speak to my parents in Queens and they're okay too.

The next day I take the subway to Fourteenth Street and pick up Damon from my sister's apartment. It's a relief to have him back with me. We walk south but stay clear of Canal Street, where a security cordon has been set up with soldiers and army vehicles. The air is dense, fetid.

Damon looks the same but seems oddly marginalized, as if the crisis has diminished his footprint. Even in the subway, a state of emergency prevails. The cops wear white masks with carbon filters while travelers eye each other warily.

"How were things at school?" I ask as we board the train. "Did people panic?"

"Not really," Damon says. "We heard a boom and then they came and told us about it. Everybody stayed pretty calm, except kids whose parents work in the towers."

"Doesn't Jon and Kirsten's father work in one of the towers?"

"Yeah, but he's an architect, so when he saw the first tower get hit, he bolted, even though they told people to stay put. He escaped just before the second plane hit and walked over the Brooklyn Bridge all the way home in a daze."

"Good for him!" I say, then add, "We're all in a kind of daze, D-man."

My son looks at me. "Didn't you show me an article on this, like, a month ago?"

"Yes, people knew they were planning *something* but not on this scale . . ." I nudge him. "Maybe now you'll start reading the papers?"

Back home, Shealagh and I note how subdued Damon seems. He tiptoes by us like a pale bird, making tentative inquiries in a muted voice.

"He's not the main focus. Something bigger has our attention," Shealagh remarks.

Damon helps his siblings adjust, especially Sam, who saw the smoking towers from his class window. He invites Sam to his room, a rare treat. They have long chats, play Doom, and listen to Coldplay. Damon even allows six-year-old Miranda to join as they huddle over cards and board games, forming a stable, self-contained sibling crew.

I feel relieved because everyone in my family is safe. Of course, no one can predict the psychological fallout on the children. An entire generation will grow up remembering this date. Not just the devastation but the fact that we, their parents, were rendered so helpless and vulnerable. Why couldn't we stop this? What else can't we protect them from? Is there a limit to our power, and thus to our authority?

I feel this acutely with Damon, who stops by for increasingly serious talks. He turns his gentle, searching blue eyes on me and analyzes my face, as well as my words.

"Could they attack New York again?" he asks on the first Sunday after 9/11, when I return from Ground Zero on my bike. We sit in my study as I towel down.

"Sure," I reply. "But the Pentagon attack worries me even more. Because you can never protect every civilian building but we have only one national military headquarters—and it seems to have been penetrated with remarkable ease."

"No one's talking about that," Damon says. He's reading the papers daily now.

"No, it's too upsetting. Just like why we didn't foresee the global nature of this conflict. Remember my military tour in July?" I point to an F-16 photo on my wall.

Damon nods. I got him souvenirs from all four armed services.

"During one briefing, I asked a four-star general if the military was worried about the rising tide of anti-Americanism I saw whenever I went abroad. This general dismissed my question as irrelevant, too far below the radar to merit a serious answer."

"Why would he do that?" Damon screws up his features.

"Beats me . . . But I thought of that general today, when I rode my bike over the Manhattan Bridge and went to see firsthand what they'd done to our beautiful city."

"And you wouldn't take me with you!" Damon chides. "I can ride now, Dad."

"I know, D-man, but it's still too dicey. Place is like a toxic, bombed-out war zone, with army troops in battle gear, sewage-filled streets, and rescue workers sifting for human remains. And it stinks! I had to take shallow breaths on my bike not to puke. Site's still smoldering five days after impact!"

"Wow," Damon says, rapt. "You find your friend and his family?"

"I tried but their building was roped off and they weren't in the queue to go back in . . . It was surreal. People held signs with names of relatives and handed out photos of the missing. Like a displaced persons camp after World War Two!" I scowl.

"You sound angry, like it's personal," Damon observes.

"That's how it feels, like a violation. This is my city, and I know all these streets and lanes intimately. When I drove the night shift as a cabbie, I used to tuck the sleeping city into bed every night . . ."

"That sounds cool, Dad, I'd like to try that!" Damon says.

"Maybe one day you will." I smile at him. "Though today, D-man, all I could do was jump on my bike and get the hell out of that cesspool! My one consolation was cycling back over the Brooklyn Bridge, which was completely deserted—not one vehicle or pedestrian along the entire span! I stood up in the saddle at the crest, alone under that great filigree of cables, with a clear sight line to the statue and the harbor mouth."

"I want to come with you next time!" Damon cries. "Can I? Please, Dad!"

I hesitate but Damon's ardor is irresistible.

"Okay, I'll take you. But only after things improve, including the air quality."

"Cool. Thanks, Dad." Damon beams and deftly pockets my IOU.

I continue conversing with Damon and trying to make sense of what happened when I receive an e-mail from a friend saying that his father, a top official in the fire department, rushed into one of the towers just before it collapsed. Although I know that several hundred firefighters and rescue workers have died, not to mention thousands of civilians, this is the first victim I am acquainted with, and suddenly all the talk of bodies and funerals is personal and real. This man was not just my friend's dad but also the grandfather of two of Damon's childhood friends, Kelsey and Siobhan.

"I have some bad news," I tell my son in his room. "Billy's father ran into the southern tower to rescue his men, and he never made it out . . ."

Damon's face drops and his eyes mist over, while I begin to get a glimmer of understanding for a tragedy whose true dimensions I can never grasp nor adequately explain to my own children.

Chapter 10

Two weeks after 9/11, I am sitting with my wife and three children in Temple Beth Emeth for the Yom Kippur service, the holiest date in the Jewish calendar and the one day we attend synagogue. Because I hope to have Damon Bar Mitzvahed in June, I have joined this congregation, paid dues, and tried to act more observant than I am.

I make the kids dress up, which means no T-shirts or sneakers. Damon wears stiff black shoes that squeak heavily as he walks and an open-necked blue shirt that shows the tip of his midline scar and buttons tightly across his belly. His unruly shock of red hair is combed and wetted down, and he glistens with pale, reproachful handsomeness. Sam and Miranda, two beautiful if bored children, shine in their clean outfits, and all three kids look like flowers ablaze with color in this dour ecclesiastical setting.

We are listening to a thunderous sermon about the unprecedented terrorist attack on U.S. soil when word comes that Shealagh's father has died.

Philip Rosenthal was eighty-four and living in Germany, so we did not see him much. But he was a complex, outsize figure and the only father Shealagh has known, and his death is a shock to us all—and another blow to Shealagh, still recovering from back surgery.

We are not especially close to Shealagh's family. Her parents are separated; they live in Europe and have led largely self-involved lives. Shealagh's mother, in particular, has not treated her daughter well. But Shealagh's father, a celebrated industrialist and politician who publicly disinherited his children and joined the Socialist Party under Willy Brandt, rising to secretary of state, has reached out to her in his latter years, and Shealagh has made her peace with him. His overtures to our family, especially to Damon, have been genuine, and he and I have a mutually respectful if wary understanding.

On getting the news, we quickly return to our house and check on flights to Germany. While Shealagh calls her family to discuss arrangements, Damon stops by my study, a notebook and tape player under his arm.

"Can I go to Germany with you?" Damon asks, his face full of urgent tenderness.

His request takes me by surprise, even though he's gone with us before.

"Let's wait and ask Mom. We want to be sensitive to her and her family."

Damon nods and I ask him about the tape. He explains it's an interview he did with his grandpa for a school history project. "I also wrote a class essay, 'My Grandfather,' and worked out a family tree." He opens his notebook and shows me the material.

Philip Rosenthal's life intrigued Damon. A Catholic who joined the Hitler Youth at fourteen, ignorant of his father's conversion from Judaism, Philip had to flee Nazi Germany for England when the Gestapo appropriated his father's china company. After boarding school in Broadstairs and rowing at Oxford—the same college, Exeter, where I would later meet his daughter—young Rosenthal tried joining the British Army to fight Hitler but was rejected as a German national. So he enlisted in the French Foreign Legion, where the most action he saw was with the woman who convinced him, belly with child, to make the first of his five unsuccessful forays down the aisle. After many attempts, he finally escaped the legion and its lifetime indenture. He drifted in England and then returned to Germany, where, aided by his family name and significant reparations, he reclaimed his father's china firm and led it to new heights during the German postwar economic boom. He was also elected to parliament as a proponent of worker participation, joined the cabinet, and became a leading statesman and celebrity.

"It's good you got him on tape," I tell Damon. "He told many stories and even if some were self-mythology, he was a fascinating guy and a real embodiment of history."

"With his own castle and pool!" Damon's eyes twinkle.

The family lived in a 1740s *Schloss* modernized into a sleek mansion with contemporary art. Damon favored the Party Room, converted from a former stable into a *La Dolce Vita*–style cavern featuring an indoor pool, alcoves, recessed lighting, and a vaulted ceiling. Every year Philip organized a big fireworks display in the front courtyard of the *Schloss*. The dazzling spectacle attracted many denizens of the small china-manufacturing town where he ruled like the revered local prince, with a flamingo-fronted factory designed by Walter Gropius, state-of-the-art amenities for workers, and streets named after him and his father, also called Philip.

"It was cool going on walks with Grandpa because everywhere we went people pointed to him and he pretended not to notice," Damon says. "But I think he liked it."

A big, handsome figure with a touch of the white-haired John Huston, circa *Chinatown*, about him, Philip walked around the *Schloss* in a flowing djellaba and sandals and slept on a sand floor under tented fabric with artificial stars. He climbed the Himalayas, flew his own plane, and walked, swam, or rowed across ten European nations in a two-decade odyssey he proudly charted on a huge map in the *Schloss*.

"Grandpa did a lot, but I don't think he had many friends," Damon says quietly.

"No, but he was very fond of you. And he loved that your name was 'nomad' spelled backward," I remind Damon. "It made him feel closer to you, since he saw himself as a wanderer. That and the fact that he had a heart murmur as a boy."

"And he introduced me to pig's trotters!" Damon grins.

Shealagh wanders into my study, red eyed, and says her siblings have decided that no one is bringing children, so we can't take Damon. She's still in shock.

"You gonna be okay, Mom?" Damon instantly forgets his own disappointment.

We leave the kids with my parents and fly that night to Germany, meeting up in the *Schloss* the following afternoon.

Only the immediate family is invited, as stipulated by Philip, who's planned every detail of his postmortem in the Teutonic way. There will be no funeral or public ceremony. No trace of religion of any kind. He wants to be cremated and the ashes, housed in a black porcelain

Rosenthal urn, lowered into the ground under the beech tree in the front garden of the *Schloss*. He's written his own epitaph—at once pompous and true—and had it carved on a headstone with only the date of his death left blank: OF PORCELAIN THIS SO-CALLED KING KNEW LITTLE. HE LEARNED MORE FROM HIS SOCIALIST BROTHERS AND FELLOW MAN AND FROM ROWING.

His death is on the front pages and on television. The chancellor issues a statement, as does Rosenthal China. But we keep the family end very small and private.

Shealagh, her three siblings and their spouses, and her older half sister attend. Philip's devoted executive assistant, PR handler, nurse, companion, onetime lover, and caretaker oversees things, aided by and occasionally clashing with his eldest son.

Shealagh's mother, not on the invite list, crashes the gathering. She's technically still married to Philip even if she decamped for London decades earlier. The *Schloss*, once celebrated in designer magazines as the home of an innovative, world-class company, is crumbling now. Philip had donated it to the firm in a typically grand gesture, keeping a small flat for himself. But the renowned china company, formerly the product of true vision and a unique, rigorous aesthetic, has since been sold and debased, and Philip ousted. Marginalized, even mocked, by crass salesmen and bean counters, the former CEO and founder's son was consigned to a tiny, decaying remnant of his onetime kingdom.

I've been to very few funerals and Philip is one of the first people I am close to whose corpse I behold. When I see him laid out in the casket in his custom-made brown suede jacket with his sparse white hair and his willful, prominent, and subtly curved nose—a medieval portrait worthy of Rembrandt—I also see his carefully obscured Semitic roots and I understand him in his full historical dimensions. It's a dramatic revelation, as if death has swept away any last illusions, and it makes me appreciate the monumental project of self-invention and determined adventure that was his life.

I draw lessons for myself but also for Damon, who has a part—a physically recognizable part as well as specific character traits—of his grandpa in him. Because I like to imagine myself the founder of a new line—I harbor big dreams for my family—I see Damon as *my* Philip, the scion whose father started things but who took them to new heights. So as I gaze at my son's grandfather, I look into the future as well as the past.

But mostly, as I stand by the casket, I am filled with sorrow and speechlessness at the mystery of silence, of no-moreness, that is death. It's hard to believe that Philip, such a dominant force, whom I loved sparring with, is gone. After comforting my wife as best I can, when no one is looking, I wipe away my own tear.

Chapter 11

Shortly after returning from Germany, oppressed by sadness and the lingering national doldrums, we decide to stride forward and, in the spirit of Philip, initiate our own family walkabout.

Growing up, Shealagh hiked through most of Germany, Italy, and Turkey, joining her father for large sections of his European peregrination. Many of her school vacations were commandeered by his odyssey—especially when he wanted a press photo—but she also has fond memories of these times spent together as a family.

We've considered a U.S. variation of this Continental theme before, but now the time seems ripe. And we know that Damon, a poor runner but a tireless anaerobic hiker, can walk his siblings into the ground.

We decide we won't march straight across America, at least not on this first go-round, but instead we will limit ourselves to the mid-Atlantic region. We'll start from Brooklyn, pass through Manhattan and the Bronx, and continue upstate along the Hudson. All distances will be covered on foot or on bicycle. Each section of the journey will begin where the previous part ended. After a few segments, we'll need to drive to our starting-off point and leave the car. We'll do it on weekends, holidays, summers, whenever the opportunity presents.

Shealagh's back remains an issue but she is game—it's her family tradition and her dad we're honoring—as long as I promise not to race ahead.

The kids, fresh from their outdoor triumphs in Skye and cognizant of the homage to their grandfather, readily agree to our plan. On the last day in September, a blustery Sunday, the five of us don comfortable shoes and light jackets, stuff a backpack with sweaters and water bottles, and walk to the end of our street, entering Prospect Park by the Vanderbilt playground. We skirt the still blue lake, pass two lumbering horses on the bridle path, and climb past Lookout Hill, where scouts scanned for German U-boats during World War II. A stream of cyclists, runners, and Rollerbladers zips by as we round the corner by Bartel-Pritchard Circle, where a new multiplex and cafés attest to the area's gentrification. Everyone in the family seems primed for this historic inaugural march.

Damon takes the lead by my side, with Sam hot on our trail, as we traverse the meadow's perimeter, crunching leaves and twigs. Miranda ambles with her mother, two handsome Victorian ladies on a nature tour. The terrain is flat, and we make good progress.

I keep my eye on Damon as he whacks tree trunks with his latest sword-branch. He wears a gray hooded sweatshirt emblazoned with the fiery words NO FEAR and at first he appears energized. But soon he begins to dawdle. He veers off to thump trees and loiters, appearing distracted.

By the time we reach the northern end of the park, Damon clearly lags and is struggling to keep up. Shealagh flashes me a worried look as we wait for the traffic light by the intersection. The light turns green and we cross to Grand Army Plaza. Now Damon appears in distress. I point the kids to the big triumphal arch and walk over to Damon.

"What's up, D-man? You feeling okay?"

"Yeah, I just need a minute to catch my breath . . ." He waves me off and walks away with hands on hips, looking pale and listless.

Shealagh wanders over to me, half-accusing. "What's going on?"

"I don't know," I reply. Sam and Miranda pretend to study the victorious bronze charioteer crowning the monumental arch. "He seems tired, out of breath."

Shealagh shakes her head. "That's not like him. We haven't walked that far and it's only the flat bits so far. He can usually go for hours."

I sigh. "He hasn't been himself for a while."

Shealagh stands with arms akimbo, catching her own breath. "Maybe he's dehydrated. He didn't drink that much today." She unzips a water bottle from my backpack and approaches Damon. He takes a perfunctory sip and hands the bottle back to her.

"I'm okay, Mom," Damon says with a halfhearted teenage smirk.

He doesn't look okay, but we grab more downtime in the island plaza, with cars streaming in about us. I spot a small bronze bust of John F. Kennedy.

"Now, there was grace under pressure . . ." I show Damon the inscription and we discuss our thirty-fifth president, whose assassination when I was in third grade marked a black day like 9/11 for my generation. Damon gets swept up in the historical drama and his eyes gleam. Even his color starts to return.

"Come on, let's go," he says after a spell, as if we've been holding him back.

We cross the wide roadway and head down Flatbush Avenue. It's busier here and a little grungier but it's mostly downhill, with frequent rest stops for Damon at the traffic lights. He uses them artfully, catching his breath on each street corner. We make for the Brooklyn Academy of Music, maintaining a semblance of purposefulness.

But both Shealagh and I are nervous now, our excitement at this inaugural family outing marred by our anxiety about Damon. We can sense his unease, the uncharacteristic hesitation in his step.

We go slower and stop at a candy store, hoping to revive him.

Sam and Miranda can feel something's off. They too begin to flag. They grumble they're tired and bored. A few blocks later, Shealagh starts to falter. I can't tell if it's her back, her asthma, or her concern about Damon, but everyone's losing heart.

I try to keep them all moving, like the group leader prodding his straggling, dispirited charges. This is not the communal, milestone-setting march I had in mind. It's not going well. But I'm desperate to keep my family on course, any course, before they give up and call it a day.

Everyone perks up as we approach the great spidery span of the Brooklyn Bridge. We ascend slowly along the elegant steel structure, letting Damon linger at various spots on the promenade, until we reach the crest, a windy crow's nest.

A small, excited crowd mills at the top. Three weeks after 9/11, the city remains under lockdown, but irrepressible signs of life appear from this sweeping height. We stand on the deck of a great ship, lashed by a sharp ocean breeze, and savor the spectacular vista of Lower Manhattan and Upper New York Bay. Damon grins between the soaring cables and lofts outstretched arms. His hair flaps wildly in the wind and his eyes sparkle as he's buffeted from all sides. Sam and Miranda come alive, galvanized by the gusty heights and by their giddy brother. Shealagh and I beam.

Only the absence of the Twin Towers jolts, like an erasure from the skyline.

When we reach the Manhattan side by city hall and the wind subsides, we can smell the foulness from Ground Zero. An acrid pall still hangs over the wounded city.

We turn south along the East River. The waterfront area appears spectral, semi-deserted. Damon starts to drag again, and we all feel the gloom.

We find a restaurant by South Street Seaport and try to replenish ourselves with a big lunch. But even the food does not quite fill the void. Looking around the table at my family, I realize we've gone as far as we can. Sam and Miranda are ornery, the air quality is suspect, and Damon looks pale and out of sorts. His mother is not faring much better.

I go to hail a cab while they wait inside. There are no taxis and I walk for miles by the icy water, my fingers bitten, before I finally find a cab. I try not to lose heart as we ride back across the river. We didn't go as far as I'd hoped but at least we clocked the first few miles. And we need to sort out Damon's problem before resuming.

Back in the house, Shealagh offers Damon her asthma inhaler and shows him how to use it. Damon inhales, awkwardly at first, but then he gets a few good puffs in and the bronchodilator appears to take effect. His breathing eases and he starts to unwind. By evening, he seems okay again. He does his homework, watches TV, and hangs out with me.

I'm relieved Damon's problem seems concrete and remediable. He's had allergies before and this may be a natural progression. More and more children have asthma, especially in urban areas. His mother has it, so there's a family history. And we know from Shealagh's experience how to treat and manage the problem.

But both Shealagh and I concur that since it's Damon we're talking about, he should see a doctor right away, just to be sure.

Chapter 12

We take Damon to Columbia Presbyterian Hospital to see his cardiologist, Dr. Constance Hayes, who has overseen Damon's case since he was three days old. A diminutive woman with short gray hair and austere features, Dr. Hayes is an accomplished professional who is caring but cautious and spare in manner, giving the term "tight-lipped" new meaning. But she is conscientious and kind, her recommendations are usually first-rate, and she has rarely steered us wrong. Now she listens to Damon's latest problem and suggests we see a pulmonologist she knows.

We meet with the lung specialist, who gives Damon a thorough exam and tests. He confirms that Damon's breathing problem appears to be asthmatic but reminds us "'asthma' is an umbrella term covering many symptoms." When we tell him about Damon's enlarged liver and his heart condition, he explains that pressure on the diaphragm—from the liver, the heart, or other stressed organs—"can cause or mimic the airway constriction that is a hallmark of asthma." This wouldn't change Damon's treatment for now but could suggest other, confounding factors at work. He prescribes a bronchodilator and an antihistamine and tells us to keep an eye on things.

Shealagh gives her son a few more lessons and helps him administer the new regimen daily. She makes sure he always carries his inhaler. The therapy seems to work, and Damon's breathing difficulties subside. The problem appears under control.

Damon is in eighth grade now, engrossed in the challenges and excitement of a new semester. Sam is in third grade and Miranda has started first grade. The next week, Sam is due to see a doctor about a minor procedure. Shealagh asks if we can defer Damon's checkup because he's just seen Dr. Hayes and our calendar is tight. But, reversing our roles, I insist Damon keep his appointment because I retain a bad feeling from the summer I'd like banished.

Shealagh gets Damon the same date as Sam. I have several meetings that day, so she'll take Damon for his usual tests in the morning and I'll come up from the office after. We have Damon's checkup down to a routine, but we've never met Sam's doctor, so he's the main event.

On the day in question, my last meeting runs over and I arrive at the hospital a few minutes late, just missing Dr. Hayes. She was called to the OR, but not before revealing to Shealagh disturbing new test results for Damon.

"What exactly did they find?" I press. My wife looks very upset and is doubly constrained because Damon and Sam are in the waiting room nearby.

"They think it's something called PLE," Shealagh says in a low, fraught voice. "He's not keeping protein in his body."

"Never heard of it . . . What's the treatment?" I ask, assuming a new medication.

"Dr. Hayes says they'll see if they can fix the problem in the cath lab or redo his original operation, but otherwise he will need a heart transplant."

"What?" I shake my head in disbelief. "Hold on! How do we go from 'He's doing so well' in one checkup to 'It's all falling apart' in the next? Where did this *come* from?"

"That's what Dr. Hayes told me," Shealagh says. "I was too upset to ask questions and then she had to go. Maybe you can get more out of her." She stifles a sob.

"Okay, I'll talk to her." I don't want to let it go except we can see Damon and Sam in the adjoining room, playing with Sam's action figures. The boys can see us too.

Sam's doctor calls us in and I sit through the meeting in a daze. All looks good for Sam and his routine procedure, but it makes the contrast with Damon even more incredible.

I've had my concerns about Damon since the summer, but not on this scale! He goes to school every day, participates in sports and extracurricular activities, parties and horses around with his friends—he leads a full and active life. How can everything just *unravel*? Without any warning from Dr. Hayes, whom I grill on every occasion?

At our last checkup, Dr. Hayes told us how proud she was of Damon's progress. She stood by the upright scales with arms crossed over her white lab coat, beaming at his development. As he sat on the paper-lined exam table with his shirt pulled up, Dr. Hayes listened to his chest and lungs, as well as his latest exploits, with a big smile. She is fond of our son and delights in his success in the world, like a benevolent if slightly stern godmother, which is how we've come to regard her.

Troubleshooting as usual, the biggest worry I could come up with on that last checkup was whether, as Damon reaches puberty, his anomalous blood flow could affect his sex life. Dr. Hayes, a thin, reserved woman, blinked at me and checked Shealagh before acknowledging it's a valid question. She told us she'd look into it and get back to us.

From such mundane concerns to this life-threatening crisis seems too great a leap. I refuse to panic until I know more. I page Dr. Hayes, but she's still in the OR. I redial several times, without success. Reluctantly, I go home with Shealagh and the boys. I can't let Damon see how rattled I am. He looks to me for guidance and can read my moods as well as I can read his— maybe better, since his survival depends on it.

In his room, we listen to the Top Ten on Z100 and discuss his upcoming exams.

"I'm thinking of going out for Model UN," Damon proudly confides. He suspects nothing, as far as I can tell.

Up in my study, I consult a medical text on PLE and browse the Internet. I don't like what I read, but I have no definitive data or diagnosis yet. Although Shealagh has more formal scientific training, she lets me take the lead on Damon. I've written a couple of medical books, I work with top scientists and researchers, and I'm relentless in my digging. I also successfully shepherded both my parents through health crises.

I have one basic rule: if we can't understand an issue or a medical approach makes no sense to us, it's the doctor's problem, not ours. No mumbo-jumbo. We must always know exactly what's going on so we can help ensure the best decisions are made. The most capable physicians supply the clearest explanations—equally clear about what they don't know as what they do—and only the mediocre take refuge in obfuscation or omniscience. I tell myself that once we have more facts, we'll sort this out.

I finally set up a phone appointment with Dr. Hayes while on a business trip in Los Angeles. I clear my morning schedule, hang a DO NOT DISTURB sign outside my door, and sit on the bed with pen and pad, perching anxiously by the phone. I can feel my heart hammering in my chest as I wait for the appointed hour to call.

I need to hear straight from Dr. Hayes and to know things are not as bad as I imagine. I cannot grasp how the same voice that has seen us through two open-heart surgeries and countless medical difficulties to the verge of young adulthood, the same voice that has bantered with us about skiing and schoolwork and Damon's plays, the voice that's been so full of optimism and encouragement about my son and never, not *once*, breathed a word about the possibility of a new disease—which, if he has it, has been developing for some time—how this same voice could so suddenly change its tune.

But Dr. Hayes, after pleasantries notably more strained than usual, does not have much good news for me. She explains that PLE, or protein-losing enteropathy, is a very serious illness that develops in about 10 percent of children who've had Damon's Fontan heart operation. The albumin count—albumin is the critical protein molecule that keeps vital components flowing inside the vessels—plummets, and all the vital proteins necessary for the functions of life leak out of the body. If the leakage cannot be stopped, the patient will eventually "starve" to death. No one really knows what causes PLE—though many suspect a link to higher pressures in the heart—nor has anyone found a cure.

But before assuming the worst, Dr. Hayes says, there are many things we can do.

First, they will take Damon to the cath lab and see if there is any obstruction that could account for his PLE-like symptoms. Sometimes it's a simple problem doctors can correct on the spot—in effect, a false alarm. If that doesn't work, they'll check if the original Fontan surgery is starting to unravel. (Damon has a Gore-Tex patch in his heart, made of the same material as my winter coat.) If there is a flaw in the repair, a Fontan "redo" could fix things. Then we can try various therapies—diet, drugs, injections, minor surgery—culminating in a heart transplant if nothing else works.

There seem to be multiple variables and approaches, so I press Dr. Hayes on data and outcomes, much of which she cannot supply. The disease is rare, the patient population small, and the published literature scarce. Yet even surfing the Net, I tell Dr. Hayes, I noted many papers from the U.S. and abroad, so it can't be *that* uncommon.

"Yes," Dr. Hayes says, "PLE is known and recognized, if poorly understood. It's complex." She offers to send me a recent paper on it. "I rarely recommend scientific articles to patients' families, but because of your background, I feel you can handle it."

I thank Dr. Hayes but ask why she never hinted to me before that anything like this could happen. "Haven't I always asked for more information about my son?" I say.

Dr. Hayes tries dancing around my question but I force her to go back to Damon's last checkup—and to all his previous checkups over the last nine years.

"Surely a condition like this does not occur overnight but develops gradually over many *years*?" I say. "The albumin is a liver count. Could PLE be connected to Damon's enlarged liver and the protruding belly we've asked about for several years? What about the recent slowdown in his growth? Could PLE also explain his asthma-like symptoms? Even his hernia? Why didn't you ever give us *a hint* about this possibility?"

There is a long silence on the other end. "Damon was doing so well and I was so encouraged by his tremendous success that I didn't want to believe it *myself*," Dr. Hayes admits. "Until his last albumin count went so low, and it became undeniable . . ."

I'm dismayed by what I hear even though I know Dr. Hayes is a caring doctor—it's her excess of concern, rather than unconcern, that led to her behavior. And she still has hopeful options to offer us, which we desperately need.

Dr. Hayes and I dwell on the best-case scenario and toss around the possibility of a quick fix in the cath lab. Dr. Hayes has seen this work before but we won't know until we go in and explore Damon's anatomy. We agree to schedule the catheterization without delay. Maybe we can head this thing off now. And even if we can't resolve it all in the cath lab, we can always repeat the Fontan. Damon responded so well to the first operation—he's had nine great years!—this must bode well for a second repair.

Dr. Hayes agrees we still have many options. As we pull back from the brink and prepare to end our conversation on a brighter note, I suggest that maybe this whole thing is manageable and will soon blow over. Dr. Hayes hears what I'm trying to do—hasn't she tried to do something similar?—but this time she will not go that far. She repeats she remains very hopeful but she believes this is a "significant" development.

The word sticks in my craw and makes me queasy. I want to ignore it and roll back the clock to where we were before I ever heard this dread news, to return to the triumphant narrative of Damon—his name means "he who conquers" in Greek—that we have all recited like a heroic epic since his birth.

But Dr. Hayes, perhaps cognizant of my recent criticism and not wishing to compound it, will not give me this satisfaction. Despite all my transparent efforts to downsize the crisis and reduce the alert level, Dr. Hayes repeats in a dry, all-too-practiced voice words that sound more chilling for their bland, clinical understatement:

"I believe this will be a significant event in his life."

I hang up the phone, still reeling, and stagger to the louvered windows. The room spins and shakes around me. I grope for the blinds and open them.

Outside, the California sun still shines and the palm trees sway.

The world carries on as before.

But underneath my feet, deep cracks and fissures appear. I shiver and hear someone who sounds suspiciously like myself begin to sob and scream.

"No!" I yell, slamming the wall and listening to my own wailing as if it came from another. "You can't take him from me . . . No, I won't let this happen! No, no, no!"

I barely recognize the deranged person howling inside my body but he seems to know more than me, as if a deep-buried and long-suppressed nightmare has returned.

My firstborn son, Damon, age thirteen, has been diagnosed with a severe, life-threatening illness. His congenital heart impairment, once believed successfully palliated, has erupted into a full-blown, potentially fatal disease!

There are many steps and hopes and therapies and trials along the way—and I'm going to explore and exhaust every one of them, and invent some of my own—but at that moment, the bottom falls out, and I stare down into the abyss.

I have a beautiful family, a loving wife and three wonderful kids, a nice home, good friends, a satisfying job, my own creative work and ever-rising prospects . . . I have a great life, but in that instant, it all turns to shit.

The original diagnosis occurs on October 11, 2001—exactly one month after the tragic terrorist attacks of 9/11. But now, for me and my family—and for the person whom I love with all my heart and soul, for Damon—the terror really begins.

Part II

Chapter 13

The week following my conversation with Dr. Hayes is like a powerful but invisible aftershock that pursues me from California back to New York.

No one else in the family understands yet how grave things are. And I fear saying anything until I know more and can prepare them better.

I pore over the scientific paper Dr. Hayes has sent, a multicenter study that aggregates much of the available data on PLE. I track down the original sources and references and read everything I can get my hands on.

All the peer-reviewed literature in all the best medical journals, though couched in staid jargon, seems to reflect a similar bafflement bordering on helplessness:

- "Protein-losing enteropathy (PLE) is an enigmatic disease with significant morbidity and mortality seen after the Fontan operation. It is unclear why its onset occurs months or even years after Fontan surgery."
- "PLE, defined as severe loss of serum protein into the intestine, occurs in about 4–13% of patients after the Fontan procedure and carries a dismal prognosis with a five-year survival rate between 46% and 59%."
- "PLE after the Fontan operation is a life-threatening complication that may be refractory to medical treatment. Preventive strategies and new therapeutic approaches are necessary."

I refuse to get discouraged and focus on treatments that have worked. I analyze all the therapeutic possibilities and outcomes in the literature, including any anecdotal data, and follow every footnote. I do my own calculations and make a list of options, arranging them in order of least intrusive (diet supplements, oral medication) to most intrusive (assist device, heart transplant).

I know that I will see things more clearly at the beginning, before anyone has raised false hopes or muddied the facts—and before the need for shielding myself and my family overtakes reality. I am single-minded in using hard statistics to understand the odds. I can always search for unheralded treatments and unconventional approaches, encourage or devise new solutions myself, or hope for miracles or at least a break, but I need to know what we're up against.

What we are up against is a devastating, little-understood disease with no known cure. It kills 50 percent of its victims within five years and 80 percent within ten years. And because no one has checked Damon's albumin for several years, and because Shealagh and I have observed what turns out to be PLE symptoms for an indefinite period, I don't know how long ago the illness started or how much of Damon's time it has already consumed.

I talk to half a dozen pediatric cardiology experts across the country who've dealt with PLE. I consult many other smart doctors and scientists I know. The generalists voice more optimism than the specialists, who, when pressed, admit they do not really understand this dread illness or how to cure it. But they all have their preferred treatments, each of which has worked for *some* people in *some* cases. Because the disease is rare and data scarce, I make a note of each case and add any new therapy I don't already have, be it standard or experimental, controversial or not, to my growing list.

I will deploy this master list, built up and refined over time, like a series of fortifications thrown up against an advancing enemy. The list gives me a rough battle plan to follow and a semblance, or illusion, of control.

My scientist friends with medical backgrounds, like Jeffrey Friedman, a leading molecular biologist at the Rockefeller University, and Robert Ben Ezra, an accomplished cell biologist at Memorial Sloan-Kettering Cancer Center, initially try to reassure me. I mustn't overreact. This is the twenty-first century, with molecular medicine and biotechnology, and medical care advancing by leaps and bounds. They'll look into PLE for me, talk to their expert friends, and return with an answer. Invariably, they call back and speak in more careful, subdued tones. This is a very tough illness with an uncertain prognosis.

Perhaps the hardest thing in those first days, after I've begun to grasp the grim parameters of this disease for myself, is how to convey the news to Shealagh and to Damon. I've accepted that I am breaking down inside—I feel emotionally paralyzed all day and twisted up all night, and I cry at odd moments—but I know how to continue functioning in the world. I do not know how Shealagh and Damon will react or how to broach this subject with them. And then there are Sam and Miranda to explain this to . . .

I want to tell Shealagh everything immediately and to share the terrible burden with her. We have always been full partners regarding Damon's care. But Shealagh has suffered a succession of unspeakable blows within a very short time—back surgery, her father's death, and now Damon's diagnosis, absent the dire statistics I've just learned—and I feel unsure about her frame of mind. Her best friend, Sonja, a physician who assisted her over the summer and now helps me research PLE, warns against upsetting Shealagh with too much depressing information. But we both agree she must know the big picture right away.

On a Friday morning after the kids have left for school, I invite Shealagh for coffee in the downstairs kitchen. It's a bit chilly for my taste because the door to the backyard is flung open, but Shealagh prefers fresh air at any temperature and I want to make her as comfortable as possible. I rub my arms and blow into my cupped hands by the dishwasher.

"Wear a sweater if you're cold, silly," Shealagh says in her pragmatic, English way.

"I'm fine." I fill the coffeemaker with filtered water from our sink and grind up the coffee beans in an automatic grinder that whirs and roars. Shealagh waters the heather and the flowering cacti on our windowsill with a copper watering can. Then she wipes down the counter with a sponge and deposits an empty milk carton in the recycling bin.

We cleave to our rituals, avoiding the subject at hand. Shealagh knows I must give her an update on Damon but she has not pressed me and seems content to stay in the dark. As she settles into a high-backed chair around our rustic kitchen table, I consider letting things slide. My wife looks fragile and tense in her soft lamb's-wool cardigan as she pencils in Miranda's Irish dance class on the monthly calendar. All she wants is the routine of parenthood, the daily satisfaction of bringing up her children. I'd do anything to spare her and maintain our hard-won equilibrium, but I know—we both know—that things have already deteriorated, and a reckoning is overdue.

I finish brewing the coffee and heat the milk in a giant china mug, as Shealagh likes it. I join her at the trestle table, our legs touching under the broad surface.

I look into Shealagh's wary face with its remarkable pale blue eyes—palely luminous, like the sky—as I start explaining what I've learned: how serious PLE is and how little understood; how there are various things to try but no consensus on a cure; how we confront a very formidable disease and will have to marshal all our resources to beat it.

I summarize the papers I've read and relate my conversations with numerous doctors and scientists. I describe the situation as delicately but accurately as possible, because we must be clear-eyed if we hope to persevere. It's tough, awkward going. I can find the silver lining in the darkest cloud, but first I have to tell Shealagh how overcast it really is.

"So basically, no one really understands why the Fontan circulation breaks down and why the body starts leaking protein from the gut," I say. "But it can't go on indefinitely because he needs the protein to grow and thrive."

"But he was doing so well!" Shealagh cries. She understands the medical information but it still doesn't make sense. "Why is this happening?"

"I don't know." I cover her hand with mine, trying to cushion the blow.

My wife trusts me to protect her and take care of things and now I must let her down, even hurt her. I feel culpable, as if I'm not keeping up my end of the bargain. And I feel shocked all over again, as if I am just learning the truth anew.

"My best guess is that it's related to the original congenital heart disease—remember how severe Damon's was? And that the Fontan is only a temporary fix, despite what they told us," I hazard.

Shealagh looks as if she's seen a ghost, and suddenly it feels as if time has collapsed and the past thirteen years have been erased.

We are back to the dark days of Damon's birth . . .

Shealagh's labor and delivery goes smoothly and out pops a handsome, fair, eight-pound, two-and-a-half-ounce baby boy with big hands and big feet and a gorgeous full-lipped smile. He looks well formed and capable.

The first two days are blissful, with mother and child bonding at the breast. The proud father dispenses cigars and rushes back to the hospital from work. Everyone in the family rejoices.

On the third day, we discover our newborn has a serious heart problem. The slower heart rate detected in utero is the result of a malformed heart that does not deliver sufficient oxygen to the body.

The doctors snatch Damon from his mother and rush him to the neonatal intensive care unit. He is placed inside an incubator. The room is filled with many premature, tiny-sized infants encased in similar apparatuses, struggling for survival. Damon, full-sized and pale skinned, stands out.

We watch our newly quarantined baby get extra oxygen from a high-tech helmet that squats on his head and sends a steady spray of mist wreathing about his nose and mouth. His oxygen saturation, which should be 98 percent, hovers around 72 percent before the Olympic Oxyhelmet boosts him to 90 percent. A pulsing red sensor attached to his tiny foot sends a stream of data to an overhead monitor, which flashes continuously.

Three-day-old Damon lays inside a clear bubble, separated from us by modern technology, a pint-sized astronaut marooned in his own world. We slip our hands through little portholes to touch him, but this only brings home how distant and sealed-off he is.

Shealagh suffers withdrawal, shock, grief. Her newborn is suddenly a captive of the medical profession. When they come to lance Damon's heel for a blood sample, his mother wants to hold him but they won't allow it. He must remain inside the incubator and we must step back and let the technicians proceed. As the long needle pierces his skin, an outraged Damon starts to cry behind his solitary barrier. We stand at a distance and watch the big syringe fill with bright red blood as the plunger pulls back. The forlorn cries of our exsanguinating infant in his caged apparatus pierce us. Shealagh, blocked from going to comfort her distressed baby, breaks down. I lead her out of the ICU, propping her up.

Shealagh, so ready for motherhood, is crushed. She can't establish a bond with her newborn and may only nurse him at strict intervals set by the ICU. To keep her milk flowing, she must sit on a stool and pump.

Meanwhile, we hear about Damon's pulmonary stenosis, a narrowing of the artery leading to the lungs that prevents the blood from receiving enough oxygen.

We are told of his atrioventricular (AV) canal, a hole in the heart that sends blood back to the right chamber, so it must be pumped again, raising pressures.

We learn that, best case, Damon will need a major operation in four to five years, and another procedure much sooner if he develops any sign of blueness.

The doctors, explaining that many of Damon's organs are reversed, inform us he has no spleen and will need daily lifetime medication. We are crestfallen until they return an hour later to report they've "discovered" a spleen on his right side. So we are spared this extra cross to bear and feel, perversely, lucky.

Finally Damon is discharged but Shealagh cannot take her baby home. She must relinquish him to another hospital for more tests. My heart cringes as I watch my young, nursing wife on the steps of Brooklyn Hospital, her arms empty, while they place her baby in an ambulance bound for Columbia Presbyterian Hospital. She sobs inconsolably in the sunlight as the ambulance pulls away.

I feel my wife's suffering more acutely than my own, because my powerful feelings for Damon have not yet developed—fatherhood remains largely an abstraction to me—and I don't understand that this little pale infant with his reddish tuft of hair will become the center of my life. It is Shealagh's privation, her harsh and unnatural introduction to motherhood, that affects me most deeply.

But sometime during those first weeks, a change comes over me too. I watch my newborn son as the doctors tell me he will always have a heart defect and never be like other children. I am overwhelmed by his complex congenital heart syndrome and devastated by our misfortune. Shealagh and I both enjoy robust good health, and there is no trace of any illness resembling Damon's on either side of the family. How could this happen to us?

I take in all the bad news, I listen to the gloomy prognosis. But to my eyes, this child still looks beautiful and full of life. Damon lays there, a sweet, thoughtful-looking infant, placid but supremely alert. He's primed for engagement with the world. And he's ours; we made him. Already, Shealagh points out how he sleeps like me, right arm draped by shoulder, left hand poised by jaw.

I conclude that nothing we've heard from the doctors, daunting as it may sound, precludes ultimate victory. We have a fighting chance and together we can beat this.

And for thirteen years, we do.

Damon undergoes two successful open-heart operations, thrives and succeeds beyond anyone's imagination.

Now Shealagh casts her eye to the refrigerator, settling on a recent photo of a beaming, sunburned Damon fishing off a boat on Cape Cod. Nearby is his certificate of excellence from karate with a raised gold seal.

"He's going to be okay?" Shealagh says. "There are effective treatments against this disease, right?"

"Yes," I reply. "We have lots of things to try. And many people make it. But the numbers are not great." I look down at the floor, then across at my wife. "We need to face that—and then we can figure out how to beat PLE."

"But Damon is not a number," Shealagh says with unimpeachable authority.

"No, exactly," I reply. "He's extraordinary, he's our amazing Damon."

Shealagh takes it very hard but nothing can rival Damon's reaction when he learns that he will have to go in for an unexpected procedure the following week. Shealagh tells him about it when she picks him up one evening from theater rehearsal. Damon asks why he needs a catheterization and Shealagh mumbles about problems that showed up on a previous test. She promises his father will explain it to him back home.

By the time Damon walks into the house, he knows something is wrong. The look on his face as he marches into the kitchen to confront me is excruciating to behold: anger, fear, bewilderment, accusation, and pleading vie across his boyish features. He dumps his heavy backpack by the door but his shoulders stay hunched, as if flexing against a great, unjust weight. He strides forward with his wide gait and slams his cell phone, MetroCard, and play script onto the counter. The top page flutters to the ground. A gentle, supremely rational boy, he can barely contain his fury at this incomprehensible turn of events.

Damon can't yet grasp what's happening, but he knows it's bad and that it doesn't fit any template we've previously discussed. He says not one cross word to me but his reproachful look effectively screams in my face: *This wasn't part of our game plan, Dad! What's going on?*

My son's look pierces me. I've been his coach and his mentor from the start, and together we've developed a true collaboration and a careful winning strategy. But now we've run into a fierce hurdle I could not prepare him for because I knew nothing about it. By choosing not to warn me about even the *possibility* of such a setback—believing we were better off *not* knowing— Damon's doctors have undermined my role and made me shirk my obligations to my son.

As we go up to Damon's room, I try to explain what's going on. Damon has matured and possesses a first-rate mind. He also has a diagram of the human heart pinned to his wall and a model skeleton standing atop his dresser, so I assume he'll want all the details.

"We believe it's related to your original heart problem," I say. "Your body is losing protein because the heart isn't pumping enough oxygen to your cells."

"Will I need another operation if the Fontan isn't working?" Damon asks. He doesn't look happy but at least he's thinking clearly.

"If it's PLE—we're not even sure yet—then we'll have to try various things. An operation is the last resort. But you've been through worse, and you'll get through this." I try to reassure him by drawing on his past record of success.

"Will I have to miss school?" Damon focuses on practical matters.

"No, not now. But it's complicated, so we'll have to keep our eye on it."

I'm ready to tell him more—all I know, in fact—but it turns out I'm wrong about my teenage son's inclinations. Damon extracts the gist of his problem from me but he decides early on not to immerse himself in his own medical case. He's more interested in attending school and participating in theater workshops and being with his friends. He doesn't want to learn all the details of his illness or the history of PLE or the latest research, but trusts me to manage these things for him and to report back any major developments.

It's a decision that surprises and even disappoints me at first—I respect Damon's ability and believe he could help himself, and even assist me with his insights—but it's a decision whose wisdom I learn to appreciate over time.

Damon just wants to lead a normal life.

Chapter 14

The morning of Damon's catheterization Channel One reports snarled traffic, so after seeing Sam and Miranda off on the school bus—we tell them Damon has a routine procedure—we leave our car in the driveway and take the subway in.

Shealagh packs two oversized bags, one with Damon's things and one with hers. A devoted mother ready to serve her son in any capacity, she is the designated hospital overnighter. We both bring work, knowing the drill.

We take the F train, each immersed in a different section of the paper as we sit with our luggage. At Jay Street–Borough Hall, we switch to the A train.

Damon wears frayed black shorts and a pale green T-shirt with palm trees on it. He looks a tad drawn—I note a small raccoon blotch under each eye—but otherwise he appears in decent shape. The Zyrtec he's been taking for allergies has reduced the puffiness in his face, and his belly seems less protuberant. His red hair gives him a bright luster even in drab surroundings.

Damon soon grows bored with the paper—he reads it dutifully but the daily habit has not quite taken—and pulls out an *Animorphs* series book. The cover shows five kids who morph into animals and fight evil with enhanced powers.

"You know, there's a theory that the structure of the modern human brain still retains traces of our ancestral evolution," I tell him. "It says we have remnants of a snake brain and an early mammal brain, like a cat, which means we are not so distant from our animal past . . . So there may be a scientific basis for such tales."

"Yeah, I know, Dad." Damon gives a dreamy, cunning smile. He's familiar with this idea, even if just now he's more interested in escapism than realism.

We disembark at 168th Street and pass the newsstand and the peanut vendor before entering the giant hospital complex and going up to the third floor.

"I feel a little nervous." Damon smiles awkwardly, as if it's just hit him.

"You've been through this twice before, when you were much younger." I touch his back.

"And both times you sailed through with flying colors," Shealagh says.

We sign in; Damon gets the standard checks and is told to prepare. There are no changing rooms available and Damon is too self-conscious to change in front of his mother, so we find a private bathroom down the hall. I help him slip into his hospital gown, noting how his abdomen seems marginally less swollen. I attribute this to two new medications prescribed recently. From my reading, I estimate 25 percent of patients with PLE can resolve their symptoms with medication alone, and I pray that Damon will fall into this category.

I carry his clothes as he pads out in thin gray slipper socks and a green gown.

Dr. Donnelly, the head of the cath team, comes to talk to us before the procedure. She has polished manners and is eager to begin. But first I want her views on fenestration: creating a small opening between the chambers of the heart to relieve pressure, which has reputedly resolved many PLE cases.

"We've heard it's effective and can even be done in the cath lab," I say.

Dr. Donnelly smiles. "We'll be proactive if we find anything small to do but the primary purpose of this procedure is to gather information."

Dr. Donnelly says they will likely go in through Damon's neck rather than the groin because the veins around Damon's groin are blocked from his previous catheterizations. Damon moans at this and becomes visibly agitated. I press Dr. Donnelly for alternative access points but apparently there are none. She promises they will numb the neck area before entering and give Damon additional sedation so that he remains "comfortable."

"How long do you expect this procedure to last?" Shealagh asks tensely.

"Two hours if we only take pictures, but longer if we need to do anything."

We accompany Damon to the cath lab, a dark, chilled, cavernous room. The nurses tip him from the gurney onto a flat board encircled by huge swinging steel arms housing imaging equipment that feeds into a bank of large, overhead monitors.

Damon lies twitching on the narrow bed, restless and uneasy. He is wary of being stuck, so they give him numbing cream. But the resident who tries inserting the needle misses Damon's vein several times, sending him into a paroxysm of squirming. Shealagh squeezes his hand and I stroke his arm, glaring at the fumbling resident, while Damon continues to wriggle and yelp like a recalcitrant puppy on the vet's table.

A Jamaican technician seizes Damon's lower body to steady him. A big, gentle man, the Jamaican needs to tape his genital area but Damon is too riled to lie still. He's also too embarrassed. Shealagh squats by his head, whispering that she can't see anything and his privacy is protected. I try guy talk—"It's a homemade jockstrap, D-man!"—as I help the Jamaican to stabilize my writhing son, heartsick at his frail thrashing but quietly thankful the technician is male.

Damon continues to wiggle and twist against this ignominious violation. I've rarely seen him so wild. He kicks and bucks. I wince as I hold his legs down, hating myself for the role I'm forced to play. Better me, I rationalize, than an impersonal pair of hands. But it's humiliating, for both of us. The Jamaican applies three strips of tape, diapering my teenage son, and I quickly let go of his legs.

"No, I don't want it!" Damon cries as a nurse finally gets the needle in.

Shealagh and I are told to exit the OR but Damon pleads for us to stay. He's unusually skittish and clingy and we don't want to leave him in such a state.

I stroke his hair. "Hey, D-man, forget where you are and think of something nice. What would you most like? I'll get you anything you want . . ."

He's so upset I'm not sure if he's following me, but then Damon suddenly pipes up. "Can you have Lachlann fly in for my Bar Mitzvah?"

I smile. "You got it."

It's a brief respite before multiple, crisscrossing hands attach wires and sensors to his body, sticking him like a pincushion. Damon whimpers and again begs us not to go. We ask to stay until his eyes close but the OR staff won't hear of it. They must put him to sleep in stages, and we must exit so they can begin.

Shealagh and I harden ourselves and kiss him good-bye. Damon cries as we leave the room. Shealagh waits until the door closes before daubing her tears while I try to suppress the grisly image of Abraham sacrificing Isaac as I leave my son alone on his altar bed. I tell myself the biblical story turned out well—it was only a test, after all—but it feels like scant consolation.

Shealagh and I spread out in the waiting room and buckle down with our diversions: chitchat, reading, phone calls, coffee. After an hour, we grab a quick bite and hurry back to our stations. There's no telling when Damon might get out.

I work until Shealagh, under great stress, falls asleep on the couch beside me. I move to the plastic chair, giving her room, and continue reading proposals.

After three hours, I begin to grow restless. Usually, if it's taking this long, a nurse comes out with a progress report. But we still haven't heard a peep from the cath lab.

I page Dr. Hayes, Damon's cardiologist and still our go-to person at Columbia. Her assistant says Dr. Hayes is in the OR but will get back to me ASAP.

At some point, Dr. Hayes materializes, hands tucked demurely inside the pockets of her white coat. I rise and give her a searching glance.

"Everything so far is okay," she says in her small voice.

I let out a sigh. We chat and I explain that Shealagh, sleeping on the couch below us, has had a terrible few months. We agree she should not be disturbed.

Dr. Hayes reports that Dr. Donnelly, a cath lab veteran, feels Damon looks "surprisingly good" and is "impressed" by his overall condition.

"They haven't found anything yet." Dr. Hayes smiles softly. "We're hopeful they've caught any problem he might develop early enough so it's manageable."

Dr. Hayes also discussed the case with Dr. Hohrdoff, head of the whole cath lab, and he agreed that Damon's hemodynamics looked "wonderful."

Dr. Hayes sounds almost chipper, as if she's trying to cheer us both up.

I'm pleased to hear good news but ask Dr. Hayes if we hadn't perversely hoped to find something *wrong* that would explain the PLE, so that we could fix it.

"Bad news leading to good, rather than vice versa, which is what I fear you're telling me?" I explain.

Dr. Hayes turns grim. "Yes, it's true," she sighs, as if on a separate sub-ject. "No one knows why these children with perfect pressures go on to develop PLE."

I wince. "So we're back to square one?"

Dr. Hayes doesn't answer, but such is the temptation to extract hope and seek solace that I find myself focusing on the positive aspects she's empha-sized—Damon looks good and his numbers are good—even though I know it's not so simple or straightforward.

It's not simple because Damon lacks a working ventricle to pump blood returning from the body to the lungs, so his body must maintain artificially high pressures *continuously* just to let this blood reach the lungs. And even with higher pressures, the fluid sometimes backs up and leaks into other organs, requiring even higher pressures in a vicious cycle. So even "perfect pressures" for a child with a Fontan would be abnormally high for you and me, and may not address the underlying problem.

But I don't dwell on such counterintuitive facts as Dr. Hayes departs— I cleave to the positive and share the good news with Shealagh when she wakes. My wife nods but starts to worry as more hours pass without a word. At five P.M., the receptionist leaves and the hallways empty out. Someone turns off the lights.

"What's going on? Why hasn't anyone come to update us?" Shealagh asks fretfully.

I page Dr. Hayes and try her assistant, but I only get voice mail. I scam-per across the dark, deserted floors and yell along the empty halls but all I hear is my own echo. I too start to fret. It's twilight, and we're in a very weird zone.

Finally, well after seven P.M., Dr. Donnelly emerges in scrubs and tells us all is well. I note she's refreshed her makeup. She quickly sketches a dia-gram of Damon's anatomy and shares two findings: Damon had developed some collateral veins, which they coiled off, and this should improve his saturation; and they noted a very small fenestration from his first surgery, sug-gesting some mixing was already occurring, so a new fenestration might not provide much additional benefit.

"Otherwise," Dr. Donnelly reports, "all was fine and Damon tolerated the procedure well. Absent his cardiac anomaly, we found nothing wrong with him."

"So there's no identifiable problem you can fix?" I point out.

"Yes, from the cath lab point of view, Damon is in good shape," Dr. Donnelly says, sidestepping my question. "You can go see him in the recovery room now."

I thank Dr. Donnelly and follow Shealagh into recovery.

Damon lies behind a half-drawn curtain, encircled by monitors. He looks wan but dogged, his plume of hair a pale, diluted crest across the pillow.

"How are you, sweetie?" Shealagh says as we rush to his side.

"Okay, but it was pretty rough," Damon says. His eyes are groggy and bloodshot and his mouth turned down.

Our son reports he was awake for the entire procedure and experienced acute discomfort and distress. When they inserted the catheter, he was aware of being pierced and could sense the wriggly tube snaking through his veins. He felt a stinging sensation when they injected contrast dye in his arteries and a burning nausea as the hot dye spread to his heart. His body cramped from lying still so long. And he felt physically abused and morally ignored as they manipulated his body.

"Once when they hurt me, I cried in pain and they told me to be quiet . . . I thought I imagined it but when I did it again, they yelled, 'Stop talking!'" Damon says with ashen incredulity.

I have to stifle my own anger. Damon is stoic and rarely complains, so it must really have been bad.

By eight thirty P.M., we're out of recovery and up on the floor. The nurses enter constantly to monitor Damon. He must lie flat and use the chamber pot.

Shealagh unpacks and, like a good mother, tries to make our room more homey. We check in with Sam and Miranda, then find a movie on the overhead TV. Shealagh wanders up the hall—she knows all the hiding places—and returns with crackers and cheese and soft drinks, plus extra pillows and blankets. We sit around Damon's bed, eating, watching the movie, and making a small party of it.

After the film, I pull the chair-bed out for Shealagh. While she goes to change, Damon and I chat. He is still weak and sore but I detect the glimmers of a comeback on his face. I describe the initial catheterization results and relay to him the positive news Dr. Hayes emphasized to me. Damon asks when he can return to school and I say as soon as he feels up to it, which seems to satisfy him.

Shealagh returns in a long T-shirt nightgown with her skin scrubbed and her thick hair pushed back by a velvet hair band. Her myopic blue eyes look lost before she adjusts to the makeshift hospital accommodations. I dislike leaving her alone in such surroundings but they only allow one parent overnight and Sam and Miranda wait for me at home. And I know that Shealagh is steadfast and will do whatever is required for her children.

I linger for a spell, wondering why an exploratory test Damon has undergone twice before felt so harrowing this time, before I kiss my son and my wife good night and ride the subway back to Brooklyn.

Chapter 15

It takes Damon longer than expected to bounce back from his catheterization, as if the sharp and protracted medical probing he underwent has disrupted his basic equilibrium, the secret bargain he's struck with his body.

At least that's what I tell myself, because the doctors have no explanation.

He comes home the following day and goes straight to his room to rest. Shealagh, too, is exhausted from her labors and retreats upstairs to our bedroom.

When I return from the office, Shealagh is napping and Damon lies on his loft bed, staring up at the ceiling fan and listening to soft music on his clock radio. I catch up with my wife and son, check in with Sam and Miranda, order dinner.

When the food comes, I place Shealagh's meal on a tray, add a glass of red wine, and carry it to the top floor. Shealagh's back is acting up and she's wiped out. But Damon, despite fatigue and lingering soreness, insists on eating with us in the downstairs kitchen. He descends gingerly from his loft bed and waddles from the middle to the bottom floor, grasping the stair rail and protecting his groin.

I sit with the kids and watch Damon hold court at the table. He slumps forward on weary elbows and is a little short-fused with his siblings—what can they know of his aches and pains, his travails?—but he's also affectionate and playful with them.

"Damon, what did you eat at the hospital?" Miranda asks.

"Hospital food," Damon says, tucking into his seafood salad.

"What's that?" Miranda misses the irony.

"Chicken, mashed potatoes, carrots—but it all tastes like applesauce."

"Yuck," Miranda cries, grinning. She and Sam delight in their big brother's return and hang on his every word and gesture.

"Mirandy, how do you like Ms. Garvey? Me and Sam both had her," Damon says.

"I know. She keeps asking me why I don't have red hair," Miranda replies, pouting.

"Because you're a girl," Sam teases. "And you're silly."

"Sam, don't be annoying!" Damon says. "Girls have red hair just like boys."

"Yeah," Miranda says. "Look at Pippi Longstocking!"

After dinner, Miranda volunteers to dash upstairs, change into pj's, brush teeth, and even forgo a good-night story if she can watch *Lizzy McGuire*. Sam and Damon groan but I consent because I connect with my daughter by watching this show with her. After Miranda goes to bed, we tune in to *The Fresh Prince of Bel-Air*. Damon likes Will Smith, and Sam likes watching with Damon.

The phone rings. It's an employee from the hospital pharmacy informing me, in broken English, of a mix-up in Damon's prescription. It sounds like a bad joke from one of our sitcoms, except it's not. The guy can't answer any of my questions, so I hang up and call Dr. Hayes, leaving an urgent message. Eventually, I get a call back from the attending doctor, who's covering for Dr. Hayes. She beats around the bush until I get her to reveal that Damon was supposed to get 1.25 milligrams of enalapril, a drug that opens the blood vessels, but instead the hospital mistakenly filled a prescription for 12.5 milligrams.

"You mean you gave my son *ten times* the approved dosage of his heart medication!" I raise my voice, though it's nothing compared to my anxiety level.

"I didn't do anything, I'm only relaying information for your benefit." The attending sounds blithely detached, almost condescending, as if she's doing me a favor. She asks how Damon is and explains the peak effect from the overdose would have been six hours ago, so we're past the danger point— assuming I haven't given him another dose. She suggests picking up a new prescription tomorrow. The doctor also warns me that enalapril lowers blood pressure so we need to watch out for dizziness or fainting. "No warm baths or sitting up suddenly. Otherwise he should be fine, though of course you must stay vigilant."

I thank the attending and hang up in dismay. I check with two physician friends who confirm the peak danger should have passed but that a tenfold increase in dosage is significant and could cause kidney problems. They tell me to keep an eye on Damon and add that such an error constitutes malpractice.

The next day, I take the morning off to be with Damon. He's still weak and dizzy but not significantly worse to my eyes. We rent *My Cousin Vinny* and laugh together. I watch him closely for signs of an overdose effect before going to work.

When I return that evening, my parents bustle in our kitchen. They have driven over from Queens and prepared a wonderful Friday-night meal, replete with Helga's homemade chicken soup, a favorite of Damon's. Shealagh is grateful for a night off.

The seven of us stand around the brimming table and light the Sabbath candles—the single ritual my parents observed when I was a boy, and one I honor only sporadically now—and then I bless my children. This is a new tradition I haphazardly inaugurated a few years ago. I read about it or saw someone do it and it spoke to me, so I adopted it.

I walk around the table and place my hands over Damon's and Sam's heads. The bright, flickering light from the Sabbath candles shines on their two thatches like the sun gilding a russet field. They bow their heads before me—Damon's is a deeper, richer red; Sam's has lighter tones—and both bask in my embrace. With my palms covering their resplendent crowns, and Miranda excitedly waiting across the table for her turn, I look at my wife and my parents and feel like the richest man in the world.

I smile upon my two beaming sons, stroke their hair, and recite the blessing:

> *May God make you like Ephraim and Menashe.*
> *May God bless you and watch over you.*
> *May God shine his face toward you and show you favor.*
> *May God be favorably disposed toward you and grant you peace.*

Ephraim and Menashe were Jacob's grandsons, whom he praised as role models, a "blessing," for the people of Israel. I've explained this to my children several times but all they know is that Dad is touching them and saying nice things about them. They understand it's part of his tradition—their mother has converted to Judaism, though no one is very observant or consistent in this house—and they grasp they are valued and loved. And that's good enough for them. For me too.

The minute I finish the boys' blessing, Miranda beckons me to her side, yanking at my arms. She looks like she might burst with pride as she helps install my hand over her crown. She bows her shimmering blond head, radiant in her solo glory, while I repeat the benediction, changing only the role model names, to the righteous matriarchs this time: "May God make you like Sarah, Rebecca, Rachel, and Leah . . ."

The candles burn and we bless the wine and the bread and sit down to eat. Damon still sags a little in his chair but he eats respectably and engages actively with my parents, two of his biggest fans. My mother, who used to help with his day care as a toddler, now accompanies Damon to the theater, and my father, who plays soccer and catch and any game going with his grandson, and who shares a penchant for telling stories and jokes and performing, is teaching him Hebrew in preparation for his Bar Mitzvah.

"How are your lessons coming?" my mother asks, smiling at her grandson.

"Okay. I'm still having a little trouble with the vowels," Damon admits.

"You've almost got it, laddie—a wee bit more practice is all you need," my father says.

On Saturday, Damon sleeps late and then the two of us hop the subway into the city. On the way in, Damon complains of tightness on his left side, from the ribs back to the kidney, and I give him a massage. I'm not sure if it helps but he thanks me sweetly.

We pick up one schoolmate, Kiri—a compact girl with a witty, tomboyish air—on Fourteenth Street, and wait for another, Keith, at Rockefeller Center. Keith's mother—she's so young, at first I mistake her for another student—drops him off by the Atlas statue before we proceed into the International Building and ride the elevator to my office on the twenty-fifth floor. I serve, in a voluntary capacity, as secretary of the New York State Selection Committee for the Rhodes Scholarship, and Damon and his friends have come to help me process the applications, which must shortly be sent to my fellow committee members. It's a labor-intensive task and I pay the kids for their efforts, but it's also a social outing and a good way for Damon, who's missed school the past three days, to catch up with his friends.

We lay out nine copies of each application on a big conference table. I stress that each file is confidential and represents a lifetime of hard work and dreams, so they must treat it with respect. But invariably, teen irreverence creeps in.

"Check out Miss America!" Keith brandishes a glossy headshot. "Is that a *halter top*? Oh, she wants to work in *global health*, so this shows she's ready to fly to the developing world twenty-four/seven and *get down* with the heat and the jungle."

Kiri smiles. She holds little truck with glamour shots but, perhaps out of gender solidarity, she shows a slick male photo that would do a politician proud.

"Would you buy a used car from *this* man?" she deadpans.

"No, but tell me what toothpaste he's using!" Keith shrieks.

Damon walks around the long table—I notice he drags a little—and inspects the photo. He grins. "That's scary." Then, beaming wickedly, he holds up a sheet.

"Another essay beginning with a hardship case that inspired someone to enter public service . . ." He flutters the paper with comical, hard-nosed skepticism. "Is that, like, the secret formula, Dad?"

I chuckle, then glance at the meager number of completed files on the table.

"Hey, I'm sure when you guys apply, you'll knock it out of the park, but how about a little more work? If we finish on time, I'll take you to the movies."

Damon returns to school on Monday though he's still not back to full strength. I drop him off in a taxi in the morning and Shealagh picks him up at three P.M. That night we go celebrate my mother's birthday at a restaurant on Smith Street, even though we worry Damon is not really up to it.

The trendy little restaurant has a "minor plumbing problem" and all night a kitchen hand feverishly swabs the floor. Meanwhile our food is late and everyone grows peckish. "Even the *Titanic* kept serving!" my father grumbles. Damon sags in his chair, exhausted. A car alarm goes off and shrieks uncontrollably. When the food finally arrives, Damon forces down a few bites and then jumps to his feet, looking queasy. Everyone stares at him.

"You feeling all right, sweetie?" Shealagh asks nervously.

Damon's mouth is sealed but he lifts one finger as if to say, "Just a minute." Then he bolts out the door. I follow him to the street and catch up just as he bends over a trash can and vomits neatly into the receptacle.

I put my arm around his shoulder. "Better?"

He leans against me, pale and weary, and his eyes roll back in their sockets.

I stroke his drooping head. "It's gonna be okay, D-man."

We return to the restaurant, clean him up, and resume our meal. Damon is game but he's just not himself. He sits there, weak and dispirited, trying to cope. I wish we'd brought along a friend for him. His big puppy eyes, so sweet and knowing, flash disconcertingly at us and then beyond us, as if registering in their objective sweep that things are awry.

We try to cheer him up but he has only one thing on his mind.

"When do we get my cath results so I can stop taking so many meds?"

We don't answer directly because this is a white lie to help him adjust to his new regimen. He must swallow half a dozen medications, some several times a day, plus vitamin pills and protein supplements and fatty oils that nauseate him and kill his appetite. Damon bitterly resents this daily ordeal and blames it for his current malaise. And I don't yet have the heart to tell him I only pray he can *keep* taking these medications so we won't need to do anything more drastic.

"We just have to monitor things and see how it goes," I tell him.

The waiter brings a cake with candles and we dutifully toast my mother's seventy-fourth birthday, but everyone feels the uncelebratory weight of the evening.

Damon continues to have a rough few weeks. When he gets home from school, he often wants to lie down and rest, highly irregular behavior for him.

One day he storms into the house and cries, "I can't breathe!" He's having an asthma attack. Once he uses his inhaler, the attack subsides, but it's a bad sign.

His disorientation persists, and for the first time in his life he experiences motion sickness. Previously, he could read for hours in a speeding car without any discomfort. Now he gets dizzy just sitting in the backseat. Even the rolling subway affects him. I worry he has lost a fundamental layer of his immunity, like a turtle or a snail deprived of its shell. His filtering defenses have been compromised and life suddenly assails him. I can't tell if it's the effects of his catheterization or if his diagnosis has accelerated things, the way naming a problem can hasten its onset.

Damon's doctors can't tell either, so we remain baffled and concerned.

In the fall, I take Damon to the entrance exams for New York's specialized high schools. Like most aspirants, Damon has practiced for this test and attended a prep course, but in the last two months he's trailed off, as with so much else.

"You can wait until you feel better to take the test," I tell Damon. "I'm sure we can get you a medical deferment and even if we can't, your health comes first."

"But I want to take the test with everyone else. I'll be fine," Damon insists.

I drive him to the test site, an immense public high school, on a Saturday morning. When we get there, hundreds of students are already lined up outside the building. The first thing I notice is how big and physically developed these kids look, and how small and pale Damon appears by comparison. As we walk along the sprawling queue, I feel like I'm bringing a child to an adult competition and console myself this is not an athletic contest. Nevertheless, Damon appears dwarfed by these strapping adolescents bursting with hormones and rude health.

He gets in line and I hand him juice and energy bars. "Don't forget to eat and drink," I tell him. I watch other parents giving similar last-minute advice and supplies, including enough number 2 pencils to repopulate a forest. I smile ruefully because while I'm normally competitive for my kids, my main concern now is that my ailing son not fall asleep during the three-hour exam and embarrass himself.

I suddenly realize I no longer care about this test—I know how smart Damon is—because I'm too preoccupied with his physical well-being and his medical, rather than his academic, prognosis. I look out at the sea of aspiring young faces, many from families with big stakes in this race, and I decide I'd gladly trade ten points off Damon's IQ with any one of them for a single point on his albumin level. Let them have their Ivy Leagues and all the scholastic laurels; I just want a healthy kid!

"You can go, Dad," Damon says. "I'll be fine."

I give him a final pat on the back—no kisses in front of this group!—and head back to the car.

As I walk off, I glance back at my son standing in the middle of this great, hulking crowd. He appears small and isolated with his protruding abdomen, and I worry I'm leaving him all alone; yet I also note how Damon maintains his own center of gravity, casual but self-possessed. Within seconds, he engages a new student and proffers advice to his grateful family. He speaks with easy authority while others, less sure, drift to him. Checking out the wider action, he nods at an attractive girl with chopped, purple hair and she nods back at him.

I smile. You'd think Damon shouldn't be here, yet here he is, on his own terms, with everyone else. He even possesses a certain coolness, in his compact, mop-headed, jeans-low-on-hips slouch. I want to tell him how proud he makes me, that in my eyes he's already passed the test, but I don't dare cheat him of this important rite of passage with his peers.

Bullhorns bark and the students file in.

I depart but return early, uncertain what to expect. At the appointed hour, Damon walks out of the building with the other kids, looking nonchalant, and casually strolls toward me.

"So how was it?" I scan him for any hint of distress or a blowout.

"Fine. Maybe a little harder than I expected." Damon looks calm and unfazed. "I had to rush at the end but I think I did okay."

"You didn't get tired?" I'm amazed at his serenity. "No special problems?"

"No, except I had to get up and go to the bathroom all the time. From all the diuretics I'm taking . . . And the proctor kept giving me dirty looks, like I was cheating. So for the last hour, I just held it in. Which was a little distracting."

"Well, congrats on getting through it, D-man. That's an achievement itself."

Now he admits he feels a little tired, and even before we get home from the test, he dozes off beside me in the car.

Although we won't learn the results for several months, Damon winds up winning entrance to Bronx High School of Science and Brooklyn Technical High School, two of the city's top three schools. It's an impressive performance, better than anyone else from his middle school.

Chapter 16

Damon gradually recovers from his catheterization and crawls back to sea level. The motion sickness fades. The asthma attacks cease. He seems more like himself and resumes a normal, or near normal, pace. Or have our expectations just changed?

One Saturday I'm working in my second-floor study, revising my five-hundred-page first novel after an initial round of rejections, when I hear footsteps pounding up the stairs and Shealagh and the three kids burst into the room. They surround me with great, nervous excitement and heavy breathing. Hushed, conspiratorial giggling fills the room.

They have a secret, a *surprise* for me.

The kids, led by Damon, push their mother forward. Shealagh carries a black Sherpa bag with nylon mesh at either end. A rustling movement issues from inside the bag.

Miranda and Sam look like they're going to explode from the suspense.

Shealagh unzips the bag and removes from it the long, reddish-brown neck of what appears to be a large, lively rodent. Everyone looks expectantly at me.

"A ferret?" I frown, trying to be a good sport. I recall once discussing with the kids getting a rabbit or a guinea pig but never a ferret. "Aren't they a little wild for house pets?"

An awkward silence, followed by laughter.

"No, Dad. It's a dog!" Miranda reproaches me on everyone's behalf.

"A *dog*?" I study the tiny creature. It's under four pounds with a smooth-coated body, muscular neck, pointy ears, and docked tail. "Doesn't look like a dog."

"He's a *miniature pinscher*," Damon informs me with a bright-eyed look and stilted pronunciation suggesting he's just learned this fact for himself.

"He's a cross between an Italian greyhound and a dachshund, a mini-pin," Shealagh says, a mite sheepishly. She knows she's on shaky ground but she's counting on mitigating circumstances. We used to have a real dog, a Gordon setter named Ophelia who died when Damon was five and whom we all adored. But Shealagh and I had agreed, or I thought we had, that the family wasn't ready for a new dog. And when we were, we'd choose together.

"Please, Dad, can we keep him? Please!" Sam is near tears. He's never had a dog—Ophelia died shortly after his birth—and he's clamored relentlessly for one this past year.

"Mom and I will walk him," Damon says, as if they've rehearsed this. "Every day."

"And clean up after him." Shealagh delivers her lines, smiling.

"Oh sure—" I start to express my skepticism, but I don't get to finish.

"You won't have to do anything, Dad, except maybe let him out in the morning because you get up first," Miranda chimes in.

"And he's so little we can take him on the plane to Skye," Damon says.

I pause. Given recent events, it seems churlish to deny anyone, especially Damon and Shealagh, any opportunity for joy.

"His name is Freddie!" Sam announces, sensing vacillation on my part.

"Freddie is a purebred Kentucky gentleman," Shealagh adds with her plummiest English accent. "He comes from a very distinguished Southern family."

"His father was called Little Red Flame," Damon says, his eyes twinkling at me.

"We have a certified pedigree from the American Kennel Club," Shealagh boasts wryly. "He has a most impressive lineage stretching back many generations."

"Yeah, that's why he was so expensive!" Miranda blurts.

"He's not *that* expensive . . . ," Shealagh says defensively.

"Yes, he is. That's why you had to sneak back into the house and get more money," Miranda reports with oblivious precision.

Damon gives a toothy, embarrassed grin while his mother tries a broader perspective. "We could breed him. Mini-pins are very popular. And his pedigree is compiled from official stud book records so his offspring would fetch a handsome price."

"I don't want to *breed* Freddie." Damon looks horrified. He picks up the puppy. "Unless *he* wants to. Huh, Freddie?" The dog snuggles against him.

"Not now, he's far too young," Shealagh reassures Damon, eyeing Freddie's microscopic breeding equipment. "Anyway, it's just a suggestion."

"Who came up with his name?" I ask, impressed by the pace of events.

"Damon did," Sam replies.

"But I saw him same time as Damon," Miranda asserts.

"We went to Little Angels for haircuts and the pet store is just across the street," Shealagh explains. "But we had *no intention* of buying a dog when we left the house."

My wife always cites original motive as a moral indicator, even a defense, whereas I tend to focus more on outcome. But now it seems the outcome is clear. I've rarely seen my family so excited and united. And we've certainly had enough bad news.

As Damon leans his head against Freddie's coat, I note how they form a match, as if cut from similar cloth. "They have almost identical coloring—that same brownish-red shade," I remark.

"Yes!" Shealagh senses victory. "Freddie's official pedigree color is *rust*."

Damon cradles Freddie, posing for a dual shot. Not for nothing he's an actor.

"This woman walked into the pet store and saw Damon sitting on the floor and holding Freddie and she said we *had* to buy that dog because the two of them looked so alike, as if they belonged together." Shealagh smiles. "Almost like they were related."

"Well, don't exaggerate," I say, admonishing her.

Miranda tries to help, tactlessly. "They're both kind of small."

Damon winces. "That's not what Dad meant."

"Damon's a lot bigger than you!" Sam assails Miranda and defends Damon, a twofer.

"He's bigger than you too," Miranda retorts, more from rhyme than reason.

"Okay, guys. Relax." I blow the whistle. "Let's enjoy what we have."

A pause. Sam leans in shrewdly to me. "That mean we can keep Freddie, Dad?"

"Please, please pretty please, Dad!" Miranda begs.

"Come on, you know you really like dogs," Shealagh coaxes.

"Yes." I sigh. "But he's a *ferret*." I pick up the tiny creature in one hand, holding him aloft as he swipes at me with his mini-paws. "Freddie the ferret," I dub him.

"No, Dad, don't say that," Miranda pleads. "He's a dog." She rescues Freddie from my hands but then almost drops him until Damon intervenes with a surer grip.

"A cute ferret?" I offer.

"No, he's a dog!" They drown me out in unison, feigning offense even if they realize the tide is turning in their favor.

"So how about it, Dad?" Damon speaks up in a manly tone but beseeches me with big eyes.

I flash back to Damon at four, dawdling with Ophelia on our little postage stamp of a beach on Indian Lake in the Adirondacks. It was before his second surgery, so he was less active, but he would sit all day on the sand with his dog, building things and playing by the big, tranquil lake. Ophelia, with her lustrous black-and-tan coat and floppy ears, was both beautiful and vain, but she also made a loving and loyal guard dog. She'd watch over Damon and bark at anyone or anything that moved across the lake or approached from the road. Damon would stroke Ophelia's pretty head and pet her silky wattles—we called her Pouch for the soft undulation beneath her chin—and throw sticks into the water that she fetched in her stately manner, lovely head held high above the surface as she paddled primly along. She was a good-sized Gordon setter, much bigger than Damon, but she had a way of wriggling on her belly and making herself small to accommodate him and insinuate herself into his embraces.

Now minuscule Freddie cocks a cropped ear and watches me with shiny, alert eyes.

Damon presses me. "Can we keep him, Dad?" His mother stands silently behind him, plaintiff, judge, and head of the ambush party that surrounds me in a tight circle of love.

"Do I have a choice?" I smile and throw up my hands, stroking Freddie's head before I move up the evolutionary ladder and muss my elder son's hair.

"Yes!" Damon pumps his fist into the air.

They break out into cheers and applause and I receive a cascade of free kisses, including a sloppy, wet one from Freddie.

Chapter 17

Damon continues to function reasonably well under his new regimen and Dr. Hayes professes satisfaction with his progress. She finds the decrease of his ascites—fluid retention, most notably in the belly—"very encouraging."

But I've learned not to drop my guard and I no longer trust any single voice on Damon's illness. Everything we are seeing could be real improvement, as we devoutly hope, but it could also be the relentless pattern of PLE, with minor progress at the margins unavailing against the core onslaught.

One of the first people I turn to for guidance is the Columbia surgeon who performed Damon's original Fontan operation nine years earlier. Dr. Jan Quaegebeur, or "Dr. Q" as he is known, is an internationally renowned cardiothoracic surgeon who trained with Dr. Fontan himself. Dr. Q, a Belgian, is among the top people in the world in his field, he operates a hundred times a year with an amazing success rate, and he enjoys a quasi-cult following. We can vouch for his extraordinary skill and the masterful surgery that gave Damon an excellent quality of life, at least until he developed his most recent problems.

However, not unlike other high-powered surgical stars, Dr. Q manifests a self-assurance some might construe as arrogance. He is very hard to reach, especially now that we're not scheduling an operation. I'm advised not to bother the great man, that it's out of his hands now.

But I'm on a sacred quest and I can't afford such advice. I keep calling and leaving messages, making it clear to Dr. Q's underlings there's no way he can avoid me. As Shealagh points out, Dr. Q owes us—and her personally, she feels—an explanation. After Damon's successful Fontan procedure, the supremely confident surgeon breezily told my wife to go home and have a good life, her son was fine and our troubles forever behind us.

"He laughed at my worries and promised me everything would be okay from here on, and I believed him!" Shealagh cries.

But now everything is *not* okay and we need to understand from the person who knows Damon's anatomy best what exactly went wrong and how we can fix it.

Eventually, when it's clear I won't stop, Dr. Q returns my call.

"I'm sorry Damon is not doing well but I doubt it's PLE, which is extremely rare," he says preemptively.

"Excuse me, but if ten percent of Fontans now develop PLE, it may be uncommon but it's not rare," I reply, upset at his dismissiveness. "You can't pretend you never see it."

"No, this ten percent is exaggerated. And among *my* patients, it is rare!" Dr. Q declares. "Damon's pressures are very good, so he shouldn't have developed this problem at all. And Dr. Hayes is still unsure what is causing it. I think you're overreacting and things may not be as bad as you're making them," he chides. "Why not follow Dr. Hayes's protocol and give it a chance? I'm sorry, but there's nothing more I can offer you."

I'm surprised by Dr. Q's defensiveness and hasten to assure him I'm not questioning his performance, which everyone acknowledges was first-rate. Rather, I'm asking him to help me understand, and try to solve, my son's cardiac problem. A problem that bears all the symptoms of a progressive, and potentially calamitous, case of PLE.

The Fontan, I propose over Dr. Q's objections, gave Damon nine great years, but now it's failing him. Is it possible this operation provides a wonderful but temporary respite from the underlying cardiac anomaly? That in future it will be seen as a bridge therapy, and a more permanent cure is required? And if so, what would he recommend as the next best treatment for a patient like Damon, whose Fontan has clearly expired?

But Dr. Q cannot, or will not, follow me here. He won't accept that Damon has PLE, as if admitting this might somehow taint the reputation of his brilliant procedure. "We do not know what Damon's problem is," he asserts with an adamance bordering on hostility.

Nevertheless, because I still crave any glimmer of insight from this world expert, I ask Dr. Q about fenestration, which shows a promising outcome in the literature. He says flatly, "It doesn't work." I tell him about the Mayo Clinic and Children's Hospital of Philadelphia, which reported several PLE cures from fenestration, and he says: "If you believe that, maybe you should take your son *there*." I mention other treatments, and he's equally dismissive.

"Damon should continue with the diet and meds," he insists.

"Yes," I say, "but what if they *don't work?*"

Dr. Q repeats, with the same stern disapproval, that I should not leap to conclusions. "We do not know what is going on, so why assume the worst?"

"Because it's my son and I'm worried about his *survival.*"

"Don't exaggerate!" Dr. Q admonishes me. "Things are not at this stage. Dr. Hayes does not believe Damon's life or anything like that is at stake."

"But what if his life *is* at stake?" I say. "Do you know any way to *stop* PLE?"

Dr. Q gives a long sigh. "If Damon continues to deteriorate, and if none of the drugs helps, then the only way to stop PLE is a heart transplant. But that is way down the line . . ."

I feel my blood freeze but force myself to confront this now. I ask Dr. Q about the outcomes for a heart transplant, for which surgery he's also celebrated.

"It's far too early to consider such an option!" Dr. Q chides. "Damon, if he ever comes to it, is at least two to three years away from a transplant, so why discuss it now?"

Two or three years is like *tomorrow* for me. We are talking about my son's *life*, and the specter of such radical surgery and the alarming deterioration it prefigures horrifies me now. But for Dr. Q, with his daily lineup of patients, it must seem like eons away. He appears to think sequentially, in terms of his day-to-day tasks, and to avoid such out-of-sequence speculations. In fact, he seems offended that I'm posing the question at all. Now I'm just a hysterical parent wasting his time, and he wants to get me off the phone.

"I'm busy, I must go," he announces.

"PLE kills fifty percent of its patients within five years and I'm not going to let my son just drift away!" I tell him.

"I don't believe this fifty percent figure—statistics can be used to support anything. But you can do what you want, I have to go now!"

There is a tense silence as Dr. Q retreats into his remote treetop and

I consider cutting him down to size. It's not his self-importance that bothers me but his inability to live up to his reputation. He seems to take little responsibility for his former patient, now that he's not a success story, and even denies his problem. Here's a man who's internationally feted and richly rewarded for his surgical specialty—he earns millions of dollars a year, with all the perks—yet he can't seem to face up to the technique's limitations.

I'm so irate I'm ready to track down the legendary Dr. Fontan himself—I've learned he's retired in full laurel to his vineyards in France—and threaten to expose him, with his protégé, unless he can explain this imperfection in his legacy!

But, wisely, I count to ten and suppress my indignation. My sole objective is to help Damon, and each action must be analyzed in those terms. While I hope at all costs to avoid a heart transplant for my son, if ever I must go that route, Columbia is a pioneer in heart transplantation and Dr. Q is a leading transplant surgeon. So I still may need Dr. Q in the future and antagonizing him now is counterproductive. I swallow my anger and thank him for his time and his help.

At the other end of the spectrum, around this time I get an introduction to Dr. Alvin Chin of Children's Hospital of Philadelphia (CHOP). Chin is a pediatric cardiologist who grew so frustrated with the lack of knowledge about a single-ventricle, Fontan-type circulation such as Damon's—and the debilitating problems, like PLE, he kept seeing at the bedside of these children—that he switched to bench science to grapple with this disease.

A professor of pediatrics and biology at the University of Pennsylvania School of Medicine and an attending cardiologist at CHOP, Dr. Chin has lobbied for more federally financed research into this poorly understood disease. He believes more scientific knowledge at the molecular and cellular level holds the key to progress.

From the outset, Dr. Chin readily admits what I've observed but what every other medical expert seems intent on denying: that no one knows how to treat PLE because they don't yet grasp its basic mechanisms or causes.

"We don't even have an animal model for this disease, which is the gold standard in scientific medicine!" Dr. Chin says.

Dr. Chin believes the incidence of PLE is higher than reported and that many top institutions such as Columbia pretend they never see it because they regard it as a blot on their reputations and an impediment to luring patients. He also thinks PLE will increase as the young adult Fontan population in the United States more than doubles in the next ten years.

Dr. Chin and I begin a regular e-mail correspondence that will last several years and constitutes a veritable tutorial on PLE, cardiology, and the modern practice of medicine. Our common goal is to help Damon and crack the PLE code, and Dr. Chin educates me as needed:

> In the late 1980s, the prevailing attitude was, If we get a bit better with the technical aspects of the single ventricle surgical procedures, and if we offer the surgery in infancy rather than later childhood, the long-term sequelae like PLE will vanish. This attitude had worked for all other congenital heart defects . . . Needless to say, essentially ignoring the problem did not work in the case of single ventricle. It will take an extraordinary individual to mobilize an Apollo Project–like effort in this country.

In preparation for our first meeting after months of cyber-contact, I send Dr. Chin Damon's complete medical records. But he keeps asking for *more*: echo reports, Holters (heart monitoring data), growth curves, and all protein and albumin readings since his Fontan. We discover no one has measured Damon's liver function for years, so we can't tell if his levels have been low for a long time or if the drop is more recent. The startling gaps in Columbia's records—no other hospital tracks this either—convince Dr. Chin to begin measuring liver function more frequently at CHOP.

In January, Shealagh and I drive with Damon to Philadelphia to meet Dr. Chin. It's a bleak, wintry day, made starker by our hurtling across slippery bridges and icy highways. Shealagh's back still acts up and she gripes I drive too fast. We are both tense and bicker along the snow-blown turnpike while Damon, the object of all our anxiety, sits unperturbed in the back, blithely listening to CDs on his headset. He loves music and is an old hand at tuning out his squabbling parents.

Dr. Chin is gentler looking and more soft-spoken than I pictured from his sharp, iconoclastic e-mails. He gives Damon a careful physical exam and speaks to him in a warm, respectful manner. As Damon removes his Salk T-shirt, he reveals thin upper arms and a pale, distended abdomen crisscrossed by blue veins. Dr. Chin nods sympathetically.

"That's his liver wrapping around his middle like a belt." He touches Damon's belly tenderly. There's something reassuring about Chin, even when he explains troubling things, and we all respond to his calm handling of Damon.

"The liver is full of fluid that's backed up from his high pressures because his heart has to pump so hard to get blood to the lungs," Chin says as he probes Damon's abdomen with sensitivity.

"But his belly is less swollen. The Aldactone seems to be working," I say.

"Yes, but it may not be addressing the protein loss—it's a diuretic that's drying him out. He's peeing out fluids, but this does not mean his PLE is better."

"Oh, I see." I try not to show my disappointment.

Dr. Chin says one also needs protein for growth, which may explain why Damon's development has stalled. Damon, listening closely, suddenly pipes up.

"I used to be one of the shorter kids in the class but now I'm the shortest."

Dr. Chin gives a poignant nod. "Well, Damon, we've seen growth hormone help with some PLE patients," he says, and I watch my son perk up.

We agree to look into this and keep an open mind.

After listening to Damon's heartbeat and taking his pulse, Dr. Chin informs us Damon has a "slow heart rate." He warns this could be a problem—but one that CHOP has effectively managed in several similar cases with "a pacemaker."

I wince and sense a kindred shudder from Shealagh but Dr. Chin assures us a pacemaker can be implanted via a simple procedure using long leads so Damon can grow, while the battery "lasts eight to ten years." This bionic tidbit does little to allay our unease, even when Dr. Chin says it can improve cardiac output.

"In that case, you can put in the electrodes now but hold off on the external generator box, so we don't initiate pacing until you're ready," Dr. Chin says.

I glance across at Damon and realize how hard this must be for him. Although he chose to stay in the room with us, this doesn't mitigate the blow. I recall how upset I was when they told me I had to wear eyeglasses as a kid—I quickly opted for contact lenses—and now my son has to confront *this*. It doesn't seem fair. Shealagh also looks riled. Her father had a pacemaker implanted, but not before his late sixties; Damon is thirteen.

We agree to explore this further but we remain deeply skeptical. In fact,

Dr. Chin will never persuade us to go this route, despite his best efforts. He is a wonderful mentor and a trusted adviser, but we always do our own research and solicit input from many sources before making a decision.

The area where we find almost complete accord with Dr. Chin is fenestration.

"Fenestration is not always a solution," Dr. Chin admits. "The benefits last five years on average—though some people are still good after ten years—but it's the most consistently effective therapy against PLE. And it's not as invasive, irreversible, or dangerous as a heart transplant. We've had many successes with it."

"Won't it make me more blue?" Damon asks, recalling Dr. Hayes's concern.

Dr. Chin nods. "The trade-off for punching a hole between the chambers of the heart is some blood mixing. So you will see greater blueness and lower oxygen saturation. But this does *not* necessarily mean you'll have less energy, because the oxygen deficit may be offset by a more efficient liver producing higher levels of protein that yield *more* energy. Plus, you won't have PLE!"

"It's the safest, most effective weapon we know," I tell Damon. "It comes up in all my literature searches. And Dr. Chin has seen it work for many patients."

The key, we all concur, is not *whether* but *when* to try fenestration. How long do we give less intrusive approaches to work? We won't risk cutting Damon's oxygen unless we must, but we can't wait too long. We agree to revisit by summer.

As the meeting ends, Dr. Chin talks to Damon about graduation and his interest in theater. When Shealagh leaves to show Damon to the bathroom, I find myself alone with Dr. Chin for the first time. He tells me what a nice family I have and how bright Damon and Shealagh are, and I commend his bedside manner and his clear medical explanations. Then I lean forward and look him in the eye.

"So what do you think now that you've seen Damon in the flesh?" I smile. Despite our long exchanges, until today Dr. Chin has only viewed medical records of my son and heard about him secondhand.

Dr. Chin pauses, weighing his words. We've been sharing thoughts and ideas very freely, but now I see him trying to reconcile this openness with my being the boy's father.

"I think he looks about the same as other PLE patients I've seen," Dr. Chin says.

I feel a sharp letdown and suddenly realize I'd wanted Dr. Chin to tell me what I heard at Columbia: that Damon looks too good for PLE and it's all a big mistake.

Dr. Chin is my second opinion—in the next months, I'll solicit a dozen more expert medical views—but he is confirming, in the most diplomatic manner, what I've dreaded.

Chapter 18

Weekdays I rise at four forty-five A.M. to write, stealing a few quiet hours in my study before we get the kids up for school and ourselves off to work. The energy consumed as I sit in a chair and cogitate over a keyboard in my sealed chamber generates so much heat and sweat that I must strip down to my underwear, even in winter, while the windows fog up like steamy portholes. When Shealagh barges in to tell me my time's up—ideally carrying a fresh cup of coffee—she is assaulted by the humid, tropical heat and the sight of a semi-naked, wildly oblivious man. She throws open the windows, laughing at the human "steam furnace," and reminds me to put on some clothes.

Only now, it's no longer Shealagh but Damon who first enters my hothouse at dawn. Damon has such an exacting diet with so many pills to swallow that he needs extra time in the morning, and we take turns trying to give him a hand.

He knocks with a light touch and slips unobtrusively into my study around six A.M., perching on the wicker chair by the door like a polite bird. "Hey."

"Hey, D-man." I swivel from my desk and check the state of his puffiness, which is most pronounced in the morning. He checks me out too, ignoring the familiar nakedness but scanning my book-lined shelves and project-strewn desk.

"How's the novel?" Damon asks. He knows I've cut it and resubmitted.

"Good. I've got some real interest, more than I had before. We'll see."

"Cool." My son is pleased for me. He believes in my unheralded creative work, making him special indeed. "So what you working on now?" He cranes toward my laptop.

Among the papers, I spot a copy of Dr. Chin's lab results, stating, *Damon's PLE and liver dysfunction are quite severe.* I quickly turn the report facedown.

"I'm outlining an idea for a new novel—a heist with a moral rationale—and storyboarding that film about Grandma and Granddad." I point to my camcorder.

"You gonna show the film at their party?" Damon asks.

"If I finish on time." I'm making a short film about my parents for a fifty-second wedding anniversary party planned for the night before Damon's Bar Mitzvah.

"Getting close, huh?" Damon chuckles. He still has lots of prep work.

We've decided to carry on with both events, even though we planned them before Damon's diagnosis, which has altered everything.

Shealagh and I debated whether we were putting Damon under too much pressure but he insists he's up to it. He regularly attends Hebrew classes and Bar Mitzvah lessons while keeping up with his schoolwork, extracurricular activities, and social calendar. He may be a half step slower but he's as focused and determined as ever. He's even resumed karate class, after an eight-month hiatus.

"It's still fun," he says.

Taking a cue from Damon, we've decided not to make any concessions to his illness unless we have to. Even my parents, thrilled with the idea of their party, offer to let me put it off, fearing we may be taking on too much. But they've had their own ups and downs and I've wanted to do this for them for a long time. I also know that if we start to give up on a normal life, we're done for.

"Hey." I tap my wristwatch. "It's time!" We shuffle down to the kitchen. I prepare breakfast while Damon feeds Freddie, then jogs with him in our backyard, exercising them both. That sly ferret-dog, who craps under my desk and chews the heads off Miranda's Barbie dolls, is a godsend for Damon.

"How you feeling?" I ask Damon when he comes back in, flushed and panting.

"I get a little more tired than before, but otherwise I feel okay," Damon replies.

I count out his morning meds on the counter, laying out the pills in a white eggcup: enalapril, Aldactone, Zantac, Adeks, calcium, baby aspirin. The Lasix and Zyrtec are for the evening but now he also must swallow a big spoonful of greasy MCT oil, which contains medium-chain triglycerides for easy absorption. To help it go down, I give him a glass of orange juice. Then I peel a kiwi and slice an apple for him.

"Thanks, Dad," Damon says, using the sweet, palatable fruit to chase down the pills.

While Damon sits on a high stool at the counter and gets through his meds, I cook him a soft-boiled egg, which he spoons avidly from the shell. The news plays quietly on the TV above the counter.

Damon often requests a second egg, which I happily supply. Once, when I'm by the stove, he gets up for the salt, stepping on the low, mobile platform that lives on the kitchen floor, a ridged booster step for little Miranda. He notices I'm watching—I dislike the step, which trips me up and reminds me of his dependency—and he turns to face me.

"Ever since the doctors started talking about how I haven't grown, I suddenly feel small," Damon says huskily. His eyes moisten and I wonder if he's going to cry. Shealagh says he puts on a brave front for me but she gets more tears. But now Damon's mouth turns wry. "I'll be one of the smallest Bar Mitzvah boys ever. Tom Thumb at the Torah."

"You'll be fine, Damon," I assure him. "And you'll be a man, more than I can say for many people twice your size."

As the Bar Mitzvah nears, Damon and I plan to meet at Brooks Brothers to buy him a new suit. The store is on Fifth Avenue, by my office, but Damon is late—he's coming up from school—so I stand out on the sidewalk and look for him. The ceaseless press of humanity, which I pass unthinkingly every day, suddenly looks daunting. This is a special day—I recall when my father bought me my Bar Mitzvah suit—and I want it to go well.

After scanning the throng and trying his cell, I finally spot Damon on the street. He's unmistakable, even in this dense crowd: a pale, compact, ginger-haired boy motoring forward at a surprisingly vigorous clip, like a speed-walker with a battery pack strapped to his back. He swings his arms like pistons. The minute he recognizes me, he breaks into a smile and slows down, shutting off his engine. We walk into the store arm in arm.

In short order, we pick out a classic dark suit, a couple of dress shirts and silk ties, then throw in a pair of new shoes. We go to the fitting room, where a natty man with a tape measure bends over Damon. The jacket only needs minor alterations but the pants must be recut at the waist. The tailor, humming an aria and exuding cologne, wields his measuring tape with silken dexterity, makes a few brisk chalk marks, and previews the final product in the full-length mirror:

"What a handsome boy. He look like a prince, a young lion!"

The night before the Bar Mitzvah, we host my parents' anniversary at the Century Club. Many relatives and close friends join us, flying in from many countries. But the most exciting arrival for Damon is Lachlann, who materializes from the Isle of Skye with his wiry hardiness and gorse-bush accent.

"Och aye, let's get smashed!"

Now the two young rascals cruise the stately reception hall, set with a dozen handsome tables, a screen, and a podium. Damon looks sharp and jaunty in his dark new suit. He greets guests with confident aplomb, then sidles up to me at the projector.

"Hey, Dad, you nervous? Grandma said they love that you're doing this for them, she just hopes it won't be too embarrassing." He dims the lights for the film, which begins with a 1949 map of Europe and the theme music from *Casablanca*. My father as a scrappy, leather-jacketed youth with cigarette dangling from mouth in old sepia photos has always conjured up Bogie for me, while my mother, a tall, striking European blonde, bore a real likeness to Ingrid Bergman.

But it's my parents in their unglamorous seventies, sitting together at their Rego Park kitchen table in a tight two-shot, who are the heart of the film: Robert, grayer and stouter, more like Edward G. Robinson than Bogie now, in a burly cable-knit sweater. A nimble athlete, a pleaser of ladies, and a witty, well-defended, warm-hearted Glaswegian, born in Budapest, with a decade of pioneer work in Israel and then a business career, at first highly successful and then less so, in America; and Helga, still beautiful and dignified, and still tragic and self-dramatizing, with high cheekbones and her long, stately nose in the air, a little sadder about the eyes, and a little rounder, a survivor of cancer and of Leipzig, Germany, where the Nazis wiped out her entire family. She escaped with her brother on the Kindertransport to England, where she met Robert, in Liverpool, from whence they journeyed, via France and Italy, to a kibbutz in Israel, marriage, and children, and then, by chance, to America. Now wearing a vivid red turtleneck and mauve lipstick, she fluffs her thick, frosted hair with die-hard female vanity, an elegant and eloquent woman, upright, vicarious, and true.

They sat side by side for hours—I taped them over several months, from across the kitchen table where I ate my meals as a boy—and they spar, bicker, and one-up each other, rolling their eyes at the camera and expressing the frustrations and self-justifications of a long marriage: "A lifetime or a life sentence? A little of both," Helga quips. But somehow, as they talk about their upbringing and their own parents, the impact of momentous historical events on their lives, and their meeting, courtship, and subsequent marriage, culminating in two children and three grandchildren, one of whom is Damon, whose sharp gaze I can feel beside me, the years peel away, and part of the mystery of love is revealed.

The film is followed by laudatory speeches. My parents are royalty for this one night, which pleases me greatly, and appropriate homage is paid.

Damon, Sam, and Miranda are last to speak and marched up to the front by a take-charge Damon. Their mere appearance at the podium brings smiles and murmurs of delight.

As Sam and Miranda hide behind him, squirming and giggling, a decidedly mature Damon lowers the microphone and speaks about the three kids' close relationship with their grandparents and how they were always there, "Especially," he says, "when we wanted to get away from our own parents." As the crowd laughs, Damon displays a keen appreciation of time. "I feel this has been a pretty long week for me, but for my grandparents' marriage, it's been two thousand, seven hundred and four weeks, one hundred and eighty thousand days, twenty-seven million minutes, or one point eight billion seconds."

Flashing a big smile, Damon wishes his grandparents a happy anniversary, then beckons his siblings to follow suit as they've all rehearsed. "Okay, guys, now!"

Shy, giggly, dashing Sam sidles up with rubbery limbs, juggling his assigned words like a hot potato, which he quickly tosses to the audience before darting back. But gap-toothed, golden-haired Miranda is stymied because she's too short to reach the podium. Without a pause, Damon bends down and heaves his sister in her blue sash dress right up to the podium mike.

"Happy anniversary, Grandma and Granddad!" all three kids blurt in unison.

Chapter 19

The day of Damon's Bar Mitzvah begins badly.

It's pouring rain, a washout, which will not only impede our preparations but augurs poorly for the turnout. We still have several hours of setup in the synagogue's banquet hall—they needed it for another function the previous night—and it must be ready by ten A.M.

Even more upsetting, Damon had a rough night. He says he feels okay now, a big relief, but his face has swollen up, making him appear more frog than handsome prince, and his body drags, dampening his ebullience.

"It's rotten luck because all eyes will be on him today," Shealagh says.

But the day improves. And under Shealagh's direction, we transform the banquet hall with bright hangings, fine chair coverings, fresh flowers, and balloons—hundreds of colorful balloons in thick clumps and bunches, rising from the tables and descending from the ceiling. We finish by draping bold rainbow streamers and kites, throw in a popcorn machine, karaoke, raffle balls, candy, and wrapped gifts, and the room looks ready for a party and Shealagh's idea of "jollification."

Upstairs, the majestic if somewhat faded turn-of-the-century sanctuary of Temple Beth Emeth v'Ohr ("House of Truth and Light") fills up with nearly two hundred and fifty of our guests plus regular congregants. Key members of my family fly in, as do all Shealagh's siblings. And most of our close friends make it in from points far and wide, along with many neighbors and local friends. Even the sun, miraculously, makes a belated appearance.

We enter the sanctuary from the rabbi's office behind the podium. Damon looks sharp in his dark new Brooks Brothers suit, a little less frog and more prince. A bright blue silk yarmulke rides high on his crown and a striped prayer shawl adorns his shoulders. He shuffles through a folder with his key papers—speeches, blessings, prayers. He looks nervous but totally focused and ready.

I sit on the stage in a high, carved armchair with a scalloped crest, facing the congregation, and listen to Damon, his back to me, recite the first of innumerable blessings in praise of God:

"The Lord is the earth and fullness thereof, the world and they that dwell therein . . ."

I normally don't have much patience for this stuff but since Damon's diagnosis, I keep a more open mind and search for clues everywhere, much as I scan the medical literature. So now when Damon reads "Who shall stand in God's holy place?" and answers, in his high, clear, and firm voice, "One that hath clean hands and a pure heart," I *know* that my son qualifies. I look up at the ark and tell whoever is minding the store that there is no one better or purer to receive "the blessing of the Lord and justice from the God of salvation."

I emphasize the word "justice," shaking an imaginary finger up at the tabernacle.

Rabbi William Kloner, regal in long black robe and gold braided prayer shawl, commands the congregation to rise. Damon climbs three steps and opens the hammered bronze doors of the ark, revealing a large and a small Torah book under a gleaming light. Rabbi Kloner hands Damon the small Torah and carries the big Torah, the crown jewel, to center stage. The rabbi prods Damon, who is cradling his junior Torah just under his chin, and Damon recites from the prayer book.

As the congregation's singing rises to an ecstatic pitch, Rabbi Kloner and Damon descend from the stage. They march up the aisle carrying their respective Torahs like two beaming Moseses, young and old. Members crowd in to touch the mantle, using bare fingers or their prayer shawls, then kiss the holy spot. The two figures return to the stage, unsheathe the Torah, and roll open the parchment. As Damon chants from the Torah, his mastery of the material is unmistakable. Once, toward the end, he stumbles but recovers so seamlessly few realize he's tripped up. He never loses command.

The performance is impressive to us not just because of Damon's diagnosis but because he was rejected as a Bar Mitzvah candidate by the first two Park Slope synagogues we approached. The rabbis felt one year was not sufficient time to prepare. At least *three years* were required, during which one had to be a paying member of their congregation. When I explained that Damon was a trained actor who could learn major parts in weeks, and that my father and I could help him with the Hebrew, it did not matter. Nor did they budge when I said, without specifying Damon's medical past, that timeliness was a factor.

It surprised me that at a time when a majority of American Jews have assimilated and synagogue membership is flagging, they would refuse us, but they did. Rabbi William Kloner, our final try, was also wary about any appearance of a shortcut. However, being a navy chaplain and lifelong student of history, as well as a Reform rabbi with an aging congregation, he was more sensitive to the "survival of the flock" argument. He did not say yes right away but agreed to let us try it out on a "let's see if he's as good as you say" basis.

As Damon finishes singing, Rabbi Eric, the younger, second-in-command rabbi, praises his "phenomenal" job and takes Damon to the side, offering him a personal blessing that no one can hear.

I am handed the Torah while Damon recites more blessings, until Rabbi Kloner removes the weighty scroll from my arms, where I confess it's growing heavy, and places it back in the ark. Following this consummation, I am sent from my privileged perch back down to the congregation, where I take my place beside Shealagh, Sam, and Miranda.

Damon now delivers the talk on his Torah portion, focusing on the Ten Commandments. He reminds us that even this document is based on a "photocopy," the original lying somewhere at the bottom of Mount Sinai, smashed into a thousand pieces.

"So no one," Damon says with a twinkle in his eye, not even Moses or the Israelites, "likes rules." Yet rules, or a "single set of uniform laws that uphold absolute values and principles," are essential if people want "to live together and avoid chaos." Accepting rules means "you accept responsibility for your actions" and the fact that "you don't live alone."

As Damon speaks, alternately playful and serious, I note how his eyes lift off the page and scan the room. He has undeniable presence and a natural eloquence, but I'm also struck, now that I see him head-on, by his pallor and the lingering puffiness in his face. I tell myself to relax and enjoy his triumph. Even at three-quarters strength, Damon shines.

I tune back in as Damon concludes: "I still plan to enjoy myself and to make my life into something original, but I accept the Ten Commandments as a moral code to guide me as I go forward in the world to find my own place."

Downstairs, after the kiddush, the party is in full swing. Jolly music plays while wide-eyed children wander through the billowing, festooned banquet hall as in a wonderland, tugging at the coiling ribbons that stream down from canopies of bright balloons. Our seating chart quickly gets jettisoned as people plunk themselves down wherever. Miranda and her cousins Lucas and Harry spray over seat name tags with cans of Silly String. Only my parents' elderly friends, who have trouble standing, quickly find their assigned seats and tuck into the food.

Damon, happily dazed, accepts handshakes and greetings as he makes straight for his friends, a multicultural assortment of young teens sprawled across three tables. Kyle is there, barefoot in a strapless black dress with her hair swept off her neck. Daniel, an old friend from music school, hovers awkwardly because he doesn't know the other kids. Brenda, a big, precocious blonde, finds Jason, a math whiz, two pals from elementary school. Keith leads the middle school contingent, a sharp figure in dress slacks and tie, while Kiri has cleaned up nicely, even if she still wears pants. Most of the other girls are dolled up in party dresses and gowns. It's a month before graduation, and they are excitedly trying things out, showing off new outfits and makeup and hair. Maddy, a leggy six-foot classmate, bends down to kiss Damon, towering over him even more than the other girls. But Damon takes it all in stride, accepting embraces from a bevy of admirers.

Damon hands his skullcap to Kirsten, who wants to try it on, then removes his prayer shawl too, unwinding as he realizes this part of his day is over now. He snaps his fingers, glances at his sea of friends, and breaks into a wide smile. "Party time!"

The master of ceremonies, I make the rounds and check that all is in order. There's food and drinks galore and representatives from all stages of our lives. Everywhere I turn, I see people I like, people who matter to me. It's an amazing turnout. Yet even with all these special people here to celebrate Damon's coming-of-age, and even with all the decorations and the champagne and the music, I cannot quite shake my lingering sense of fretfulness.

Shealagh sidles up in her willfully giddy party mode and instantly recognizes my thoughts as we share a silent high five at bringing this whole thing off. My wife shoots me a pleading look and shoves a glass of wine in my hand. Since our CHOP visit, I've taken Damon to three more hospitals across the country.

"Have a drink, you look too sober!" Shealagh says, as much for her sake as mine.

And I do have a drink, several in fact. I notice my second son has already exchanged his tie and jacket for a blue T-shirt he wears inside out, while Miranda, pretty in a pink dress with a big bow, snaps photos with a disposable camera and interviews adults about life.

I take the mike by the karaoke machine and call up family and friends to toast Damon. When it's my turn, I talk about Damon's incredible courage, his beautiful mind, and his unbelievable messiness, three areas with little in common except, perhaps, that he's already surpassed me in each. In citing his courage, I glancingly address the elephant in the room—most of the guests know nothing of his diagnosis—remarking that Damon was born with congenital heart disease, so his whole life has been a battle, and he's far braver than he realizes.

Then Damon graciously thanks everyone. "And it's great to see so many of my friends show up, it's so cool, you guys, even if I know you mostly came for the food and the gift bags."

Damon speaks with ease and panache and this crowd adores him, but I can't help noticing again that something's off. There's an odd catch, a furry thickness, in his voice, and a faint, rabbity twitch about his nose.

After Damon, Shealagh, the grand event designer, raises her champagne glass and toasts her son's wonderful courage and amazing character. Then in time-honored tradition, his school friends, aided by assorted adults, place Damon in a chair and lift him off the ground. They form a snaking line and raise him above their shoulders, clapping, chanting, and swaying.

The stomping and pounding grows wilder, and the surging crowd more frenzied. The boy on his throne is small and light and the mob intoxicated with its massed, heaving power. The pack hurls Damon into the air with intensifying force. He must hold on to the flying chair to keep from falling off. His disheveled mane bobs up and down, his jaunty shoulders flop, and he bounces hard on the seat, soaring above the heads of the celebrants.

It looks like he's losing his balance, but he isn't. He's having the time of his life.

Chapter 20

"In middle school it was all about fitting in, but in high school you have to find your own way . . ."

In June, Damon graduates from the Salk School of Science in a ceremony held at the First Avenue campus of New York University School of Medicine, a Salk affiliate. By virtue of his size, Damon leads the processional of sixty students down the aisle as Elgar's "Pomp and Circumstance" issues from a solo trumpet. The teens look alternately mischievous and somber as they fan out to their seats. Damon wears a purple silk graduation gown while the long horse's-tail tassel on his mortarboard swishes merrily. He plops down one row in front of Keith and turns around in his seat, smiling puckishly.

"Hey, Keith." Damon points his disposable camera at his friend, who is a foot taller with a brash buzz cut, and Keith swivels his head. "Gotcha!" Damon grins and shoots.

We listen to inspirational speeches and student poems. When the awards are handed out, we're surprised to see Damon repeatedly called to the stage, winning prizes for academic excellence, for leadership, for writing, and for science. He marches to the podium in compact triumph, lit by a luminous smile and his own warm spotlight as his classmates cheer.

After the mortarboards go sailing into the air, Damon hugs friends and bids farewell to teachers.

It's a proud day for us all, but the normal, bittersweet joys of graduation are marred by our abnormal anxiety about what the future holds for our son. Damon's protein levels have not budged, despite daily medications and a strict diet.

"He hasn't improved, so what do we try now?" Shealagh asks that night.

"It's between heparin and fenestration," I reply, and list the differing views of four hospitals we consult with closely: Columbia, CHOP, Boston Children's, and the Mayo Clinic. "Heparin is less invasive, so we'll probably try that first."

Shealagh sighs. "Oh well, I guess we're not going to Skye this summer!"

"We can't. And no sleepaway camp for Damon either," I say ruefully.

I still remember waiting for the returning camp bus on Damon's maiden outing the previous summer, wondering how he'd survived in such a close, unrelentingly physical environment for a whole month. I was worried, so I kept my eyes peeled on the door as the kids poured out of the bus. There was no sign of Damon for a long time, and my anxiety mounted. But the instant he appeared at the top of the bus steps and stood there with his shaggy, unkempt new swagger, I felt elated. I took in his blazingly defiant, sunburned face; his sinewy, mosquito-bitten arms; and the proud, faintly rebellious smile on his cocky lips—that heady flowering of freedom and new powers that summer camp can confer on a boy—and I knew he'd held his own with his peers and tasted true independence for the first time.

"Hey, D-man. How you doing?" I gave him a brief hug as he stepped down.

"Good," he said in a more mature, aloof voice. "Very good!" He grinned.

But now we cannot let him return to the six-thousand-acre mountain playground in Frost Valley, New York, much as we'd like to. Fortunately, instead of camp, Damon sets his sights on auditioning for New York University's Looking for Shakespeare summer theater workshop. It's part of the Educational Theatre division, where graduate-student teachers direct an ensemble of thirteen-to-eighteen-year-olds to create and perform an original adaptation of a Shakespeare play. The production takes place at the historic Provincetown Playhouse.

For his audition, Damon prepares two soliloquies, modern and classical. He also gets an improvised scene to perform. "I don't think I did that well," Damon says as we exit the theater on MacDougal Street. The program is a notch up from any stage work Damon has done before but I also wonder if his condition has started hindering him. But two weeks later, a letter arrives saying he's been selected for *Cymbeline,* making him among the youngest actors in the program.

Damon attends the workshop five days a week, and on weekends as the production date nears. Each session includes warm-up exercises, stretching, vocals, and ensemble-building activities run by the gifted stage manager, Krista, who turns out to live on our Brooklyn block and becomes Damon's friend. The directors cast Shakespeare's *Cymbeline* and then create a contemporary frame story where each actor writes a new role based on his or her character.

Damon quickly establishes himself. He learns all his lines and then helps others with their lines. When no one else will do it, Damon dons a pair of antlers and hangs upside down off a broom, playing a dead deer. "I don't mind except my arms get a little tired," he tells me. He befriends several actors and hangs out with the cast after rehearsals. Afternoons, they go down the street to the Olive Tree Café and eat Middle Eastern fare while doing loud, wicked imitations. "They almost threw us out today when we got a little rowdy," Damon says with a smile.

On the first Friday in August we drive to the Provincetown Playhouse, where Eugene O'Neill and Edna St. Vincent Millay debuted their work. A bold, graffiti-strewn urban backdrop sprawls across the stage.

In the frame story, Damon plays Raven, a pizzeria owner mediating between rival tribes. Amid the strutting gang members who tower over him in do-rags and leather, Raven, in checked apron and brown fedora, exudes quiet authority and calm reason. "Oh, sorry," he jibes, "is fighting the only thing you're good at?"

In *Cymbeline* proper, Damon enters grand, eliciting laughter and applause as he rises through a trapdoor and emerges in full regalia as Zeus the Thunderer on the back of an eagle. He sparks great mirth with flamboyant, deadpan godliness.

After the show, one woman so admires Damon's performance that she gives us her card and invites us to consider letting him join her small acting company.

"He's very castable. You should let him develop his talent," she advises.

As we watch Damon clasp hands and bow onstage with his fellow actors, grinning in bright costume and makeup, I'm struck by how natural he looks in this setting, like a bird that can only display its full plumage in a native habitat.

"Did you enjoy it?" Damon asks in the car after, invigorated and hungry for feedback. "What'd you like most? Was the frame story okay? What didn't work?"

After we've supplied detailed critiques of his performance and analyses of all the other cast members, Damon also solicits our views on the directing, writing, staging, and costumes.

Two days later, we're back at Columbia for more tests and visits.

In the morning, Damon goes to the X-ray department, where a radiologist conducts an upper gastrointestinal series. The aim is to see if there's any problem in his digestive tract that could account for his protein leak. "It's unlikely but you want to rule out any possibility, especially a treatable one," the GI expert advises. The test is unpleasant but Damon hangs in. We'll get the results in two or three days.

After the test, we go meet with a pediatric endocrinologist. Discussing delayed growth with an adolescent boy is a delicate matter under any circumstances, and we've already had one bad experience at Columbia, so we're uneasy about this meeting. But the reserved-seeming Dr. Mary Horlick quickly impresses Shealagh and me with her up-to-date knowledge and unobtrusive empathy. Which doesn't mean seeing her is a pleasant experience for Damon, only that Dr. Horlick makes the best of a very tough situation.

"Let's get your exact weight and height, okay, Damon?" Dr. Horlick has Damon remove his sweatshirt and sneakers before stepping on the digital scale, then measures his height with a state-of-the-art stadiometer. Although I know there's been no progress, I hold my breath as Dr. Horlick adjusts the sliding headpiece over Damon's crown. She takes three different measurements in her thorough and meticulous way, but each time we get the same read: fifty-six inches. It's as if Damon is stuck and can't get past that ceiling.

"Dr. Chin suggested a bone-density test if we're considering heparin and growth hormone," I mention, wondering how she'll react to outside advice.

"Yes, and a bone-age scan too." Dr. Horlick nods. "I have a lab at St. Luke's where we can test him. We'll also want a full blood workup for Damon's hormone levels."

"That's just a blood test, right?" Shealagh asks as Damon watches keenly.

"Yes." Dr. Horlick pauses. "But to get a full picture of Damon's status, I also need to give him a physical exam, including a manual check of his testes." She winces for us. "I promise it won't hurt, and I'll make it as quick as possible, but there's no other way!"

I've forewarned my son and he looks resigned if very leery.

Dr. Horlick chats with a nervous Damon about school and other activities, then asks with an apologetic smile if he can change into a gown.

"Okay." Damon swallows. "But, Mom, can you, like, wait outside or something?"

Shealagh is thrown but only for a second. "Of course." As she leaves the tense room, she does not look totally unhappy, and I watch her exit with a mix of emotions.

Damon changes into a loose green gown and lies back on the exam table, looking pale, apprehensive, and excruciatingly self-conscious. I make small talk as Dr. Horlick dons thin surgical gloves and approaches Damon's side. She lifts his gown and gently probes Damon's testes with one hand while holding a string of numbered wooden beads in the other. The beads, arranged in ascending order on a rosary, correspond to testicle size, and testicle size "correlates directly with puberty and developmental age," Dr. Horlick explains.

"Oww!" Damon jumps and squirms as Dr. Horlick, who's being very careful and correct, palpates his privates. She's totally professional but there's no escaping what's happening and I cringe for my fourteen-year-old son, whose entire body now seems fair game for probing. Previously, when a more insensitive doctor gave him a digital rectal exam, Damon cried, "It's not fair!" and I feel a terrible, guilty helplessness at his continuing ordeal.

Dr. Horlick finishes and seems almost as relieved as Damon as she covers him back up. "You can get dressed now," she says thoughtfully. I open the door for Shealagh but she's gone. I go down the hall and find her sitting by a sunny window with a coffee and a pastry, trying to create a small oasis for herself. It's all very hard on my wife, and I hesitate before breaking in on her.

"Well, Damon," Dr. Horlick says once we've all reassembled in her office, "you've officially entered puberty!" She smiles at him in his jeans and sweatshirt. "You're at the earliest stage but it's definitely started."

Damon raises an eyebrow at this unexpected sign of progress and Shealagh and I pause to savor it too. But we also know what's *not* happening.

Dr. Horlick explains that Damon's development remains "nascent"— she points between the second and third beads on the chain—and the "major cascade" of hormones and other pubescent markers has not yet begun. "But this is a good thing," she says, "because it means you still have time to develop and catch up once full puberty kicks in."

She seems pleased but warns there is only a finite interval or "critical period" when normal growth is possible. "After that, the growth plates close and are replaced by solid bone." To boost Damon's chances of benefitting from this narrow window, Dr. Horlick suggests we consider growth hormone. "Results vary, and you'd have to vet the idea with Damon's cardiologists before proceeding, but the downside is minimal, and I've seen kids shoot up half a foot in ten weeks," she says. "I think it makes sense to try it for Damon."

Damon's eyes light up. It's the best news we've heard in a long time.

Food is much on our minds these days. With Damon's albumin levels still too low, he must eat three high-protein meals daily, plus two protein supplements. I'm stricter and less forgiving than Shealagh about it. When he sleeps past noon on weekends, I worry he's already missed a meal and we must play catch-up. I morph into the food police, demanding a daily inventory of his dietary intake and verbally frisking him when he comes home.

One day he calls me at four thirty P.M., after theater, and asks if he can go to Jon's house.

"Sure," I say. "What'd you eat for lunch?" He usually has a bite at the Olive Tree.

Damon hems. "We went to a fast food place today, so I didn't eat anything."

"What!" I cry. He's losing protein nonstop, so he must refill himself constantly. "By now you should be on your *second* supplement and you haven't even had lunch!"

"I didn't want to eat bad food," Damon says, both defensive and defiant.

"Damon, I give you extra money so you can always buy good food, whatever it costs . . . You've got to stop screwing around and take this diet more seriously!"

I still let Damon go to his friend's house—it's summer and I want him to enjoy himself, after all—but I demand he return for dinner so I can make sure he eats properly.

He comes home late and sits down with us at the table but says he doesn't have an appetite. He looks tired, pale, and sulky. I feel for him but insist he at least eat his chicken, a good protein source. By now, he's *two* meals behind, and I won't take no for an answer.

I keep the pressure on while we sit at the table—"Come on, Damon, three more bites!"—until he jumps up, makes a retching sound, and bolts from the kitchen as if to vomit. I follow him to the bathroom, filled with remorse, and place my hand on his back as he leans over the sink and opens his mouth, gagging. I hold a bucket under his chin.

Now I've really gone too far, and I feel ashamed of myself.

But Damon's attack passes and he keeps his food down. It's possible he exaggerated to teach me a lesson. Regardless, he's won the argument, and I leave him alone about eating for the rest of that day, wondering what to try next. I can see the protein leaking out of him daily, and I want desperately to plug the leak.

Damon still has his spirit, which manifests in surprising ways.

One day we're in Prospect Park, playing a makeshift game of soccer, with an oak and jacket for goalposts. It's Miranda and me against Damon and my father, who used to play semiprofessionally. My father still likes to kick and head the ball and he still has fancy moves. But at seventy-five, with high blood pressure, a previous mild heart attack, and extra pounds, he runs out of breath and is less fleet.

I was never as adept as my father at this game but my relative youth gives me an advantage, and Miranda and I take the lead and dominate. But Damon surprises us with his skill and tenacity. I often have to run to Miranda's aid to stop Damon, who powers past her and heads for our goal. Once, I allow Damon to score as a reward for his impressive efforts, and Miranda screams at me.

"No, Dad! You let him do that!" She must win and won't tolerate any laxity.

But Damon doesn't need much slack. Even when I stop him and recover the ball, leaving our goal unattended as I run upfield, he comes right back after me, chasing me the entire way. He just *won't give up.*

Once, as I near the goal and feint left to fool my father, Damon sneaks up from behind and steals the ball. It's a brilliant move, and I'm impressed. But Miranda doesn't share my admiration. "No, Dad, get it from him!" she cries, egging me on until I run Damon down and steal back the ball. Damon puts up a furious fight, refusing to relinquish his prize, until I overpower him. He kicks at my legs, livid, and screams as I advance with the ball, elude my father, and score.

Shealagh comes by and Damon complains he and my father are getting creamed. So Shealagh joins Damon's side, altering the dynamic. Now I must cover the goal closely and poor Miranda is overwhelmed by three bigger players. I can't stop them either, and they go ahead. Everyone is satisfied now, save for Miranda, who yells, "Three against two isn't fair!" I tell her she's playing great, but she's still upset. So I rush out and score on a booming kick, making her smile. But mostly I'm stuck guarding the goal and we have no offense, so our fate is sealed.

We've been playing for a long time and it's getting dark, making injuries likelier. I'm also worried about my father, who's panting, so I suggest we stop and go for dinner. Shealagh agrees and my father says he will accede to the majority.

I'm picking up the jacket that delineates the goalpost when Damon storms over.

"Why are we stopping?" he demands, irate.

"Because it's dark and it's late and we've all had enough," I reply evenly.

"No, let's keep playing!" He kicks the ground, fired up. "I wanna play!"

"Listen, D-man. My father's tired, I'm tired, your mother has other things to do . . . We had a good game. You played a terrific match."

"No. I want to play more!" he snarls. "We were just starting to do well."

"Hey, you *won*," I say, surprised by his anger. "You defeated us."

"No, you stopped trying, Dad. Play more!" Damon is seething, his adrenaline is pumping, and he refuses to be mollified. He's taken the game far more seriously than I realized, and he still wants satisfaction. Miranda, too, gets into the act and bawls, insisting we play on. Shealagh tries to reason with them, as does my father, to no avail. The two children kick at the grass and wail.

I'm amazed at how overwrought Damon looks, how choked with fury. It's so unlike him. Yet as I watch my son continue to fume and curse, sputtering uncontrollably, I can't help but be impressed. There's such an incredible fighting spirit beneath his tantrum. He's already mobilized for war.

I decide to refrain from any further reprimand, because I wish to preserve that spirit. Even if it's misplaced here, this fieriness will serve him well in future contests.

Chapter 21

We haven't been to our country house in over a year, so when we get there the first priority is cutting the weed-choked, waist-high grass that overruns our Catskill Park property. The deer and field mice carry ticks, and we don't need Lyme disease added to Damon's ills, nor our own.

"Can I help, Dad?" Damon watches me rev up the old mower and don goggles.

"No, I want you inside with the others until I clear the area." I make him go back in.

The house, a two-story modified cape, sits on a terraced lot with a stone wall, a garage, and a writer's shack, all nestled between a brook and a hilly forest. Damon stands in the family room and tracks me from the big picture window while I mow down the meadow. As soon as there's a path, he runs out in boots and long pants and trails me, raking the cuttings into black trash bags. He feels excluded if he cannot lend a hand.

"I got it, Dad!" He helps me lug the bags to the compost heap behind the garage.

Meanwhile, Shealagh has us get the house operational. We switch on the water pump and water heater, clean out mouse turds and spiderwebs, activate the fridge and fill it with groceries, and buy coupon books for the town dump.

We're almost done when we find a dozen wasp's nests on our property.

"They're everywhere!" Shealagh cries. Damon once had a severe allergic reaction to a hornet sting, so we call pest control to come clear the hives.

With our house functional, we head down to the Olympic-sized town pool by the fairground. Damon leaves Sam and Miranda at the gate. All three of our kids are water rats and can frolic for hours in the pool, but today Damon wants to pass the diving test before his friends come up for a visit.

Damon trundles over to the water with an impish smile. His body above his red trunks is pale and tubular, with skinny arms, a sloping belly, and a zipper scar down his chest. Unabashed, he takes a running start and hurls himself full-tilt across the pool, letting out a booming cry. His eyes glitter as he tumbles downward, yodeling fiercely in the giddy, free-falling moment before impact. Then he crashes with a thunderous splash. His large head drops like a stone and drags his body down with it.

When he resurfaces after a breathless interval, Damon's wet hair shimmers like a crown and his features glisten.

"Whenever you're ready," the lifeguard tells Damon. He must swim halfway across the pool, tread water for one minute, then swim back.

Damon nods, steeples his hands before his chest, and begins. He doesn't swim so much as paw and grope his way forward with both arms while jerking his torso and legs. After each spasmodic lunge, his weighted body begins to sink to the bottom. You can see his patient, smiling face as he drifts underwater and calmly waits to stop sinking, exuding mirthful bubbles. It's hard to grasp how he can ever resume buoyancy but each time Damon manages to return to the surface. He swims like a seal on land, rolling up and down via ill-suited flippers but making undeniable progress.

Damon reaches the halfway mark and begins to dog-paddle. He appears to be struggling as he tilts his head back and gasps. But he stays afloat, grinning as the water laps his purple lips.

"Okay, you're good." The lifeguard signals his minute is up.

Exhausted but sensing victory, Damon swims back in the same awkward hodgepodge, except the transition between rolls and lunges is smoother. He knows he's going to make it now, and he's more confident in his undulations.

He reaches the end of the pool and taps the ledge, glancing over his shoulder for the official result. The guard gives a thumbs-up.

"Heya! I can dive off the big board now," Damon says exultantly.

That evening we celebrate Damon's fourteenth birthday at a local eatery, Mr. Willy's. It's a quiet affair, especially after his Bar Mitzvah and graduation, but it suits our mood. Back at the house, Damon sets up his "movie theater" and sells tickets and refreshments before introducing a film for our screening pleasure.

One day we pack the kids and their friends in the Eurovan and go tubing in the Delaware River. We get a brief "mini-lesson," then everyone grabs a life jacket and an inflated rubber tube and heads down to the rocky banks of the river.

There's a long, flat stretch before you hit the rapids and the water suddenly drops. Shealagh ties Miranda's tube to hers, so she's secure, and paddles calmly downstream with her daughter in tow, while Sam flails away.

Damon has the most trouble getting started. He rocks fruitlessly from side to side while his friends, after spinning in circles, gradually work it out and slip off downstream in their tubes.

As Damon's efforts grow more frantic, his tube tips over and his life jacket, which he deliberately left untied, slips off. It's broad daylight but I'm watching a nightmare. I paddle over at top speed and yank him out of the water.

"You okay, D-man?" I wrap the life jacket around him and pull it tight, snapping the buckles. He's shaken up and so am I. "Listen, I understand about independence, but this is going *too* far. You've got to keep this tied on at all times!" I help him back into the tube.

Damon is ashen and silent. I'm struck by the panic on his face. He got a real fright, rare for him, and he's also embarrassed and very angry with himself. He's not doing well—his disadvantage is showing—while his friends have all streaked ahead. Plus, he's got his father, whom he needs to defy and impress, on his case.

"Use your limbs as paddles," I advise. "You can make this work, I promise."

"No, I can't, because I'm too short to reach the water," Damon says, sulking.

"Don't use your size as an excuse, I know you can do this!" I show him how to position himself in the tube for better leverage.

Damon begins to move, then stalls out again. It's just not happening.

"Okay, I'll help you get to where your friends are. It's easier out there."

I place my feet in Damon's tube, he grabs on to my legs, and I backstroke with my arms. It takes a moment to coordinate, but soon we're cruising downstream and everything around us is in motion. The trees on the riverbank whiz by.

"Yeah!" Damon smiles as we gather speed, breaking his long inertia. He perks up as we overtake other tubers, relishing our swift passage over the water.

We're racing when we pass Sam, still floundering. He spots us and throws a fit. "Why are you helping Damon and not me? It's not fair! I'm younger. Help me!"

Sam protests bitterly until I drag him along too. Not only is everyone staring at us—Sam's sharp voice skitters over the water—but Sam has a point.

Now I place one leg in each son's tube, and they both grab on to my ankles as I haul off. It's hard going, much harder than before. I struggle to hold the two tubes together with my legs as I backstroke furiously with my arms. It feels like we're hardly moving but the boys relish my flailing on their behalf. Slowly, I muscle us forward and manage to drag them with me. By the time we hit the rapids, I'm so focused on keeping both boys afloat in their tubes that I forget about my own, and it suddenly flips from under me. I tumble out, smacking my knee against the rocks, but am able to hold on to Damon's tube while pushing Sam's into a safe channel. The water foams and hisses about me, angrier than expected. I'm soaked and bruised but my precious cargo is dry and unscathed.

I retrieve my tube and climb back in, only to discover the electronic car key is gone from the dry pocket of my shorts! Shealagh berates me and all agree I was a fool to keep the key on me even if there are no lockers. I go inside and call a taxi so I can return to our country house for the spare key.

The taxi is late, and the kids grow hungry. But our picnic lunch is locked in the car, along with my wallet. Everyone gives me dirty looks, especially Damon, who's still chafing over his tube troubles. I convince the on-site shop to let us start a tab but tussle with Damon when he opts for a big bag of tortilla chips.

"There's nothing healthy here, so I have to eat junk food!" Damon argues.

Two hours later, when I return with the car key, Damon's mood has lifted. He's been practicing all afternoon, and he's finally got the hang of tubing.

He's devised his own system, which consists of lying flat on his stomach in the lower end of the tube with his legs dangling over the edge while his hands seize the side grips. Now he can use his small legs like propellers, kicking and churning with surprising efficiency as he motors along and drives the tube at will. Soon he's outracing all his pals and scooting down the rapids with abandon.

It's a wondrous sight, a grinning boy in a purple life jacket bouncing giddily in a bright orange tube that tosses like a cork on the dark green Delaware River. Damon is borne by the swift-running current, racing fearlessly for new thrills.

After his friends leave, Damon and I prepare to go camping in our forest.

"Can I come?" Sam asks at the last minute. I'm pleased at his interest but promise him a separate outing. This is my traditional one-on-one birthday excursion with Damon.

We pack a tent and sleeping bags and throw in food and water before heading into the family woods. I haul the tent and supplies while Damon carries a light knapsack on his back, a canteen on his belt, and a bow and arrow in hand. We spot spent red cartridges gleaming amid the ground vegetation. The previous owner leased the land to hunters, and deer-tracking platforms still dot the area.

"You won't let them hunt on our land, right, Dad?" Damon scowls.

"That's why we have No Trespassing signs." I point to the yellow posters on our trees, though I worry more about my children getting shot than the deer.

We've hiked a distance and Damon is not quite his energetic self, so we find a nice carpet of fern and some flat rocks and put up our gray, four-man tent. Inside, it's low but roomy. We unroll two pads and two sleeping bags, unzip the rainfly, then step back out.

"Don't leave any food," I remind Damon as I hammer a tent peg with a rock. "Put anything edible up in that tree, away from the tent. In case of coyotes . . ."

"Or bears, right, Dad?" Damon lets out a grim chuckle. He's heard all about the recent freak attack in our area. A black bear wandered into a bungalow colony and stole a five-month-old baby from her stroller on the porch. The mother, hearing cries of "Bear!" pushed her two other children into the house and rushed to her baby, but the bear had already made off with the infant in its mouth. The father chased the bear with rocks but by the time the bear dropped the baby and ran back into the woods, the infant's neck and head injuries were too severe and it died. Authorities later shot the animal, claiming bears didn't attack humans and they couldn't remember a similar case in thirty years.

"That was a total anomaly," I tell Damon. "Bears usually avoid humans. But this bear was probably habituated to people because they were leaving food out."

"Gee, Dad, that's reassuring . . . Okay, no food in the tent!" He hands me a bag, which I knot and hang off a tree.

We muck around in the woods, hurl stones, climb boulders, spot rabbit and deer, and pick strange flowers and fungi. Then we take the bow and arrow and practice shooting. I mark the target on a tree and demonstrate with the first shot. Then I let Damon try.

He holds the powerful recurve bow by its molded grip and inserts an arrow into the built-in arrow shelf. I assist Damon as he pulls back on the taut drawstring and releases. Although the first arrow falls short, he immediately senses the tremendous force in his hands. "Cool!" He smiles at me.

Damon grips the bow and shoots a dozen times, until he's hitting the tree with ease. He has a sharp eye and a steady hand and his brain calculates quickly. And because there is no cardiovascular component, Damon lacks any impediment.

Dusk falls fast as we head back to camp. Unsure of our whereabouts, we stumble through the alien woods until our tent crops up like a sudden outpost. We prepare our fire on an incline, away from the tent. As I hold a matchbox, Damon asks if they really used to start fires with rocks. "Sure." I smile at him and grab two stones, rubbing them repeatedly together. I manage to elicit a few puny sparks but fail to ignite a leaf before Damon takes pity on me and says, "It's okay, Dad, I get it!"

Reprieved, I strike a match and toss it in. The fire catches nicely and is so warm and consoling, I decide to keep feeding it. We're in a clear area, and it feels like an assertion of our humanity in this forbidding forest.

Damon watches intently as the flames leap into the sky. I keep a sharp eye on the surrounding forest as I continue stoking the fire until I feel the flesh of my cheeks burn and my dungaree-clad thighs bake. I turn to warn my son but Damon stands right behind me, riveted by the conflagration. The wild flames lick his bright hair and scorch his rapt features.

"Careful!" I say, even as I recognize my own reckless fascination in his eyes.

I let the fire die down, then open two cans of baked beans and pork with my Swiss Army knife. I burn the food but it still tastes good. Damon watches me guzzle a beer.

"Want a pull?" I offer. He sips the beer but returns to his ginger ale. We break into a bag of sweet white marshmallows but after burning or dropping one too many, we eat them raw. Then we go piss under the woodsy stars.

We slither into our sleeping bags, zip up, and huddle with our heads on either side of the center pole. The dark forest beyond comes alive with mysterious night creatures and night noises. I turn on the flashlight and place it facedown, trapping a bright ring of light, and tell Damon the eerie buzzing and yowling is the animals' nightly chatter—we're on their turf, after all. Damon finishes his pills, and we chat until we hear the furtive stirring of branches and a loud *snap*.

"What's that, a bear?" Damon cries, and for a moment I wonder too.

"Not likely, D-man." I again explain how unusual the recent attack was. "Besides," I growl, thumping the rolled-up jeans under my head, "I have a big, sharp hunting knife with me, so no one's gonna mess with us."

Damon chuckles and relaxes and we talk by the glow for a long time, covering many topics, from family and visiting friends to bears and books.

Damon is growing up and our relationship is changing. He's more independent-minded and oriented more toward his peers, and also dealing with the isolation of illness. I'm a smaller part of his day-to-day world. But our bond is deep and unshakable.

I kiss his forehead and turn off the flashlight. "Night, D-man."

"Night, Dad."

I wake up once in the still of night and grow alarmed when I can't see Damon in the pitch-black tent. I sit up and cock my ear but I still can't detect any evidence of him. Could he have gone outside to pee?

I unzip the flap and peer into the forest but it's equally dark out there and I can't see or hear a thing. I withdraw back into the tent. Where is he?

I reach over and grope in the empty darkness, my heart pounding, until my hand brushes the edge of a sleeping bag that has rolled into a dip. I palpate the mummy shell, which feels vacant, until I work up to something solid, squeeze and identify a human leg. It's small but I'm on the right track.

I reach over and locate a shaggy head, then tenderly touch Damon's slumbering face to confirm his presence.

Otherwise, he remains hushed, still, and completely undetectable in the dark.

It's amazing how silently and self-effacingly my son sleeps.

Chapter 22

In the fall, Damon enters Brooklyn Technical High School, New York City's largest public high school and one of the nation's leading magnet schools. He leaves the safe hothouse of Salk, with a student body of two hundred, for a sprawling twelve-story institution that occupies a square city block and houses five thousand students.

"My God, it's like a college!" Shealagh says. "Tech," as it's dubbed, boasts a wall of famous alumni, including two Nobelists, and a university-style system of majors. It might bewilder any kid with a freshman case of jitters, let alone a life-threatening case of PLE.

"Bronx High School of Science has half the students," I remind Damon.

Shealagh objects. "It's three hours a day on the subway! Too far from home."

"What about private school?" I ask Damon, not for the first time.

"Nah, I don't want to be one of those private school kids." Damon frowns. "And Tech's cool. I want to go there!"

Shealagh gets dizzy just going on the tour, while I'm more familiar with the setup because I also attended a vast New York City public high school. But I was healthy and full-size, whereas Damon is one of the smallest kids to ever walk through the heavy steel doors on South Elliott Place. His light complexion and hair and eye color make him even more conspicuous: 75 percent of Tech is non-Caucasian.

"I don't need a special elevator key," Damon scoffs. He's intent on a normal school experience and refuses any preferential treatment, arriving ten minutes early so he can walk up to his classes on the huge, teeming staircases. He's just as adamant about participating in all aspects of physical education.

"That kid never even had surgery!" Damon says of a boy who sits out each gym class due to a minor heart problem. Damon disdains medical excuses and performs every drill and completes every exercise, even when he's lapped on the track and comes in dead last on the mile run.

"Damon Weber?" The gruff coach doesn't even check his roster. Besieged by parents during our first mass conference in the chaotic gymnasium, he explains it's too soon to know the names of his hundreds of new students. Yet our son, not exactly varsity material, has already caught his eye.

"Damon's got a great attitude. Tell him to keep it up!"

It's another story with math, where Damon has failed two tests and is struggling. Partly it's the poor preparation at Salk, plus stiffer competition at a specialized math and science school. And it's never been Damon's best subject. But partly it's also the teacher.

"He never explains a thing," Damon says. "He just expects us to know it."

I come prepared to lock horns with the teacher but the sly old fox spots trouble a mile away and totally disarms me with his shrewd patter and practiced geniality. We agree to get Damon tutoring and let him catch up in the next term.

At first, Damon doesn't have a single friend at his new school and he struggles to find his niche. It's daunting. But he's naturally sociable and outgoing. In the school cafeteria, he sits at the senior table, where he strikes up conversation with the older students. But he's still a solo act.

"What about the theater program?" I ask. "You always make friends there."

"Yeah, if I could only find where it is!" Damon sighs. Theater is so irregular and so low-profile, it takes Damon weeks to track it down. Finally, he locates the tiny drama club in the vast, labyrinthine institution.

He auditions and immediately lands a part in the big fall play.

"I'm Dr. Chasuble in *The Importance of Being Earnest!*" Damon proudly informs us. It's a feat for a freshman and provides his first real opening in the Tech social scene.

Damon's daily homework load increases steeply at Tech, and he stays up late to get it all done. Shealagh, a semi-insomniac, worries about Damon's lack of sleep. She stays up with him, helps where she can, and makes him soups and late-night snacks. She cajoles and pesters him to knock off early until Damon, in exasperation, quips, "Mom, you're the only parent in the world who tells their kid to *stop* studying and *not* do their homework!"

Damon still has a full regimen of pills and supplements to swallow. But now he also starts daily heparin injections. It takes about one hour of prep time each night, and there's a lot of waiting-around time, which I try to help alleviate.

"Want to watch with me? I'm screening a doc we commissioned," I tell him.

"Yeah, just give me a minute." Damon retrieves from the closet a big box with all his "fixings." First, he disinfects the injection site with alcohol swabs. Then he applies a yellowish smear of anesthetic cream to his abdomen and covers the cream with a thin patch of cellophane, which he fastens with a makeshift belt. Normally he'd kill the next hour while waiting for the cream to numb his skin but tonight he joins me downstairs.

"Hey, Dad, this your show?" He settles near me on the sofa. "What's it on?"

"The impact of the genetics revolution—fifty years since the double helix."

"Cool," Damon says. We watch together until the cream has done its work. Then Damon unwraps a fresh syringe and needle and inserts the needle into a small ampoule of heparin. He retracts the plunger and fills the syringe with the clear, straw-colored liquid to just the right level, flicking it to ensure there are no bubbles or floating particles.

Then, with a determined sigh, Damon jabs himself.

The needle is tiny but it pierces the skin and leaves dark bruises on the surface. Damon becomes proficient and the technique routine, but there's always the flicker of insult at having to stick himself, and an angry band of discolored marks along his abdomen.

After seeing Dr. Hayes and others at Columbia—they advise that he should take the heparin for three months before expecting results—Damon heads to our local pediatrician for his regular checkup.

Dr. Satish Tandon, who also treats Sam and Miranda, has a solo family practice around the corner from us. People bring their kids with colds and coughs and rashes, and to get their shots and fill out school health forms.

Dr. Tandon always wears a tie and is polite and unassuming, with a big poster of Barney and lollipops for the kids. He's also a first-rate doctor and diagnostician whose thorough competence we've learned to appreciate.

Today, Dr. Tandon puts Damon on the height scale and informs us he's now fifty-six and a half inches, meaning he's grown half an inch since before the summer. This normally falls within the margin of error, but Dr. Tandon is precise, and it cheers us to think Damon has finally broken through that ceiling. Maybe he's about to break out in other ways.

"You saw it too? I prayed it was a pimple!" Shealagh chuckles over the tiny red blemish we both spotted on Damon's face. We scan avidly for any sign of puberty's onset. I'm hopeful but wary, recalling how Damon once complained of growing pains in his shin and we all felt excited until I read, with a pang, that shin pain was a symptom of PLE.

"His liver feels larger and harder than before the summer," Dr. Tandon observes. Using a tape measure, he confirms that the liver now protrudes eight to nine centimeters below the rib margin. In May, it was three to four centimeters, so this is a significant increase.

"This July," I now recall in dismay, "a GI guy in Boston estimated the liver at six centimeters. Which would confirm your read, and the idea of a progressive enlargement . . ."

"But Dr. Hayes said nothing about it at last week's visit," Shealagh notes.

"Still better to follow up," Dr. Tandon says. "There's a good liver man at Columbia." He gives us the name of a Dr. Stephen Lubritto, whom we go see.

Dr. Lubritto, short, round, and fast-talking, says the enlarged liver could be due to fluid overload, which diuretics can reduce. But it could also be a sign of "pump failure," which only a heart transplant can fix. "Let's hope for the former," he says.

By November, when Damon and his pals come to my office to help process the annual Rhodes Scholarship applications, I observe it's his reliable old gang and no new friends from Tech are there. All the kids have shot up except for Damon, who appears slight and pallid by comparison. I notice his hands and wrists look thin, almost diaphanous. But nothing seems to deter his ebullience. We make a party of it, going out after with all his friends to the Hard Rock Cafe.

Kyle also stays very much in the picture as Damon enters high school. One night I invite her and Damon to a play at a theater I'm affiliated with. It's a chilly evening and I tell Damon to take his coat. Kyle wears a jacket and dresses in multiple warm layers while Damon is clad only in a sweatshirt; he has the sniffles—he's been battling a cold for weeks—and looks pale and worn. But my son stubbornly resists and refuses to bundle up.

"Damon, I'm not taking you without a coat!" I finally say. I'm sympathetic but I can't allow teen fashion or rebelliousness to override serious and pressing health concerns. Teed off, Damon resentfully takes the coat and tosses it in the car.

We drive into the city, get snagged in traffic, and park blocks from the theater. It's curtain time, so we make a run for it. A biting wind cuts down the avenue and knifes through us. I clutch my coat collar and glance at Damon to see how he's coping, when it hits me he's wearing only a sweatshirt!

"Damon, where's your coat?" I realize with a sickening jolt he must've left it in the car. And it's too late to go back, or we'll miss the play. "Don't tell me . . . !"

"I took it with me, like you said." Damon stands looking innocent.

"You gotta be kidding!" I feel like a fool for taking my eye off him but I always try to give my son extra space with Kyle, and in our rush, I blew it. The frigid air stings us. "I can't believe you deliberately left your coat behind!" I yell.

"But I wasn't cold," Damon replies defiantly as the icy wind lashes us.

"Goddamn it, Damon, it's fucking freezing!" I blow my stack. What I don't say, in deference to Kyle, is that he's a very sick boy with a compromised immune system, and we can't afford such games. Even as I chastise him, I want to wrap his frail, stubborn body in my arms and shield him from the cold. He's so vulnerable. But all that comes out is my shrieking anger. "*I won't stand for this bullshit, Damon!*"

As I detonate, I become painfully aware of my own shrillness and loss of control. The ceaseless anxiety over my son's health has taken a toll on my nerves, and I can hear the raw, unnatural strain in my voice. The words explode from my mouth, angrier and fiercer than I intended. Damon reacts in a frozen tableau, glaring silently and bitterly at my dread authority. I've long been prepared to find every age-appropriate emotion, hatred included, in his eyes, and in my calmer moments, I even consider it my paternal duty to give him obdurate steel against which to toughen himself. But this outburst is unplanned, unpleasant, and mutually mortifying. Kyle looks like she wants to crawl into the ground.

We make it to the theater and dash to our seats as the xylophone chimes its last reminder. Kyle sits between Damon and me, a sweet buffer, but we're all so overwrought that at first it's hard to concentrate. Several times, I hear Damon try to muffle a fitful, hacking cough, a disturbing form of vindication I don't need.

But the play is surprisingly engaging, and by intermission we're all swept up in the tale and have almost forgotten our tiff. After, I take Damon and Kyle backstage and introduce them to the actors. The male lead talks shop with Damon.

We leave on a high note and walk down the street to a good restaurant. Kyle is impressed by the high-ceilinged room with its live menu of sprawling, iridescent fish; by the exorbitant prices; and by the beautiful people. But to me, Damon and Kyle are the two most alluring people in the place.

I recall taking them to another play years earlier, when Damon was in third grade and Kyle in second. After the Madison Square Garden show, we went to Lindy's for dessert and I watched the two of them banter and flirt in the most innocent, entrancing way. They were young children without a clue about romance or sexuality yet there was something electric between them that was extraordinary to behold.

"I don't know why you make me laugh so much!" pretty, wide-lipped, eight-year-old Kyle giggled at Damon from across the table.

"Kyle, your sleeve is in your ice cream!" Suave eight-year-old Damon leaned forward and grasped Kyle's arm, lofting a handsome ginger eyebrow.

I sat mesmerized and completely invisible to them. They brought their heads closer, two kindred spirits groping toward beauty and self-knowledge.

Now, many years later, we're sitting at another restaurant, after another play. Damon and Kyle, both fourteen, remain best friends and soul mates but Kyle, who loves Damon as much as ever, does not want to change their relationship in any fundamental way. I've walked into Damon's room and found them sweetly entwined on his loft bed, and nothing can ever truly separate them. But Damon wants a girlfriend and Kyle wants things to stay as they are, more or less.

It's not been easy for Damon but he's begun to swallow his disappointment and, impelled by his natural vigor and resiliency, to look elsewhere. I've caught the rumors of a girl at Tech, and there's much I don't catch. Whereas with Kyle, Damon now affects the role of indulgent older brother and bemused confidante, which helps them both negotiate their complex feelings for one another.

This evening, perhaps animated by their surroundings, they seem freer and more direct with each other. And they retain their abiding and matchless affinity.

"Here's to the two of you." I hoist a glass to Damon and Kyle.

"Thanks for inviting me." Kyle smiles with her long ice cream spoon in the air. "I really liked the play. And this is *so* nice." She points to the elegant restaurant. "But tell me one thing." She frowns in intellectual puzzlement. "How can they charge seventeen dollars for a fruit platter—a *fruit* platter?"

"That's for the small fruit platter. The big one is thirty-one dollars!" Damon grins.

"It's not always about price," I say to the two bright-eyed friends, forever young. "Remember that certain occasions, like tonight, are priceless."

Chapter 23

In early December, Damon's blood test shows a dramatic spike in his serum protein levels, presumably a result of the heparin injections. His albumin nearly doubles, jumping from alarmingly low (2.2) to normal (3.7). The total protein, a measure of all the proteins in the fluid portion of the blood, also soars, suggesting the PLE has abated.

"Wow, this is unbelievable!" I cry, staring deliriously at the new figures. Although we started the heparin treatment with precisely this goal in mind, and although we've learned that such positive effects, when you're lucky enough to see them, tend to diminish over time, the news brings immediate joy and relief.

"That's fantastic!" Shealagh exults as we stare incredulously at one another. "It's the first time since he was diagnosed that Damon has normal protein levels."

"And it proves we can stop and even reverse this relentless disease," I say.

Shealagh pauses. "Though he still looks small, and he's still not growing . . ."

"And it still could be only a temporary blip," I admit. "But if these numbers hold up, we could climb out of this hole and get our lives back!"

Shealagh and I share a double high five. We both feel cautiously, giddily optimistic.

Pondering this sudden change of fortune, I'm struck by how everything reduces to these two key measures, albumin and total protein. Two simple, naked numbers. Which, after stubbornly refusing to budge for over a year, have suddenly rocketed into positive territory.

So I decide to jot down these two numbers on a yellow Post-it, in two columns, and to carry them with me wherever I go. I enter the numerals from a year before on the same Post-it, so I can see how far we've come:

(Date)	(Albumin)	(Total Protein)
10/2001:	2.2	3.9
12/2002:	3.7	5.8

I will keep this little yellow Post-it in my wallet, and throughout Damon's illness, I will register any significant change in the two readings on this postage-stamp-sized ledger. At the oddest times, say in the middle of a meeting or in a movie theater, I will peek inside my wallet and ponder their pattern and meaning. While Damon's medical case only gains in complexity, and the available data and inputs multiply exponentially—and while many doctors tell me to ignore such crude measures—these two numbers are my secret bottom line. For a long time, their slightest tick, up or down, will predict my mood, functioning like stock prices for investors, final scores for sports fans, or casualty figures for war generals.

Once we get the good news about Damon's protein levels, we begin to look for, and find, hopeful signs under every rock.

"Hey, D-man, why you up so late?" I ask one night when I catch him on the stairs.

"I was really *hungry*," Damon confesses, blushing. He gets food cravings and goes on eating binges. His body appears more solid, more substantial. His color improves.

Our reenergized son invites us to the Brooklyn Tech production of *The Importance of Being Earnest*. The show is held in the massive school auditorium, a 4,200-seat, two-balcony theater space, but fortunately the actors are miked.

Damon does not have one of the leads so we have to wait until act 2 for his first appearance. But the moment he steps onto the stage with his slicked-up pompadour, twinkling eyes, and pompous thumbs hooked into Victorian lapels, Damon commands our attention as the Reverend Canon Chasuble. His colorful presence, comic timing, clear voice, and superb diction make him stand out.

It's becoming clear to us that Damon is at home on the stage, liberated by his gift for impersonation, his social intelligence, and his limitless imagination. We're equally pleased to see, once the curtain descends, that he's mingling with a new set of friends. It's first semester of his freshman year and he's found his niche.

A few days later, I take Damon to the Annual Daughters and Sons Meeting at the Council on Foreign Relations. It's a chance for members to bring their high school and college age children to this renowned foreign policy enclave, a cross between a wonky think tank and an exclusive club where you can rub shoulders with world leaders and dignitaries.

I leave my office after work and wait for Damon by the neoclassical town house on Park Avenue. Shealagh has put our son in a cab and I'm apprehensive, not just about whether he'll arrive safely and on time but about whether he's up to this event.

"You sure this might not be too stressful for you right now?" I ask Damon that morning. His face looks puffy and his voice sounds reedy to me.

"Yeah, Dad, I'm really interested in this stuff!" Damon says. "I'm doing model UN and I might want to major in international relations."

Now he steps from the cab in the requisite suit and tie but everything's a little askew: the top button of his dress shirt pops open, revealing the secret pallor of his chest; an ill-knotted rep tie bunches at his collar; and his low-hanging pants droop below a distended belly. He's a study in disarray but I have to chuckle because despite his unique case, Damon shares with me a rumpled quality I recognize.

But this is a formal place, and we don't want to draw undue attention.

"Let me help you with that," I say as we walk through the detector and pick up our two name tags. I peel off the backing and lean forward to affix Damon's tag, surreptitiously trying to straighten his tie, a role we're both so unaccustomed to that Damon involuntarily flinches.

"Dad! What're you doing?" He's not sure whether to be upset or amused.

"Sorry, D-man." I attempt to close his collar, but he grimaces with such suffocating forbearance, like a mirror of my younger self, that I give up.

We are directed past Venetian doors to a formal drawing room with a bar and a table of appetizers. Damon's big black dress shoes squeak on the parquet floor. As other members arrive with their rangy offspring, I note Damon is by far the smallest and youngest-looking person in the room, and I'm ready to present his high school ID if challenged. The chairman walks over and chats with Damon, breaking the ice. Then I introduce my son to an air force colonel I know.

The bell sounds and we all file to the meeting hall for the featured speaker, a former deputy secretary of state waiting for the next administration so he can be secretary of state. He provides a good overview of post-9/11 security challenges.

Like most members, I'm pleased to be sitting here with my son as we're briefed by an insider. Beyond the analysis and insight, I want Damon to realize the country is run by people not much different from him, so he can grasp that its challenges are his, and his generation's.

Later, after a couple of confident college kids have asked questions from the audience, Damon's hand creeps up. It stays up, even when he's not called on right away. I smile, recalling the first time Damon raised his hand in public. He was four and sat on the floor amid a crowd of nattering, fidgeting tykes in his Saturday drawing class at the Brooklyn Museum. The instructor asked about a famous painting in front of them but none of the children made a sound until one hand shot up. I was impressed then, as I am impressed now, even though Damon never gets to ask his question because the session ends promptly, per council tradition.

"What were you going to ask?" I query Damon as we exit.

"If they *really* can't find bin Laden. My Pakistani cabbie said everyone in Pakistan knows where he is, but if they tell us, they'll lose their leverage."

Damon continues on a roll through the holiday season. After celebrating Hanukkah at my parents', we go for a week of skiing in Holiday Mountain, a family resort near our country house. Bavarian-born Shealagh, the ablest skier among us, has long given up on her husband, but she wants her kids to ski properly. This year her bad back keeps her off the slopes but she still instructs Miranda how to snowplow, and Sam, when he listens, how to turn.

Damon practices with me for several days before his friend Jon comes up. His lessons have paid off, and he shows great progress. One cold, bright day, Damon and I are riding the chair lift when it stops halfway to the top, and we find ourselves stalled in midair, suspended over a steep ravine. We hear the windy creak as the aerial chair twists and dangles off its solitary cable.

"How do we get down if the lift is broken?" Damon asks, laughing nervously.

"Easy. They could use a harness, a bucket truck, or even a chopper!" I shrug and put my arm around him as we both look down. Our crisp black shadows, projected onto the snowy ground below, seem to look back at us like smiling negatives.

The chill picks up but Damon is well padded and the sun keeps us cozy in our chair. I point to the purple mountains and evergreen trees and tell my son to enjoy this spectacle. Eighty feet below us, the simple shadow of Damon and me sitting together on the chair lift with my arm draped across his shoulder resembles a perfect black silhouette of father and son stamped on the snow. I find myself wishing we could hold on to this moment and stay suspended up here indefinitely.

Jon arrives and the two boys hit the slopes. Eventually, they work up to the Roman Candle, a daunting four-hundred-foot vertical drop. At first, they snowplow from side to side and sit down when it gets too scary. But slowly, they overcome their fear and ski down in one run, returning full of pride and achievement.

I watch them from Manny's Run, an intermediate trail, until I'm satisfied they're okay. Once, I'm skiing down the hill when Damon suddenly zips past, sailing by me like a confident pro, knees bent and poles tucked under arms.

"Hi, Dad!" Damon chirps with bright red cheeks as he whooshes past me. I do a few more runs for appearance's sake, but really, I'm so excited I can't wait to get off the slopes and share what I just witnessed with Shealagh.

Our grinning, self-assured son flying right past me on his skis and racing downhill with abandon!

It feels like the blessed advent of the ordinary—it feels like a miracle.

Chapter 24

"Damn! His albumin is down from three point seven to three point four," I report to Shealagh in January, after getting Damon's latest lab results from Columbia.

"But that's statistically insignificant—within the margin of error," she notes.

"Yes, but his total protein also fell, from 5.8 to 5.1," I reply. "I know it's a small drop, but the direction is backward. This is *not* good. Heparin was supposed to buy us a year or two, but its effects seem to have peaked after *three months*." I shake my head. "We can't seem to stop this thing!"

"It's too early to know. Let's at least wait for the next test," Shealagh says.

"Sure." I nod. I'm only too happy to defer the bad news, but inside, I know.

I intensify my search for alternative therapies. I continue reading the latest medical and scientific literature and talking to researchers in the United States and abroad. I check in with the half dozen leading hospitals where I've established connections. I register for an international conference on PLE. I'm open to any angle or approach and even consider enrolling in medical school or auditing targeted classes. I'm on the case 24/7.

Whenever I run into any person anywhere with the slightest expertise—a postdoc on a late-night train from Cambridge to London, a physician at a New Year's Eve party, a former classmate turned scientist at a reunion—I pepper him with questions that might reveal a link between his field and Damon's problem. But I don't explain why.

I'm careful not to breathe a word about Damon to anyone but close friends. My wife's philosophy, Tell Them Nothing, seems prudent. Damon's illness so isolates and dominates our existence, we cannot let it completely overwhelm our lives. We have two other children and many other obligations. I must hold on to my job to support the family and it's easier to maintain things on a professional level and not let our personal crisis bleed into everything. Sympathy is nice but misfortune can also be turned against you.

I violate our rule and broach the subject at work only if I think it might benefit Damon. One day, the Nobel laureate James Watson, co-discoverer of the double helix, is in my office for one of our brainstorming sessions. We've collaborated on several projects and have a good relationship. Watson is an original, if controversial, thinker, he knows everyone, and he's had ongoing medical issues with his own son, whom I've met.

"Hey, Jim," I ask, "who's the smartest out-of-the-box cardiologist you know?"

Watson squints and gawks through his glasses, still, in his seventies, a precocious spirit. "Oh, well, I know a lot more about cancer because that's what all my friends seem to get. And the Watsons don't have much family history of heart disease. We're lucky—"

"I'm looking for a maverick who works on the human heart."

"One day they'll solve the immune issues and give everyone a pig's heart!" Jim chortles. "Or build artificial hearts and implant them like pacemakers. It's just a pump, for goodness' sake!" He shrugs and flicks his hands to indicate the glaring simplicity.

"Yeah, but meantime, I need help now. It's personal and confidential—"

"Sure. I'll see if I can think of anyone and let you know."

After enlisting Watson—he never finds the perfect cardiologist but asking him helps me feel I've left no stone unturned—I e-mail a scientist in China. Then I contact an alternative-medicine guru in India.

At home, things seem to go on as before. Our lives are filled with the daily bustle of three children and the steady drumbeat of their never-ending activities, but Damon remains in developmental lockdown.

He's still outgoing and even widens his social circle at Tech. But he hasn't grown and appears paler than ever. When he sits, stork-like, on a tall stool at the kitchen counter, his skinny legs folded on the rungs beneath him resemble toothpicks. His slight lower body seems to be receding, even while above the counter, he remains a strong, active presence.

"Hey, Dad, can I go to Web2Zone for an all-nighter on Friday?"

"One of those LANsomnias?" I say, and Damon smiles. These raucous, dusk-to-dawn video game elimination tournaments have become his favorite hangout. "Yeah, you can go, long as you take an extra half dose of heparin the day before and the day after," I reply. It's good for him to have an injection-free night out with the boys, and I'm all for it.

"Thanks, Dad. I won't forget to pre-dose. Believe me, shooting a needle into your arm in a room filled with loud music is one sure way to kill a party!"

Damon's wit, always keen, now takes on a more rapier-like quality. He skewers his siblings more mercilessly than before and even, occasionally, turns on his mother. He's a teenager, of course, and still sweet at heart, but there's a dark new edge, barbed with fury that glints though at unguarded moments: "That's stupid, Mom. I'm fourteen and you're treating me like a child. Leave me alone!"

Shealagh worries about Damon constantly. Her own health suffers. She has asthma, rashes, back pain. She's depressed and exhausted. She can't tolerate the stress of her job and wants to stop working so she can be home more for Damon. She wishes to help make his life easier while creating a more nurturing environment for Sam and Miranda.

After reducing her hours and scaling back from three days to two, we agree she should stop working altogether. We'll find a way to adjust. Although Shealagh's salary has never been more than a fraction of our household income, taking it away will leave a shortfall, especially as our medical bills are increasing. I promise to speak to my employers about a raise or to find another source of income. Either way, things have deteriorated to such a point for Shealagh that we don't really have a choice. My wife is tough but our situation is off the charts.

My own state of mind at this juncture is also parlous and I feel under constant, unrelenting pressure. I walk around all day with a knot in my stomach and a clenched tightness in my chest. And there's no escape, not even at night.

I jerk awake well before my normal five A.M. rising time, and I no longer feel refreshed or restored. My brain has grabbed the minimum rest essential for survival and then it forces me back to consciousness, like an interrogation agent slapping my face.

My writing, key to my peace of mind, also takes a hit because I often must work on Damon's case instead. There's no time or space left for the deep dive of imagination. My writer's haven has turned into a business office, full of grim, mounting stacks of medical files and reports. Even when I'm not corresponding with doctors across the country and writing careful e-mails describing Damon's latest symptoms and results, or poring over mounds of new data, or setting up appointments and more tests, my mind is unquiet.

One night, I dream I'm driving a car with Damon and Shealagh sitting beside me. Suddenly we're lurching off the road and careening down a steep mountain, with a dark tunnel at the end. There's a metal railing on one side of the car and nothing on the other. I pump the brakes but they don't work and the automobile, instead of stopping, accelerates and takes on a life of its own. I yank the steering wheel and repeatedly slam the vehicle against the railing, trying to use the guardrail to slow it down. But the car only speeds up and races downhill like a runaway train until I realize there's nothing more I can do to stop it. Just before we hit the tunnel and crash in a fireball, I turn to Shealagh and Damon and cry from the depths of my soul, "I'm sorry!"

Then I wake up, coated in a cold, clammy sweat.

Around this period, while in southern Mexico, I fall into a deep, unmarked construction hole on the elevated terrace of a bar—for real this time.

It's nighttime and I'm striding ahead of colleagues to a table on the balcony when the ground gives way beneath me. I plummet down a blind, bottomless shaft in a state of complete disorientation and increasing alarm for about ten feet—which feels like ten miles, or ten years—before slamming into the rocky ground. I crash in a shattering heap but because I drop for such a long time in the darkness, I'm actually *relieved* when I hit something, since I know I can't survive if it lasts much longer. I break three major bones in my wrist and smash my hand to smithereens, but I'm lucky because my head misses an exposed sewage pipe by inches and I remain conscious.

Once I realize I'm basically okay—my shoulder is dislocated and my face and body bruised, but I can think clearly and I can move the arm—my main concern is not to worry Shealagh and the kids, and not to let this interfere in any way with my duties to my elder son.

Compared to Damon's situation, my reference point for everything, I've already determined this is a relatively trivial problem. Although I'm still in shock and looking at an operation to reconstruct my wrist and permanently insert a metal bar into my flesh followed by a year of painful therapy, I'm already a little bored and impatient with my own mishap. I know I heal well, it's my left wrist and I'm right-handed, and all my major organs are fine.

Someone drives me to the hospital in Cuernavaca, where I'm tempted to let them operate the next day. But I'm alert enough to call my friend Jeff Friedman in New York, and Jeff, who has an MD and a PhD, along with a wry sense of humor, says, "It's your hand, Doron, a complex, delicate organ involved in fine motor coordination and multiple daily tasks, and presumably you want to use it with minimal impairment for many decades, rather than dragging it around like a crooked stump for the rest of your life—so no, I don't think you should have this surgery in a rural Mexican hospital!"

We both laugh and I wind up flying back for the operation, but what strikes me most about this incident is how Damon's condition has completely altered my perspective and how blasé I now feel about any problem short of life and death. I also register how the shock of my near-fatal accident has brought me mysteriously nearer to Damon. As if descending into that dark pit and brushing up against death was a way to embrace my son and take some of his suffering onto myself.

It makes me ponder the nature of accidents. My gravest injury until now was a car accident thirteen years earlier, which closely followed Damon's first open-heart operation. It, too, almost killed me, but it also gave me a personal window onto my son's agony and the ordeal of recovery, which I thus was able to secretly share with him.

Chapter 25

Second semester freshman year in the Brooklyn Tech cafeteria, seventh period, a girl named Rebecca introduces Damon to her buddies at the corner table, and before long he is sitting and chatting with them every day.

Rebecca is cute and all the boys have a thing for her, but after a while the guys get to know each other too. Soon Damon makes a new set of friends, and this fledgling entity, "the Group," which extends to over a dozen people and will eventually overlap drama as well, becomes his main high school crowd.

Two boys in particular, Max and Zak, start hanging out with Damon on a regular basis. When I come home, they're often sitting around the computer in Damon's room.

"Hey, guys. What're you playing?" I watch as Damon and Zak battle it out on-screen, blowtorching platoons of squiggly critters across a cartoon landscape.

"Worms." Max grins, taking pity on my ignorance. He has a solid build, glasses, and black wavy hair. "Damon always beats us at this but he's not up to our level on Warcraft yet," Max says. "But he's coming on like a fiend!"

"Damon's not going to win today!" Zak yells over his shoulder. Zak also is broad-framed but he has fair hair, which he dyes in striking pastel hues. "I'm gonna be last worm standing!" Zak declares, launching a Banana Bomb.

They go into "sudden death" but Damon pulls it out with a ninja rope and a drill. "Take that, you wormling!" Damon shouts, giggling to victory.

The three friends engage in many shared activities—concerts, movies, basketball, blogging, practical joking, amateur filmmaking, experimental drinking, sleepovers—but their preferred pastime is computer video games and their preferred venue is Web2Zone, an Internet café and game room in the East Village. This bricks-and-mortar cyber-paradise boasts two floors honeycombed with hundreds of computers, PlayStations, Xboxes, and HDTVs. When I drop Damon off on Cooper Square, he walks into a funhouse of digital fantasy and thrills, a wild, 3-D world apart from reality.

The two-day international symposium on PLE that I attend is a sobering affair, as Dr. Chin warned me. A small group of scientists and physicians describe promising avenues of research and provocative leads—I attend every talk and read every paper—but the world's experts remain fundamentally baffled.

I meet bewildered family members, their faces etched with fear, who hang on every word. They describe heart-rending struggles that sound all too familiar. I note the most bold and advanced among them have taken matters into their own hands. One desperate father has had the entire bacterial floor of his daughter's stomach wiped clean and is trying to control everything that enters her system.

I return with a bleak overview but focus determinedly on the 20 percent of PLE patients who survive and how to navigate Damon through this terrifying illness. In my overnight bag are pages of notes, scientific papers, and references to pursue.

As I step into our house, still digesting what I've seen, Damon comes down the stairs, catching me off guard. "Hey, Dad, how'd the conference go?"

"It was pretty useful." I fumble around. "I learned a lot—there's good research going on—but it's still early days and there's no magic bullet yet. We'll have to keep looking."

Damon frowns. "I thought if I managed to make it past this phase and into my twenties, the PLE would get better on its own," he says in an aggrieved tone. "That once I'm grown-up, I wouldn't need the protein so much."

I wince, torn between wanting Damon to grasp his illness—he's entitled to know what he's up against—and not wishing to undermine his confidence.

"Yes," I reply, "but it's a little more complicated. Because first we have to get you *past* this stage, which we will, once we figure out the best way . . ."

Damon gives me a brooding look, as if I've sown fresh doubts. We go down to the family room, where the TV news is blaring, and I try to explain it better.

"Look, it's a very diabolical enemy, your PLE. Think of it like a murderous tyrant, a Hitler or Stalin or a Saddam Hussein"—the United States has just invaded Iraq, and everyone is baying for Saddam's blood. "We have to stop it in its tracks. We have to vanquish our foe!"

Damon screws up his features. He doesn't think of his situation in such dire terms, and he doesn't want me to either. I've hit the wrong note again.

"Okay, maybe that's going too far," I backtrack, "but you know we got a real fight on our hands, right?" Damon nods. He's okay with this. "That's all I meant."

We hang out on the sofa and watch TV together. A show comes on about the space program and JFK's famous promise to land a man on the moon.

"A new biography of John Kennedy just came out," I tell Damon. "A historian got hold of his medical records and it turns out Kennedy was much sicker than anyone knew."

Damon's eyes stay on the TV screen but his head tilts in my direction.

"From a very young age, the future president had a series of grave ailments," I tell my son, listing them: "Scarlet fever, colitis, back injury, urethritis, Addison's disease, bowel problems, weight loss, sleep disorders . . . In the White House, Kennedy was taking ten to twelve medications a day and getting six daily injections for his back. Sound familiar?"

"Really? But he looks so youthful and vigorous in photos. And so tan!"

"Yeah, he worked hard on his image." I smile. "But this is a guy who was so sickly as a child that twice they called the priest and read the last rites over him. Twice! They gave him up for a goner. And look what he made of his life."

"That's cool." Damon nods, weighing the information. "I didn't know that."

"Me neither," I admit. "But it's inspiring to see what people can accomplish despite early setbacks. How overcoming illness and adversity builds character . . . Hey, D-man, maybe one day, you'll be president."

Damon gives me a look that shows how absurd he finds this, but I persist. "Maybe that's what all this is about. Forging your character in the crucible of suffering. You're being tested . . . and you'd make a damn good president!"

"Thanks, Dad, I appreciate the vote of confidence," Damon replies tartly, "only I don't want to be president." He shrugs with complete disinterest.

"Oh." I had not expected this. It silences me, but only for a moment. "Maybe I'll be like JFK's father and I'll hector you into it."

"You can't really force someone to run for president," Damon observes. "And even you wouldn't go that far, Dad."

"Hey, didn't you admit it was my prodding that made you realize you could be an A student in middle school?"

Damon pauses. "Yes, but that was something I wanted, I just wasn't sure I had it in me. Being president sounds really boring. Why would I want that job?"

Over Easter break, we visit SeaWorld in San Diego. The most striking creature we see is a giant, glorious, gleaming white polar bear. He stretches out in his lair, with enormous, recumbent strength packed into his long body.

"Cool." Damon stands transfixed by the magnificent creature.

"Think he knows he's trapped and we've just re-created his habitat?" I ask.

"Maybe this is all he knows," Damon says. "Especially if he was born here."

"Or maybe he's biding his time and waiting for a chance to escape."

"Maybe." Damon smiles enigmatically. He pauses. "Hey, Dad, is he male?"

The question, though appropriate for an adolescent boy, catches me by surprise. I peer at the bear's powerful, fur-clad legs but can't be sure. "I wouldn't tangle with it either way. This feels like the top of creation."

Back at the hotel, Damon and Sam play-fight more aggressively than usual. Sam is a half inch taller now, and when they wrestle, Sam threatens to overpower Damon, a potentially seismic shift.

"Okay, Sam, let's start again but away from the TV," Damon says, flushed and panting but still in charge. Sometimes, when they really go at it, it looks like Sam could inadvertently hurt Damon with his wild flailing. Sam still doesn't know his own strength, yet even as he forces Damon back, Sam hesitates because he so reveres his big brother.

Back in New York, we go see Sam perform at the PS 29 All-Star Show. Kyle, in a Mickey Mouse hat, joins Damon in the school auditorium, two seasoned graduates returning to their alma mater for laughs and nostalgia. They can't believe how small it all looks now.

"That's because you're so much bigger," Shealagh tells them.

"Not me!" Damon says dryly. Several parents mistake Damon for Sam, and Damon must awkwardly explain that he is Sam's *older* brother.

Sam is on the gymnastics team and the pep squad. We watch him leap and tumble and do a slithering caterpillar roll with his teammates. At half-time, a teacher reads a poem about a boy with red hair and a strange gift and we're amazed to see a silent, athletic, and self-sufficient Sam step from the wings. He walks on his hands from one end of the stage to the other.

"Wow, I didn't know Sam could do that," Kyle remarks, smiling amid the ovation.

"Nobody knew!" Damon says with a trace of pride. "I caught Sam practicing but he kept it a secret. Our Sam is a man of mystery!"

The next day we watch Miranda march in the St. Patrick's Day parade with her Irish dance class. Normally she wears a black leotard and black skirt as she joins in a mass, synchronized display of pounding legs and clicking feet. But today she's clad in a bright green folk dress with a gold headband and carries the school banner with her friend Caroline. After, we take them for ice cream and the two eight-year-old sirens turn heads with their captivating cheerleader-type routines.

"Hey, Dad, better keep an eye on those girls," Damon warns, both playful and protective. "They were getting some pretty strange looks out on the street!"

Around this time, the Tribeca Film Festival takes place. At a reception I host following a film panel, I introduce Damon and his friends to various well-known figures, including two of the festival cofounders, Jane Rosenthal and Craig Hatkoff. When the third founder, the actor Robert De Niro, walks into the room, there's the usual celebrity buzz. De Niro, a shy, astute, and highly alert man who does not miss much, makes the rounds and greets everyone he knows, including me because of my formal affiliation with the festival. He's followed by a train of publicists and managers and photographers. I try to catch his eye because I want to introduce him to my son. De Niro is a legend, and as a New Yorker, former cabbie, and boxer, I feel a special connection to him, like about a billion other people in the world. But there are too many eager attendees clamoring for his attention, and I can't compete with the crowd.

As he starts to leave the reception, De Niro circles back and comes up to me smiling, as if we're the oldest pals in the world and he's forgotten to tell me something, which is just trembling on the tip of his tongue. "Hey, Doron . . ."

It's a generous gesture and a real star turn, an instinctive reading of the scene meant solely to make me look important in front of my son and his friends.

He *really* is a great actor.

De Niro lingers and I make the introductions. He shakes hands with Damon and his friends. The three teenagers bask in the limelight while Damon talks to De Niro about a variety of subjects until the actor has to leave for his next event.

When I get home that night, there's a message from Dr. Hayes. Damon's total protein has sunk to 4.1 and his albumin is back down to 2.5. He's given up almost all the gains he made from the heparin.

Chapter 26

"Why am I so tired all the time?" Damon cries at night to his mother. "Why do I *get* so tired?" He looks frail and sluggish and admits he can't always keep up with his friends. He runs out of energy and goes to bed early, setting his alarm clock so he can rise at dawn and complete his homework before school.

He's also taking on more fluid. We can see it in his puffy face and in the progressively more "pregnant" look of his belly, which he obscures with baggy clothes. One night I give him a massage and feel a hump of flesh between his neck and shoulder.

"Hey, what's this buffalo fat doing here?" I joke, holding the fold of flesh between my fingers. Damon becomes very self-conscious—he's sensitive about the slightest hint of anomaly—until I assure him it's not fat, just his thick neck.

But privately, I worry it's one more sign of fluid retention.

He's also getting more bouts of nausea. Partly it's the humongous pills and thick protein supplements and greasy liquids he must swallow several times a day. He walks around the house sucking on limes, his mouth a wedge of green, to counteract the sickening fatty oils.

Shealagh and I take him to Children's Hospital of Philadelphia and sit in the waiting room in a state of deep dejection. It feels like we're running in circles, unable to break the PLE chokehold. The endless maze of hospital visits only magnifies our anxiety. Damon, sitting with headphones across from us, notices our downcast expressions.

"Hey." He waves from his armchair, flagging down our attention with a slow, gentle sweep of the arm—"Hi, Mom, hi, Dad!"—and coaxes us out of ourselves with a soft, radiant smile.

We smile back guiltily at our son. His languid hand, arcing up from a pale wrist, describes a modest but grand salute, like a young member of the royal family hailing his subjects. He commands us not to forget him—"I'm right here," his luminous smile says—and promises that everything will be okay.

It's a curious and touching reversal. The sick child reassuring the anxious parents and reminding them to be thankful for what they have.

Dr. Chin examines Damon with his usual thoroughness and care and notes the textbook deterioration in his condition. Damon's liver is enlarged, with increasing fluid about the belly and face. And a dense patchwork of spidery blue veins crisscrosses his abdomen, chest, and upper arms, giving his skin a dusky, translucent fragility.

"The blue blood is sprouting new venous pathways as it tries to shortcut back to the heart in a desperate bid for oxygen," Dr. Chin tells us, gently tracing the branching veinlets across Damon's torso. "It's a sign of increasing systemic stress," he says softly.

After Damon goes to watch videos in an outer room, we discuss our remaining options, including a Fontan "takedown," followed by an attempted repair of Damon's second ventricle. "It's a long shot but it would restore a normal circulatory system for him," Dr. Chin says. At the Mayo Clinic a year earlier, I asked Dr. Gordon Danielson, a pioneering heart surgeon, about such a procedure, and he admitted it had never been successfully performed, that it would require lots of surgery—much more than a transplant—but in theory, there was no reason it couldn't be done. Now Dr. Chin gives us the name of a surgeon who "might consider" undertaking such a high-risk operation.

We also review fenestration but agree to wait a little longer and pursue other, less invasive approaches first. We call Damon back into the room and Dr. Chin addresses him.

"Well, Damon, heparin isn't helping so we'd like to try something new."

"You mean I still have PLE?" Damon says in his disarming way.

Dr. Chin is tactful but Damon is too sharp, and Dr. Chin too respectful of his intelligence, to obscure the facts. "Yes, that's why you feel so tired and why you're puffy," Dr. Chin says, adding that we have some interesting leads on treatments to modulate PLE but there's no single answer. "We just have to keep searching and find a solution that works for you."

I watch my young son, who grasps what Dr. Chin is saying, take this in. His face pales and his leg twitches, swiping the water bottle behind him, but he hangs in and meets the news head-on, agreeing to try the alternatives.

I feel deeply distressed that I can do nothing to shield my son, even though he's sitting only a few feet from me. Shealagh looks equally helpless and bereft. We're both overwhelmed and stymied but chime in with hopeful asides about the future and console ourselves that we still have many cards to play.

Among my best-informed advisers is Dr. David "Dudu" Bar-Or. A physician, biomedical researcher, and chief scientific officer of a company he founded, Dudu runs a trauma center in the Southwest while developing new drugs and diagnostics for diseases. He's not only a first-rate clinician and bench scientist with dozens of patents to his name, he's also married to my cousin Ohna. Like Dr. Chin, Dudu possesses rare breadth and is critical of received medical wisdom. He also always takes my calls and provides a frank insider's view.

Dudu has devoted much time and research effort to Damon's case and the dread mystery of PLE. From the start, he's felt the mechanism of inflammation, which his lab focuses on for its role in inflammatory and autoimmune diseases, is a key component. Now as I press him with increasing urgency, Dudu hits on a new approach.

"To control the balance of inflammation and anti-inflammation enzyme function, or to defend against any illness, you need a strong immune system," Dudu tells me. "But Damon's T cells and B cells, the key white blood cells for fighting infection, are extremely low. So I suggest we try him on IVIG—intravenous infusion of immunoglobulins."

IVIG is a blood product that supplies antibodies, or an immune boost, for people who have an immune deficiency or an autoimmune illness. Dudu has also seen it used effectively in the ER for organ failure, another way of looking at what's happening to Damon's heart, liver, and gut. In addition, Dudu believes IVIG possesses an anti-inflammatory component that theoretically could help target Damon's underlying PLE.

A literature search quickly shows others have used IVIG for PLE without harmful effects, and with some benefit. "Ideally, IVIG could reduce inflammation and keep Damon's albumin from leaking out. At the least, it will improve his general immunity and health status," Dudu says.

It sounds like it's worth a try and even Dr. Hayes does not object, though Columbia does not administer IVIG at this stage and she's not sure what good it'll do. But to her credit, Dr. Hayes gives me leeway to seek alternatives. She's fundamentally cautious but knows the limits of current treatments and shares our concern about Damon.

In early summer, after one week in Martha's Vineyard and a week in Cape Cod, Damon and I fly west for his first IVIG treatment. An immunologist colleague of Dudu's gives us a private room where an IV is started and an IV stand with an infusion bag is wheeled in. Damon reclines on a sofa—a black pillow sets off his red hair—while a clear infusion of immunoglobulins drips down from the tall IV pole and flows into his arm. I imagine healing balm from the Tree of Life but in fact, at one stage, Damon grows dizzy, his pressure drops, and he becomes nauseated. The doctor slows the infusion rate and he doesn't bump it up again until Damon has recovered. But he interprets the reaction as a good sign, an indication the compound is "having an effect."

Damon and I hang out most of the day until his infusion is complete. We watch videos, eat lunch, and banter. I help him wheel his IV pole to the bathroom. A couple of times, Damon dozes off. I watch his thin, IV-encumbered arms hugging the white blanket to his chest, his weary head rolling back as the impassive machine gurgles and clicks away.

He endures this latest trial like a pale stoic, resolute even in slumber.

I track the vital fluid flowing into Damon's veins and pray something fundamental is happening. Is it so much to ask?

Damon gets through the infusion without further incident. The doctor says he should feel better in a week, though sometimes several infusions are needed for an initial response. "Either way," he says, "take it easy for the first twenty-four to forty-eight hours until your body adjusts."

I help a relieved but still shaky Damon climb into a taxi for the airport—he wants to return for rehearsals the next day. At first, he's sensitive to every bump and lurch on the road. At the terminal, he gets a headache and he holds on to me on the automatic walkway. Inside the cabin, the bright lights blind him and he pulls his hoodie over his eyes, moaning. "It hurts . . . I'm dizzy!"

I've had a good feeling about this treatment, but now I start to wonder.

We arrive home at two A.M., exhausted. But Damon rises by eight the next morning for school because parts are being assigned for *Pericles*. I only hope he gets through the day.

He calls me at noon in the office to report he got the part he wanted. I'm very pleased for him and note his chirpiness.

"Aren't you tired from yesterday? I know I am," I say.

"No, I'm good. I think I even feel a slight . . . improvement." Damon pauses, as if digesting this himself. "Is that possible, Dad? So soon, I mean?"

"Why not?" I register a warm glow, as if *I've* just been infused. "First, even if it's a placebo effect, you still *feel* better. And you may be one of the lucky ones who respond fast."

"Yeah, Dad, but this is *really* fast."

Everyone is thrilled with Damon's early response to the treatment. We go for another infusion a few weeks later, and Damon gets another palpable lift. We decide to make the most of this good news by returning to northwest Scotland in August for a family vacation on the Isle of Skye.

Damon's improvement gives us all a boost, but we can't tell if this is the decisive turning point—he seems much peppier—or just another short-lived hope.

I make an appointment to speak to the president of my foundation about a raise. Shealagh has stopped working and Damon's medical bills are escalating. Shealagh's family won't help and mine can't, so we must look elsewhere.

My stock is high at work and I have merit-based grounds for a raise. I also have a good relationship with the president. But what's hard is dropping my professional facade and admitting I have a seriously ill son at home whose care I oversee. I've scrupulously fenced off this part of my life from the office and my larger work environment. Even my assistant doesn't know, and going public has stopped me from requesting help sooner. But now I must break cover because the situation is too dire.

As I wait outside the president's office and review my request, it strikes me that not just this crisis but my entire professional career has been shaped by Damon. It was only after Damon's birth and jolting diagnosis that I sought my first full-time job, in my thirties. Until then I'd been a freelance writer and editor, happily doing my own thing. But I needed health insurance, and would need it forevermore, so I grabbed the first thing I could, paying my dues for a few years until I'd recovered my balance. But I never resented Damon or regretted the decision. It was an honorable duty for a great cause.

My long-deferred meeting with the president goes well, or as well as might be expected. He cannot give me what I ask for but he promises to help, and he does, once he gets the board of trustees' approval. I leave the room feeling more naked and exposed, with my financial problem only partly solved, but with my faith in people—and specifically, in the people I work for—reaffirmed.

Two weeks before Skye, Shealagh takes Sam and Miranda to her sister's place in the Channel Islands. I have work and Damon has theater, so we two remain in New York. When I return from the office, we sit in the backyard, shooting baskets, barbecuing, or just hanging out. The peaches are starting to come in on our big tree but the birds are pecking the downy fruit to pieces.

"Can you believe these goddamned cheeky sparrows and redbirds!" I gripe.

"You'd be cheeky too if you didn't have enough to eat!" Damon chides. He leaves the birds extra seeds in his window feeder.

Saturday morning, I get us ham and egg bagels, then drop Damon at Barnes & Noble while I go to the pharmacy to refill his medications. When I return to the Seventh Avenue bookstore, I find Damon browsing in the theater section.

"Hey, Dad, can you help me find a good play for our fall production?" Damon asks. He's already taking a leadership role in Drama Club. "We want fun stuff that's not too hard to stage with lots of parts."

"Sure." I confidently select several classic plays and provide brief synopses.

"No, I don't think so!" Damon gives me that killer adolescent shrug, making me feel badly outdated, until I find a modern play he deigns to consider.

That night we go see a French film in Brooklyn Heights, then sit out on a narrow street fragrant with tree blossoms. The shady plane trees in the soft summer air, the muffled streetlights, and the café intimacy remind me of Paris, where I once lived. I drink beer while Damon sips an orange soda. We discuss the film and many other subjects. Damon is good company and we can talk about almost anything. I realize he's becoming a friend.

I want to invite Damon to a matinee of *Long Day's Journey into Night* but I hesitate over the subject matter. The play's mother is a dope fiend, the son a sickly youth expected to die from his illness. But I decide Damon is old enough—he already knows things I never will—and he shouldn't be deprived of great art. I want to share all I can with him.

A few years earlier, overcoming similar scruples, I took him to see a documentary about Jewish children rescued from Nazi Germany and sent to live with foster families in England. Some of these children, like my mother, who waved good-bye to their parents from the train, would never see Mummy and Daddy again. I had to balance the emotional impact of this material with Damon's need to understand his history and his grandmother's past. He was young but I took him anyway. As we sat in the Lincoln Center theater, we spotted a familiar face in the audience. It was my mother, come in from Queens for the same show!

Thus now, on a bright Sunday, I take Damon with me to see Eugene O'Neill's posthumous masterpiece. The play is long, over four hours, and it unfolds slowly. But it still astonishes with its uncompromising yet sympathetic depiction of tight-knit family members who damage one another grievously, by intent or not, within the bosom of consanguinity.

The play leaves both Damon and me feeling emotionally depleted but filled with the exhilaration of seeing a great work. It forges another strong link in our deepening bond. And by the time we exit the theater, dusk has fallen like a curtain over the city, and the long day has indeed turned into night, making us feel we must hurry home before a dark fog settles in over the spooky metropolis.

Chapter 27

In August, the whole family returns to the Isle of Skye for the first time since Damon's diagnosis two years earlier, and in the beginning, everything feels different.

The Red Cuillin and the purple moors and the blue lochs appear like a still-life encased in a glass paperweight, a beautiful but closed-off reminder of the carefree existence we've lost. Suddenly we're aware of all the things Damon *cannot* do. There's no cover or social camouflage here. Damon's small stature and strained pallor stand out against the vivid landscape.

The contrast with his playmates is even more striking. I watch Damon trail his buddies Lachlann and Jamie as they stride through the bracken or lope along the bay. He works overtime just to keep up, arms pumping, hips swiveling, and spindly legs shuffling in outsized wellies. "Let's build a fort on that hill," he says, trying creatively to slow the pace. He's similarly exposed as he runs on the soccer pitch.

"Everyone's bigger than me now," Damon says with a sigh. His friends have all shot up and developed in the two years we've been away, while he looks physically unchanged.

But Damon has changed, and not just because of his health problems. For one, he's a savvy urban teen habituated to the high school hyperactivity and cosmopolitan cacophony of New York. And Skye has little of that social adrenaline and cultural caffeine. After a few days Damon confides he misses the city. "It's okay here but there's not that much going on. I feel like I'm not doing enough."

"You'll get into stuff here, just give it time," I tell him. But privately I wonder if we did the right thing in bringing him back. We celebrate Damon's fifteenth birthday with a big barbecue, hosting a steady stream of villagers who flow from the front garden into the house and back out again. We're staying in the Pillars this time, a three-bedroom bungalow. Shealagh prefers this pebbled modern dwelling to the old croft because it's more convenient and easier to clean, but Damon and his pals feel no such constraints. They pelt the slate roof, the picture windows, and the stucco walls with a variety of glop, which they then trek through the house. I keep Shealagh plied with drink so she won't go in and see the mess.

"Och aye, that's a bull's-eye!" Lachlann gleefully spatters a windowpane.

We herd the kids into the front garden just long enough to bring out the cake and sing "Happy Birthday." The whole glen resounds with our festivities.

After Sam and Miranda have gone to bed, Shealagh and I lounge with Damon in the kitchen as he sits with his pills and a patch of Saran wrap clinging to his side. The clear wrap, with numbing cream for his heparin shot, evokes a racing bib and endows Damon with an oddly athletic aura.

Outside the cottage, all is silent. Shealagh and I belt back shots of our beloved Talisker whiskey, grown and distilled just a few miles away. Its strong, peaty warmth spreads to the solar plexus. Damon drinks ginger ale between his pills and eyes our amber-colored single-malt with multiple levels of curiosity.

"Can I taste it?" he finally asks, pushing the limits of his birthday license.

"Okay." I pour him a shot, foreseeing the outcome but loath to deny my son.

Damon swishes an infinitesimal drop in his mouth. "Omigod!" He spits it out with a bitter scowl. "You *drink* that?" He returns to his soda and gapes at us.

"Let's show Mom your photos." I scroll through images from the Agricultural Fair in Ord, where I drove Damon and Lachlann Sunday.

"These are great." Shealagh smiles at a picture of the two boys beside an Aberdeen Angus bull. She looks up. "Oh, guess who's running for governor of California? 'Ja, I'll be back—my mission is to protect you!'" Shealagh mimics wickedly.

"Wow, Mom, I didn't know you could do imitations!" Damon chortles.

"Well, there's lots about me you don't know . . ." Shealagh winks.

"I know you can't tell jokes," Damon says. "Or even get them, usually."

"D-man, that's unfair. I've heard Mom be funny once or twice," I say.

"Neither of you two clever boots can change a lightbulb. *That's* funny," Shealagh says, zinging us back.

After Damon goes to bed, Shealagh and I stay in the kitchen and discuss our ongoing concerns about our son, a topic that increasingly dominates our marriage.

"He didn't appear to get quite the same boost from his second IVIG infusion as from the first," I remark. "I'm not certain, but it didn't seem as effective."

"No, and he looks very bloated, especially when he first gets up."

Shealagh sounds very anxious, so I pull back. "But his appetite is better and he no longer gets the same fatigue. So there's some improvement."

Damon suddenly appears in the doorway and approaches me with a targeted urgency I've learned to dread. I brace myself, while Shealagh looks equally concerned, but also relieved it's not her he's singling out.

Damon unfastens the top buttons on his pajama shirt. "Dad, can you please take a look at this?" He reveals a pin-sized, reddish-brown spot on his pale chest. "Is it a tick bite?" Damon says, looking uncharacteristically rattled.

I inspect the broad, tender cavity of his twice-cracked chest and note the dot is on the suture line, below the rib cage. For many years after his last open-heart operation, a tiny wire protruded from that very spot. It was an eyesore but the wire is long gone, and what remains is a tiny pinhole. I don't believe it's serious, perhaps a minor scar irritation, but I never dismiss a complaint of Damon's, because he is his own best clinician.

So now I tap on his abdomen, searching for any other symptoms or anomalies. I note his belly is full and hard, but before I can probe further, Damon cries out because the area I'm palpating is still tender from his recent injection: "Ow, that hurts!"

"Sorry, D-man." I feel mortified by the discomfort he must bear daily and apologize before shifting to the opposite side. But I find nothing there either.

"I can't see any new problem," I say, looking to Shealagh for her view.

"No, it looks pretty much the same to me also," my wife agrees.

I turn to my son. "We'll just keep our eye on this. Okay?"

"Yeah." Damon seems satisfied, even relieved, with this homey diagnosis, as if he needed reassurance above all. Sometimes it's easy to forget how young he is.

"Give us another kiss." We send him back to bed.

We drive south and visit Philip and Catriona in their starkly beautiful coastal retreat. They always come up for August and the Skye Balls. This time, their daughter Caroline, a onetime actress, is visiting with her husband, a sculptor, and their two children. We are fond of one another and enjoy catching up.

"Damon, are you still doing your theatricals?" Caroline queries in her posh, sweet voice. She shares a birthday and a certain leonine flair with Damon.

"I just played Cerimon in *Pericles*," Damon replies.

"What fun. And did you have a colorful costume? I'll bet you did!"

Several of Shealagh's Scottish uncles show, including red-faced Rory, whose salmon fishery scheme has fizzled, so he's exploring windmills on the Isle of Skye.

"Council's offering a bloody fortune just for putting the damn things up, even if you never generate a kilowatt. We'll form a syndicate and sublease."

Damon watches him, rapt, like an actor taking character notes.

Philip offers me a Famous Grouse whiskey and a comfy chair for one of our fireside natters. He is the queen's representative in his county and thus charged with organizing her upcoming eightieth-birthday celebrations there.

"It's a public occasion so the security is quite challenging. We don't want the anti-brigades demonstrating." Philip's eyes twinkle. A very decent, dutiful man with a broad English worldview and a wry sensibility, Philip works for a multinational company in the City of London in order to maintain his land and estate in the country.

"Does the queen have a sense of humor?" Damon sidles boldly up to us, tickled that Philip talks to the queen about mundane items like guest lists.

"Yes, rather a good one." Philip nods. "But it's best to wait for her cues, Damon, before showing off one's own."

As the summer progresses, Damon starts hitting his stride, both physically—the daily habit of outdoor life toughens him up—and socially.

"Let's go to the Portree stables," Damon says. He mounts up and resumes lessons, trots and canters in the ring, and goes out on cross-country treks.

He exercises daily on the big trampoline by Lachlann's house. It's the local hangout. Damon places Miranda and Kerry in the center of the ring and bounces them up and down by jumping on the perimeter of the nylon.

He swings on a tree rope, yodeling, "Nee-yah!" He cavorts on the sandy Braes beach and splashes in the icy Varragill River.

"It's really fun but a little nippy!" Damon grins with chattering teeth.

He tries Ben Tianavaig again and despite setbacks, he reaches the summit.

"I wasn't sure I'd make it," he says, smiling, as he stands panting on the peak.

On quieter days, Shealagh sends him down to the bay to collect mussels with Sam and Miranda. Miranda can't reach the shells and Sam can't pry them loose. "Like this!" Damon shows them, yanking a hard shellfish off its slimy perch.

Sam and Miranda soon grow bored but Damon stays until the bucket is full. He carries his catch to the bungalow, leaving it out overnight so the mussels can purge. Then he helps Shealagh scrape the shells and cook a feast in garlic and wine.

My parents come for a visit. "Damon seems so much better up here. He's active all the time!" my mother notes as he climbs the ruins of an ancient castle.

I've invited my parents not just to see Skye but also to take my father to Glasgow for a tour of his childhood. He hasn't been back for sixty years. Damon surprises me when he suddenly asks if he can join us. I hate refusing him anything but I've long dreamed of making this voyage with my father, just as I took my mother back to her hometown in Germany after the Berlin Wall fell. Now my lifelong position as a son, and my effort to honor that role, seems to collide with my obligations as a father. Fortunately, Damon gets distracted by village goings-on and forgets all about us. On our return, I tell Damon that one day, I look forward to having him accompany me on a similar voyage to my roots. "You got it, Dad!"

One afternoon, Miranda and Sam are walking up from the bay when Miranda feels a sharp thistle across her ankle. She looks down and sees she's stepped on a wasp's nest! An angry swarm pours from the ground and chases the screaming children all the way into the house, where Shealagh and I do what we can. I chase the wasps from room to room, smashing them with a rolled-up newspaper, while Shealagh dunks Miranda in the bath, drowning her nemeses. It looks like we're turning back the assault but unbeknownst to us, dozens of secret invaders still lurk inside the kids' clothes and in their hair. As we relax our guard, the waiting wasps dart out with venomous rage, attacking us from every angle in a *second* wave.

Before the carnage is over, everyone in the house is nursing wasp wounds. But Sam and Miranda, riddled with painful stings, are the worst hit, and they remain in mild shock. We put them to bed, soothe their brows, and sit with them.

The only person unharmed in all this mayhem—the one wasp-allergic person who would have been most endangered—is Damon. He arrives an hour later, sauntering up from Jamie's and eating a peach in the soft, glowing light.

"Hey, guys, wassup?" He beams at us, oblivious of the tornado that's swept through. The peach juice drips down his fingers.

As summer ends, I'm struck by how well Damon is doing. Skye has worked its magic and he flourishes, as if the pristine air and sea and mountains have reinvigorated him. Briefly I consider staying in Skye and not returning.

If that's what it takes, why not?

We could treat the whole island as one big rehabilitation center, our own magic mountain. There's a decent hospital in town with emergency evacuation, the kids can go to school in Portree, I can write or teach or find other work, and Shealagh can be with the kids. We can all lie low until Damon is better. There are worse places in the world to live . . .

It's a nice fantasy but we have too many ties and obligations back home, including the most sophisticated medical care in the world.

And so, with a lump in our throats and a flutter of remorse in my own heart, we bid farewell to the blessed Isle of Skye and fly back home.

Chapter 28

"I can't believe there's no improvement!" I fume after receiving Damon's first test results in the fall. "He seemed so good in Skye, but what was the point?"

"Don't say that, he had a great summer!" Shealagh cries. "That's important."

"Of course. But his albumin is barely above two. We're back to square one."

"At least it hasn't gotten worse," Shealagh says.

"That's true." I nod. "And he's excited about starting growth hormone injections now that he doesn't have a daily heparin shot."

In November, when Damon comes to my office to help with the Rhodes applications, I'm pleased to see a whole new gang of friends from Brooklyn Tech troop in with him. They're bigger, louder, fouler, and funnier than his previous group, but they're all basically good kids. I only have to yell a few times to keep them in line. In between, they file and ask astute questions. I buy them mountains of pizza when they flag, hand out warm cash from the ATM at the end, and take them all to the movies.

"Thanks, Dad, that was cool!" Damon says on our way home. The group invigorates Damon more than any medication the doctors prescribe.

The Brooklyn Tech fall production of *Picasso at the Lapin Agile*—the play Damon and I chose at the bookstore—is a hoot. Damon dons huge red glasses, a flowery shirt, a ridiculous bow tie, and a shiny yellow jacket, sparking laughter even before he speaks. The show is a hit and Damon spends every available minute basking in the post-play glow and sharing the embraces, confidences, and intimacies of his fellow cast and crew members. But as soon as the props and costumes are put away and the group disbands, Damon starts to look poorly again. He appears exhausted and run-down and takes to his bed, missing several days of school. "I'm just a little tired," he says.

We begin to see this pattern recur. Damon limps along, barely managing to get by, but rallies for any activity involving his friends or the theater.

On New Year's Eve, while Shealagh and I go out to celebrate, Damon throws his own bash at our place. He's become quite the party giver, aided by our tolerance and large rambling house. Shealagh cooks a big pot of chili and Damon loads up on junk food and soda, while Sam and Miranda are relegated to the top floor. "You can't come downstairs!" Damon warns his siblings. He greets guests in top hat and tux, clutching an (empty) magnum of champagne. And while he doesn't quite get the crowd he wanted—teens are notoriously unreliable and certain parents strict about New Year's— enough people show to make his party a success. Damon relishes being master of the revelry.

Once again, however, as soon as the party ends, Damon's condition worsens. He gets a bad headache and misses several days of school. The bitter winter doesn't help, but it's more than that. Weakness and fatigue now seem endemic, and Damon needs a spur to become activated. Otherwise he retreats into protective inertia, a kind of semi-hibernation.

I take him to an afternoon hockey game at Madison Square Garden. The New York Rangers face off against the Tampa Bay Lightning. It's an exciting, hard-fought contest that goes into overtime. "Wasn't that an amazing shot!" I exclaim on the car ride back, turning to him in the seat beside me. But Damon is fast asleep. It's only seven P.M.

This is not only unnerving, it's completely out of character, so I know he's ailing.

One night, I'm cooking up steaks for the two of us when Damon walks in.

"It's awfully bright in here!" He blinks and covers his eyes, grimacing.

"Really? I must need the extra light for my middle-aged eyes," I joke.

"No, my headache's back. The bad migraine that made me miss school."

"Why don't you get an ibuprofen?" I send him upstairs but note his fragility. Damon returns and we sit in front of the TV, eating and chatting.

"Feeling better?" I ask.

"A little," Damon says, but it's obvious he is not himself. There's a new, scared look that flits across his face. It doesn't linger but it's still unsettling. "I get more headaches now," he states. His eyes, previously so steady, dart my way.

"Maybe it's that new globulin you're getting? You'll adjust, you always do." I try to stay upbeat, but I don't have answers. "You excited about your first trip to Sundance?"

"Yeah, it'll be cool." Damon plays along but I can feel his uncertainty and sense of siege. I blanch inside at my powerlessness to do more for him.

Our house fills with dread and unspoken tension. Tempers are shorter, bickering erupts more frequently. Doors slam and voices rise to new shrillness.

Shealagh and I have sharper exchanges with one another, we argue more with the kids, and the kids fight more among themselves.

I see exactly what's happening but don't know how to stop it. My self-discipline starts to falter. I can't write, and I don't know where to turn.

Shealagh has stopped working and is on hand to chauffeur Damon and help him in any way she can. But Damon's worsening condition causes his devoted mother acute distress. Her asthma acts up, her back gives her trouble, and she has difficulty sleeping. One day while driving alone, she is rear-ended by a tractor trailer, which flees the scene without a trace. Shealagh is physically unhurt, but our van is totaled, and her nerves are further frayed.

Sam is applying to middle school, a competitive, high-pressure process under normal circumstances. He drafts a short application essay I correct. But when Sam rewrites the essay, the revised version has new errors, which I correct again. He does a third draft but makes more mistakes. They crop up like defiant weeds that I keep yanking out.

"Go and do it over, Sam! We need a clean copy for your application."

Sam sulks but I won't let him quit until he gets it right, and he can't, or won't, turn in a clean copy. I am all the more intransigent because I won't accept that something so under human agency and control, something so easy to fix, can be botched. Sam, seething, takes out his frustration on Miranda. Shealagh tells me to let it go but all I want is for Sam to copy one error-free page. Sam throws a fit and hits Miranda. Miranda cries and hits Sam back. Damon wakes up from the screaming, puffy and upset, and wants to know what's going on.

Around this period, an old, eccentric friend picks a fight with me and in-explicably breaks off a three-decade relationship. Eventually, I learn that my ongoing crisis with Damon proved too much for him. He's dropped out of everything else—school, marriage, career—but I'd always assumed his witty amorality could not possibly apply to our friendship.

It's a betrayal that blindsides me because it comes from a seemingly safe quarter. Even worse, it's secretly aimed at my son, whose bodily decline makes my squeamish friend squirm.

But this person's readiness to ditch me despite all our history does per-versely signal me that my prospects must really look bad from the outside. I could always rely on him for a hyperacute reading of the prevailing winds.

So I gird myself and clutch my firstborn ever more fervently in my arms. I will draw deeper from my own well, rely even less on others, and spare no exertion as I scour the earth in search of a cure for Damon.

Part III

Chapter 29

Hey cine-lovers and gawkers, it's Damon reporting from the Sundance Film Festival in Park City, Yoot-ah. Just saw this kick-ass movie about 2 rock n roll bands. The director and every1 was there 4 the premiere . . . But seriously, what's with the black? It's like the only color any1 wears! Guess it stands out in the snow—but wouldn't any color? lol.

—*From Damon's blog, January 2004*

"So where are we?" Shealagh enters my study and looks over my shoulder as I work at my desk. We both feel increasingly distraught about our son's condition, but while I turn to the medical literature and the medical profession, my wife turns to me.

"I talked to Dr. Chin at CHOP and I also checked in with the Mayo Clinic and Boston Children's," I tell Shealagh, adding that I spoke again to Dr. Hayes and contacted several other hospitals, government health agencies, pharmaceutical companies, and independent experts and even followed up on several alternative-medicine leads. "If there's a solution, we'll know about it."

Among the stacks of folders on Damon's case, I've opened a thin new file I carry with me at all times, labeled "Hope." Tucked inside are the latest reports on the use of stem cells, medical assist devices, and artificial hearts.

One day in December, I spot an online reference to an article in the journal *Pediatrics* about an Australian doctor who reports he has successfully treated a young girl with PLE by patching together or "resecting" a local lesion in her gut.

If PLE is a leakage of protein from the gut, why not isolate the *exit point* of the leak, like a hole in a tire, and plug it?

Apparently, this is what a resourceful physician at Sydney Children's Hospital has done by using a special diagnostic. The test revealed a "localized, surgically correctible lesion" that doctors then repaired. This fourteen-year-old patient, who, like fifteen-year-old Damon, also had a failed Fontan resistant to all interventions, is reported to be "doing well" after more than two years!

This news makes my pulse race. It's the first *possible* break in a long time. I quickly order a reprint of the original article, pore over every word, and share it with my big-picture medical allies like Dr. Chin, my cousin Dr. Bar-Or, and my friend Dr. Jeffrey Friedman. All agree it looks intriguing and is worthy of follow-up, though Dr. Chin is less enthusiastic, and everyone urges caution as it's only one case and we don't know all the facts.

Undeterred, I start with a radiologist at NYU Medical Center who tells me, "This technique is very rare because it involves the use of radioactive materials. I've never used it myself but I know someone who might know." She gives me the name of another expert at Memorial Sloan-Kettering. He warns me this diagnostic technique has been discontinued in the United States. "You may need to go to Canada if you want to receive this treatment."

"Going to Canada is a nonissue—I would go to the moon!" I explain.

Finally, I track down the author of this paper in his native Australia, where he holds a faculty position. It seems fitting the elusive answer may lie at the other end of the world.

Alas, this researcher has no good news for me and sounds chastened.

"The patient has suffered a relapse. PLE has returned and she is in a critical state. The doctors are keeping her alive with regular infusions of albumin."

The patient apparently had struggled from the beginning, her course never as smooth as the paper implied. I'm crushed and I want to rebuke this man, but he's just a well-intentioned researcher whose idea did not pan out.

In late January, I meet Damon at the airport in Salt Lake City and take him back to Park City for the last two days of the Sundance Film Festival. We find my best friend, David, who's flown in from Seattle, on snow-laden, banner-festooned Main Street. A hale, rugged guy with a big appetite for life,

David's Rough Rider greatcoat flaps open as he leans down, tiny gold ear stud agleam, and wraps Damon in a bear hug.

The closing-night awards ceremony, a televised event, is held in the Racquet Club. We run the gauntlet of security and rope lines, are each issued a bracelet with pull-tags for free drinks, and circulate in the vast reception area. The bar and buffet are hopping.

The Sundance senior team—it's a tiny, hardworking core, with a thousand volunteers obscuring the shoestring operation—alerts me to some mysterious "good news." Ken Brecher, who runs the Sundance Institute for Robert Redford, wanders over and says, "We have a surprise for you and I think you'll be very pleased!"

"Great," I reply, mystified. I introduce Ken to Damon.

"You must be your dad's secret focus group, right?" Ken smiles. "What's your fee? I'd pay a lot to get you on my team!"

"Yeah, I taught my dad everything he knows!" Damon quips.

"Watch for your surprise!" Ken says over his shoulder as he dashes off.

We go in and take our seats. A forest of cranes, tripods, and cameras bristles at the rear while the stage is dark. A senior programmer warms up the crowd.

"Okay, guys, it's time for the Sun Dance. Come on, everybody, on your feet!"

The entire audience stands and begins to sway in freeform boogie to a joyful beat, including Damon, who leaps to his feet, shimmying and bopping as if the ceremonial spirit is calling to him directly.

The stage clears, music and lights come up, and the actress Zooey Deschanel wends her way up to the podium as the televised show begins.

I provide the play-by-play for Damon while David supplies the color commentary.

"*That* guy got the prize? He couldn't get arrested!" David wisecracks. "Stevie Wonder could see through that film . . ."

Our Science in Film Award is early, as we're still outsiders and few films qualify for our category. *Primer*, an obscure, low-budget film by an unknown first-time director named Shane Carruth, wins.

"Cool!" Damon applauds. I just introduced him to Carruth at the buffet.

The ceremony proceeds with some arresting film clips, endless speeches, and a few flashes of true art. When the final award, the Sundance Grand Jury Prize, is announced, the winner is . . . *Primer*! The Best Dramatic Film Award

is a shocker, because this cerebral thriller was shot for $7,000 with an un-
known cast yet still manages to beat out several popular, multi-million-dollar
films with major stars. As we all pose together onstage, I'm happy for Carruth
and appreciate that it's a big shot in the arm for our program.

We go to the after-party, flushed with victory, and accept congratulations
from all quarters.

The party is in full swing and I'm on a professional high when I notice
Damon has disappeared. I search the mobbed rooms to no avail, then find
him out on the terrace, standing alone under the open Utah sky with its chill
beadwork of stars.

I walk up to my son. The ski slopes are lit up for night skiing and float
above us like gleaming white staircases descending from an invisible heaven.

"You okay, D-man?" I place my hand on his shoulder.

"I just needed a little air." Damon sounds subdued. I don't like his color.

"Hey, it's late, we can go," I say. "You've had a long day with the time
change and the altitude and all the excitement . . . Let's save something for
tomorrow, okay, champ?"

"No, I want to go back in. I just need a minute." He stands with feet
apart, hands on hips.

"You sure, D-man?"

"Yeah, Dad. This is cool."

"If that's what you want . . ." I wait until he's ready, and then we both
return inside.

The party is still going strong but suddenly it seems very crowded and
noisy and has lost its appeal. My job here is done, and I'm not enjoying it
anymore.

I watch Damon circulate solo—he's a teenager and needs his own
space—but I can tell he's struggling. He wants so badly to be at this event but
he's having a very hard time.

I see his chest heave and his eyes blink. He can't find an equilibrium
point. Finally, he marches up to me. "Can we please go?"

We walk outside. I can't tell if it's an asthma attack or something else
but the cold, bracing air seems to help and his breathing normalizes. But
Damon is very upset with himself for walking out on this party. It's one of the
reasons he came to Sundance.

I worry that his illness is not just curtailing Damon's activity but is also
starting to change *him*.

Chapter 30

Yeah well they (doctors and my parents and my consent) decided to start having me do the infusions myself at home. (The infusions is the procedure that I have about every 3 weeks where they hook me up 2 an IV and pump shit through my veins 4 a couple of hours.) Anywayz they want me to do it at home now so I can have them more often *yey* and don't have 2 go into the hospital which actually is sort of better.

—From Damon's blog, April 2004

"Damon is not getting better," Shealagh remarks shortly after the Easter break.

"I know," I say tightly. We've just returned from vacation and seen the fall-off.

"He sleeps all the time, he barely eats, and he has no energy. He's fallen behind in his classes because he's missed so much school. And he looks terrible!" Shealagh cries.

We're in the kitchen and Freddie, startled by the sudden shift in tone, trots over to see what's wrong. "And that belly—I know it's his liver, but it makes him look *pregnant*," Shealagh says with a shudder. "He's struggling every day. I'm really worried about him!"

I tell Shealagh it may be time to roll the dice on fenestration since neither Dudu's anti-inflammatory drug nor Jeff's assist device have panned out. "It could buy us as much as five to ten years, according to Dr. Chin. And fenestration doesn't rule out any other options, so it seems like the safest way to go. If it makes Damon too blue, we can always reverse it and close up the hole—"

I stop as Damon walks into the kitchen and Freddie leaps into his arms. Damon's face is puffy and his eyes buggy—he just woke up—but he beams at his pooch, who wriggles and licks him all over.

"He missed you!" I smile, noting my son's chalky complexion. Even Damon's hair, overgrown, bowl-cut, lacks its usual luster. "How'd you sleep, D-man?"

"Okay," Damon says. "I'm a little cold." He rubs his arms although it's a spring day and he's wearing his bulky gray hooded sweatshirt, which makes him look even frailer.

"You'll warm up, sweetie," Shealagh says. "Can I fix you something to eat?"

"Not yet." Damon shakes his head. At every meal now, we have to convince him to eat. It's a chore or a battle, depending on his mood, but never a pleasure anymore.

"I can make you scrambled eggs on toast," Shealagh offers.

"I said not now, Mom!" Damon snaps. Then he softens. "I just woke up, I need some time." He glances around. It's one P.M. on a Saturday. "Where's Sam and Miranda?"

"Sam's at gymnastics and Miranda's on a play date," I say. "You have any plans?"

"I may go in for a tech rehearsal for *Tommy*," he says. Although we agreed Damon should save his dwindling energy for school, he got roped into helping out with the spring musical, including a tiny nonspeaking part, and we don't have the heart to stop him.

"Want me to drive you?" Shealagh says. Sometimes she gets him to eat on the way.

"Yeah, thanks, Mom." As I walk them to the car, Damon shivers in the sun and slips the hood of his sweatshirt over his head. He looks like a wraith as he climbs into the passenger side and disappears behind the high dash.

We wait for Dr. Thomas Spray, an internationally renowned surgeon, in a vacant cardiology office at Children's Hospital of Philadelphia. It's after six P.M. and the regular staff has gone home, making the place feel strangely quiet. Dr. Chin, who's brokered this visit, wants us to meet Dr. Spray not only because he's a preeminent cardiothoracic surgeon equal to anyone at Columbia but also because he's a proponent of fenestration.

"You need someone who has experience performing this procedure *and* the conviction that it works because he's seen the results firsthand," Dr. Chin explains.

Dr. Spray, cutting and stitching since seven A.M., emerges from the operating room after twelve hours of surgery. A tall, distinguished figure, he knows the details of our case and impresses us with his measured manner.

"Fenestration is not a cure-all and I can't guarantee the results, but I think it's worth trying for Damon before you go to a heart transplant." Dr. Spray gives us an earnest, sympathetic, and straightforward look. "We've had some good outcomes with it."

"You also do heart transplants, is that right?" Shealagh asks.

"Yes, and I could perform that operation for Damon, after a suitable interval, if the fenestration did not work." Dr. Spray nods. "However, I don't believe we're at that point."

"I have a patient still doing well six years after fenestration!" Dr. Chin volunteers.

"But you want to do this as an open-heart procedure?" I stare at Dr. Spray.

"Yes." The surgeon nods. "Doing it open-heart in the OR gives me better access to precisely configure the right-to-left shunt between the two chambers of the heart. The open approach also lets me put in pacing wires or other modifications as needed."

"Does that mean you'd have to open my chest *a second time* if the fenestration failed and we had to go to a heart transplant?" Damon narrows his eyes.

Everyone pauses because the patient, a young boy in this case, has spoken.

"I have the same concern," I add. "Damon's body has already been through so much . . . Mayo and Boston do it in the cath lab, without cracking the chest."

"That's why they don't get our results! It's less precise," Dr. Chin says.

"But those results haven't been published yet," I say.

"Well, I could do the fenestration in the cath lab, without opening Damon's chest, but I think the odds are better with the open-heart approach," Dr. Spray says evenly.

We leave feeling this is very complex but Dr. Spray is a world-class surgeon in whose capable hands we could entrust our son, knowing he'd perform at the highest level of the achievable. But we remain uncomfortable with the risks of open-heart surgery.

"What do you recommend?" we ask Dr. Hayes at Damon's next exam. Our son waits out in the hall, where he's updating stage directions for *Tommy*.

"I think we just have to continue with the diet and the meds," she says.

"But you agree that Damon is not getting better?" I look directly at her.

"There are increasing signs of stress on his system." Dr. Hayes's voice is strained but professional. "His condition is consistent with what we see in kids with PLE."

Shealagh and I share a look. "Then we're going to try fenestration!" I state.

"We've only seen sporadic benefits. And there's some risk," Dr. Hayes says dourly.

"I know Columbia is not an advocate of fenestration but even the multicenter study *you* gave me cited it as effective," I reply. "CHOP gets good results and has agreed to do it for Damon." I pause. "The only thing I don't like is they do it as an open-heart procedure."

"We don't do it that way here. It's done in the cath lab," Dr. Hayes says.

"So you *would* support fenestration for Damon?" I give her a sharp look.

"Well, if you've decided to go ahead, why don't you speak to Bill Hellenbrand? He's the director who oversees fenestrations here." She hands me a phone number.

I go meet Dr. Hellenbrand on my own, ready to reject him at the first provocation due to Columbia's apparent lack of faith in fenestration and its rare use there. But Hellenbrand, a stocky, fit New Englander with a direct manner, disarms me with his hands-on approach.

"Come, let's take a look at Damon's pictures." He waves me over to the computer as soon as I enter, as if he's read the playbook on me and knows to dispense with the usual blather, zeroing in on Damon's anatomy and how he would perform the fenestration. "See, I would thread the needle *here* and then try and create an opening *there*." A splash of pixilated color spreads across Damon's two upper chambers.

"So you do the procedure yourself?" I ask, surprised.

"I'm the cath lab head, I always do the fenestrations," Dr. Hellenbrand says.

"And you do it in the cath lab, and not open-heart?" I press.

"Yes. We can create the fenestration without opening him up. No need to."

"That's a relief," I say. I ask more questions and he answers each one, a clear-eyed pragmatist who's up to date on the latest research but also acknowledges gray areas.

I came ready for an argument and instead I find almost perfect agreement.

"Tell me, do you really *believe* fenestration can be effective?" I probe for weakness.

"I *know* it can be effective because I have several patients who've done well with it," Dr. Hellenbrand replies. "It's not a big number but it seems to buy a couple of years when it works. Results vary but it's one of the few things that works *at all* against PLE."

I shake my head. "I can't understand why I never heard about you or any of these patients before. Dr. Hayes always seemed so skeptical and pessimistic about trying this."

"Oh, that's Connie, she's always grim!" He chuckles. "It's her style."

"I guess so." I nod, pleased to have found someone at Columbia whose thinking aligns with mine and who believes we have a realistic shot at making this work. I bring Shealagh and Damon to meet Dr. Hellenbrand and they are equally impressed with the straight-shooting medical director. They're also relieved with his less invasive approach.

"He seems very sensible," Shealagh says.

Damon nods. "I like him."

Everyone is on board, but it's still a risky procedure. We decide to wait for Damon to finish with the spring musical.

Damon plays the youngest of three versions of a traumatized Tommy Walker in the school production of *Tommy: The Rock Opera*. Damon has no lines—he's been struck dumb—but his pale face is wonderfully expressive as he's buffeted between incompetent adults. But what I most notice, in mortifying profile, is the engorged liver that now pads his waist and swells against his T-shirt like a taboo, gender-bending pregnancy or a sorrowful gut on a young boy.

As I watch Damon take a final bow with his far taller and more robust fellow actors, I realize we can't wait any longer. My son bends at the waist with panache, draping his belly with one deft arm, while his red locks tumble forward. Temporarily buoyed by the energy on that stage, he's the picture of actorly decorum, yet he's barely holding it together. I know from his friends he's been falling asleep during rehearsals, and even now, I can see him husbanding his meager resources to stand there and look normal.

I've already had to contact the home instruction board because he can no longer keep up with his schoolwork. He's faltering, through no fault of his own. We schedule the fenestration for the first available date after his show.

Chapter 31

"Okay, buddy, now we're going to place this mask over your head—here, feel
the padded inside groove—to make it easier for you to go to sleep."

Dr. Hellenbrand turns out to be a skilled medical technician and a first-
rate physician.

He explains what he's going to do, then does it.

In Damon's case, this involves fenestration of the lateral tunnel Fontan
baffle: opening the conduit previously made to carry Damon's returning
blood to the *right* side of the heart and to the lungs, so that it now flows directly to the *left* side of his heart.

"This rerouted blood will not get rid of its carbon dioxide or pick up oxygen at the lungs, as normal blood does, but it will, hopefully, relieve pressure
on the right side of Damon's heart—pressure believed to be contributing to,
if not directly causing, his PLE," Dr. Hellenbrand tells us. "The trade-off,
if it works, is that Damon will have less oxygen but more energy—and no
PLE!"

Dr. Hellenbrand creates this fenestration—from the Latin word for
window—using a sheath catheter that threads a fine needle through Damon's

veins to his heart, where it can be imaged on a screen and manipulated to cut precisely. Once he's fashioned the opening, Dr. Hellenbrand inserts a tiny wire stent to keep the fenestration from closing. Then he checks the hemodynamics, verifies all is okay, and brings Damon to the recovery room.

The whole process takes under three hours, and Damon tolerates it well.

"I talked to Damon the whole time and explained everything I was doing, in case he could hear me," Dr. Hellenbrand says, mindful of Damon's previous experience in the cath lab. "He was fine and there were no complications."

Given the buildup and our own fears, we feel gratified by the relative smoothness of it all. Damon is still weak and groggy from the anesthesia when we see him but he also looks relieved that it's over.

"Hey, D-man, you did great. How you feeling, big guy?" I squeeze his hand.

"Okay, I guess. I'm a little tired and sore . . ." He has pale eyelids and dry lips.

"You thirsty, sweetie?" Shealagh says. "Let me get you some ice."

As Shealagh feeds him ice chips, I stroke Damon's hair. He's exhausted but otherwise he seems like himself. I even fancy I detect an improvement.

"Does he look less puffy in the face to you?" I whisper to Shealagh.

"Don't say things like that, you'll jinx it!" Shealagh reprimands me. "It's probably his preoperative fasting, or being so worn out . . . It's too soon for any real change."

Damon stays overnight in the hospital and by the next afternoon, he's back home.

What happens over the next week unfolds like a dream.

Day by day, the fluid and all the associated puffiness that has accumulated about Damon's body begins to dissipate. It goes down slowly, so initially we wonder if we're imagining it. Shealagh plays the preemptive skeptic and I too am wary of mirages and will-o'-the-wisps. We've been down this road so many times before . . .

But by day three, it's undeniable, and by day five, we're quietly cheering from the sidelines, afraid to spook the still-unfolding miracle.

Damon can't help but notice it too. There's a lighter load on his body and less resistance when he moves. He has a cautious new spring in his step and a watchful half smile on his lips. "Hey, can you guys see a difference? I feel more like . . . like myself."

After a week, his face is almost back to normal, like an obese actor shedding his fat suit. Damon's clean jawline emerges from a soft, jowly chin, his fine nose clarifies from puffy cheeks, and his blue eyes shine from buggy lids. He's a lean, handsome boy again!

And it's not just Damon's face that returns to its familiar, attractive lineaments. Damon's huge gut also starts to shrink and recede. It diminishes daily. Ten days out, his swollen belly just drops away.

The fluid accumulation around his arms and legs also evaporates, so that we see just what a skinny figure, or a "stick man," as Shealagh dubs him, Damon really is underneath all his puffiness. His essence is revealed in the form of a scrawny but determined body that has shucked off its foreign coils and returned to its boyish core.

It's an astonishing transformation—an exorcism even. I understand the hemodynamics and the medical process that's brought us here, but the whole thing seems more like a sci-fi B movie.

We cannot believe how relatively unscathed our son looks!

Our house fills with rejoicing.

We know this kind of progress can be short-lived and that we must maintain and build on it. But it's still incredible to behold. And it means the dread PLE nemesis can be rolled back, that it has a point of vulnerability, and that we have a point of attack.

The first blood tests confirm what we see. Damon's albumin climbs back over 3.0 for the first time since the initial heparin spike. But unlike the heparin, which had to be injected daily, fenestration involves a one-time fix that should hold for *years*.

Suddenly, we're almost a normal family again. We celebrate and go to Radio City Music Hall for the premiere of the new Harry Potter film.

We begin with a pre-film Hogwarts meal replete with Snape stew and Dementor cocktails, served at tables wreathed with a witch's mist of dry ice. Then we make our way across the mobbed, cordoned, red-carpeted street to the glittering Showplace of the Nation.

I run into several familiar faces as we head to our seats, which are lined with gift bags. Damon pulls out a Muggles T-shirt and tries it on over his new slenderized belly.

"Hey, Sam, do I look like Dudley Dursley in this?" Damon mugs loutishly.

"No, you look like Harry about to make Marge float away!" Sam giggles.

Miranda holds up a purple Lego kit.

"That's the triple-decker Knight Bus," Damon explains to his clueless sister.

Various celebrities march in with their families and fan out. We also see our Brooklyn neighbors.

There's a great buzz around this big premiere, but my mind is elsewhere. What thrills me is seeing my whole family sitting together in the row beside me: Shealagh and all three of my gorgeous children arrayed one next to the other, smiling and chatting and munching popcorn as if it's the most ordinary thing in the world.

They look like a poster family, and I'm aware of this irony as I introduce them to colleagues and as we just hang out in our seats and wait for the film to start. No one could suspect what struggle lies behind such a wholesome picture or how recently Damon came out of the hospital. Yet somehow we're all here today, still part of this communal event. I'm struck by how convention can take on new meaning to those who risk losing the world.

Chapter 32

The surgery might have actually worked, which would be fricken awesome!!! Maybe I've finally beaten this thing, maybe three years struggle will not have been in vain. Maybe this is finally over . . . Well of course not *over*, this is me we're talking about lol but maybe I can just be medically abnormal again without being diseased. Yeah that would be cool. Of course it's too early 2 tell for sure but things are looking up.

—From Damon's blog, May 2004

Memorial Day weekend we drive out to my friend Jeff's place, off the south fork of Long Island. Damon stays behind in the city but agrees to join us in a day or two.

Like any teenager, Damon prefers hanging out with his own friends, but this is especially true now that he gets home instruction and no longer attends classes. He still goes into Tech for after-school drama, but otherwise he's on official leave and deprived of his regular contact with the Group. And without the daily structure and myriad nourishing interactions of school life, Damon feels isolated. "I never see anyone," he complains.

Blogging and instant messaging, already popular with Damon, become vital modes of staying in touch with friends. A lifeline, and also a forum for expressing a private identity in a public space. And right now Damon is buoyant because the fluid is sluicing off him, and he just got back his first test results:

In other news: My albumin broke 3, for those of you who that means nothing to, which is probably all of you, just accept that it's a good thing and be happy for me.

In addition to his medical results, Damon has another cause for celebration:

I was elected vice president of drama club which means I get 2 direct the fall play next year!!!! How fucking kick ass is that?! I hope you all come see it but that may be asking 2 much. Anyway that should be cool, a lot of responsibility and extra work though but at least it is something I really enjoy.

After a concert and a party, Damon takes the train to East Hampton and joins us on Saturday. Shealagh drives the twenty minutes from North Haven to pick him up at the station. She looks for any opportunity to spend time with her son. It's hard for her to accept Damon's male adolescent need to push her away, even if she understands it's age appropriate.

"I know it's a phase but he's rude and treats me like his skivvy!" Shealagh says.

Jeff and I are sitting by the pool Sunday morning when Damon pads out in scraggly red bathing shorts, book in hand. He still carries his stomach like a big barrel, which it no longer is, and black marks still circle his belly, this time from growth hormone injections. But otherwise he looks more spry and ginger, a person quietly but determinedly on the comeback trail. He dips one toe in the pool, checking the water temperature, when Sam and Miranda howl for him.

"Damon, Damon, come into the pool!"

Damon holds up one hand to quell their screeching. He's become very noise sensitive. "I'll come in and play with you later, if you leave me alone now."

"No, no, come in now, Damon!" they clamor. "Play with us now!"

"If you don't stop, I won't come in at all!" Damon frightens them into silence. He settles into a canvas chair near Jeff and me and I see he's got *Romeo and Juliet*, this summer's workshop play.

"What part you trying out for?" I ask.

"I don't even know if I'm accepted into the program," Damon grouses.

"Come on. They adore you. And you've made the cut the past two years."

"Yeah, which means my audition must've really sucked!" Damon can't extract the suntan lotion so I grab the tube and squirt some into his palm. "Alums always get in, but I haven't even heard back!" Damon daubs his brow and cheeks, leaving defiant white smears on his face.

"They're just disorganized." I gesture for him to rub the lotion into his skin. "I'm sure your acceptance letter will be waiting for you when we get back."

"If you say so, Dad!" Damon swipes at his face, making an even bigger mess.

"I do say so!" I lean over and spread the cream across his face, trying to massage it in. He briefly tolerates my intrusion before pulling back.

After Damon leaves, Jeff turns to me, grinning. "He looks pretty good. You must feel relieved."

"Yeah, it's kind of unreal." I smile. "Question is, will it last? Often, you get a quick, short-term effect and then, poof, it all goes, and you're back to square one."

"But the fact that it could resolve like this at all is a positive indicator," Jeff says like the scientist-doctor he is. "Makes me think it's more like a plumbing problem that can be fixed."

"Yes, it worked," I agree. "And so far, so good. Though between us, I already worry his belly looks marginally fuller than last week, but I'm probably hallucinating."

Jeff pauses. "You're bound to get some fluctuation before it settles out."

"Yeah." I nod. "And this means I can probably take him out to Hollywood this summer to be on *Deadwood*, which he really wants to do. He's very serious about acting and my friend Milch, the show's creator, has offered him a small part."

Chapter 33

Do you want 2 see my play?

If so please talk 2 me today.

Five dollars is what they say

Everyone will have 2 pay.

(Although I get a few tix free

those must go 2 family.)

But if you think you'd rather hurl

Just know in 1 scene I'm a gurl.

　　　　　　　　　　　　　　—*From Damon's blog, June 2004*

The good news is that not only has Damon been accepted into the Looking for Shakespeare summer theater program for the third year running, but he lands the choice role of Mercutio, "kinsman and friend to Romeo." It's his biggest part yet, and he's ecstatic about it. He throws himself into rehearsals and prepares excitedly for the big day.

The bad news is that by mid-June, even before rehearsals start, the positive effects of Damon's fenestration begin to unravel. It doesn't happen overnight, but the signs are unmistakable. Damon's face and belly puff up, and his albumin drops back below 3.0.

We take Damon to see Dr. Hellenbrand, who confirms the palliative effects of the fenestration seem to be wearing off. "I'm sorry. We don't know why." He shakes his head. We assume the opening has closed over, which often accounts for a reversal. But tests show the stent is holding and blood is still flowing through the opening. Instead, Damon's system seems to be reverting to its familiar protein-losing state by deliberately offsetting the positively shifting dynamics through a perverse homeostasis.

The bottom line is that the PLE is back, albeit in milder, stealthier guise, and Damon experiences a resurgent fatigue, made all the worse by his brief improvement.

Nevertheless, despite the apparent reversal, Damon still looks better than before his fenestration. He remains well ahead of where he started and seems to be having an excellent summer. So while we're disappointed the PLE has not been eliminated, we feel heartened by Damon's improved appearance and increased energy. Maybe we've reduced the threat to a manageable level? Even a steady, noncatastrophic state feels like progress.

One afternoon, I introduce Damon to a special visitor, my high school Shakespeare teacher, Irwin Wolfson, who's flown up from Florida.

A brilliant, outrageous, and big-hearted man—his outsized, Falstaffian qualities now span a girth of 265 pounds—Irwin was one of the finest teachers and best teacher friends I had. Now I want him to meet my oldest son, who's the same age I was when Irwin introduced me to *Hamlet, Macbeth, Othello,* and *King Lear.*

Damon and Irwin sit across from one another on the green couch in the family room: my small, pale, and preternaturally wise son with his leonine head and my former teacher, still smooth skinned and sleek haired, if grayer, at seventy, with a vital, pleasant-looking face marked by dark, deep-socketed eyes.

"Your dad tells me you're a Shakespearean actor?" Irwin says in a rich, resonant, and loaded voice. The extra weight makes it awkward for him to sit, but once he's shifted his huge, egg-shaped belly over his thighs, he perches on our couch like a visiting king.

"We do one play each summer," Damon says, nodding. "*Romeo and Juliet* this year."

"One of his greatest hits, a crowd-pleaser!" Irwin nods. "You agree, Damon?"

"I can see why it's popular," Damon says as Irwin leans forward, a glint in his eye.

"Personally, I always thought *Romeo and Juliet* was much ado about nothing."

Damon grins and cocks an eyebrow, waiting to see where this is going.

"It's an early, pretty, but comparatively immature work, at least when set beside the later, greater plays," Irwin trills. "Even the great Samuel Johnson—the guy penned thirty thousand couplets; he could produce more meaningless shit than any human—found the play's strains 'polluted.' I'm guessing he meant it lacked *tragic necessity*; would you agree, Damon?"

"What about the language, Irwin, the poetry?" I protest while trying not to laugh.

"Oh, well, that's music!" Irwin nods. "Look, the man could turn a phrase. There are twenty-seven thousand words in Shakespeare. The King James Bible uses seven thousand. And I will grant you the play has its glories and riches. For anyone else, I might deign to call it a masterpiece."

Damon and I exchange smiles but Irwin just shrugs.

"It's all relative—didn't Einstein say that? Or was that my uncle Mort? Damon, you should feast on *Romeo and Juliet* as only a sixteen-year-old can. Because it's all hormonal."

"Isn't the Capulet-Montague feud relevant for people your age?" Damon asks.

"Oh, methinks an arrow doth pierce my wounded breast!" Irwin grabs his chest and guffaws. "Now you remind me of your dad, Damon, when he was my student—except your father had blond hair and it was shoulder-length. He was very popular with the ladies, as I'm sure you are . . .

"But to answer your question, young man!" Irwin switches into a high rhetorical gear. "You're asking if these two youngsters, Romeo and Juliet, beautiful and pure as the snow, are corrupted and besmirched by a tainted world with its long enmity? And if it must ever thus be so?"

Damon half-nods as Irwin pauses.

"Alas, dear sweet boy, what can I say that will neither offend truth nor violate your father's desire to protect you? The world is a dung heap and a cesspool, a contamination and an abomination, and man is aught but a little bug, a gnat, a pissant! Every once in a while someone removes the rusty pliers from our nipple and the pain stops, briefly, before the charnel house operations resume . . .

"But why take *my* word? As *King Lear* shows—perhaps the summit, as well as the summation, of human expressive achievement—even if we are fortunate to be nobly born and attain a ripe age, we must lose it all, including those we most love, and be reduced to mad, blind impotence amidst a raging, pitiless storm. Bound upon 'a wheel of fire' and stretched out on the 'tough wrack of this world.' Could Willie have made it any *plainer*?"

"Irwin was never big on free will," I tell Damon. "We argued about it in class."

"Arguing? 'Twas no argument!" Irwin booms, and turns to Damon. "Your dad just hadn't lived or lost and suffered enough to understand that what you *want* the world to be and what the world *is* are two separate things." Irwin gives me a sharp, fond look before returning to Damon. "Your father was just a callow, gifted, moderately conceited kid who thought because he could get A's and get laid, and all the happy horseshit that went with it, the world was his . . . What can I tell you, Damon, except what I tell all my students? We're just not in charge. We want to be but we're not. It is the stars—the stars above govern our condition."

"So you don't believe *anything* we do makes a difference?" Damon pipes up.

"Possibly it can make a difference, at the margins—which is where most of life transpires, so it's not unimportant—but *nothing* can change the final outcome of a single fate," Irwin says. "Eventually we all die, it's just a question of *when*. And the when is part of a larger, cosmic pattern, not vouchsafed us to see in any way, shape, or form. We must simply learn to *accept* it—and I don't care what dumb religion you believe in or how many Higgs bosons you can tie on the end of your string theory."

Irwin starts declaiming:

> Not a whit, we defy augury. There's a special
> providence in the fall of a sparrow. If it be now,
> 'tis not to come; if it be not to come, it will be
> now; if it be not now, yet it will come: the
> readiness is all.

"I like that. That's pretty cool." Damon bops his head. "Where's it from?"

"Well, I didn't write it!" Irwin declares. "I wish I had but I just don't have that kind of talent. Frankly, Damon, in all my years teaching, I never met anyone who did—"

"It's from *Hamlet*," I tell Damon, recalling that I first read the play thirty years earlier with Irwin.

"Hey, why not fly down to Florida and bring Damon to my *Hamlet* class!" Irwin cries. "I teach every Wednesday to an overflow crowd of old retired folks. Most can hardly move a muscle, but they hobble in every week on crutches and walkers to hear me parse the text. They love everything to do with sex and fucking—some things never change—and you know me, I just read the words . . . Many of my students were distinguished people once. Now all they want to know is, why doesn't Hamlet just stab the sucker? I guess everyone wants the truth in the end, if not before . . . My mother, who didn't have two cents but lots of sense, said to me, 'What's with this Shakespeare?' I said, 'Ma, he never lies to me' . . . So come on down to sunny Florida and let's see if the old fat fuck still has his fastball . . ."

I smile at my incorrigible teacher. "Thanks, Irwin. I'd love to bring Damon to hear you lecture. But summer's not good," I say gently. "Will you still be teaching Hamlet in the fall?"

"You kidding? I take two years over that play. Fall's fine."

"Cool. I've never been to Florida," Damon says.

Chapter 34

I'm Mercutio!!! Yeah it's so cool it's such an awesome role!

—*From Damon's blog, June 2004*

"Nay, gentle Romeo, we must have you dance," Mercutio declares with a smile.

In *Romeo and Juliet*, I watch my son onstage and for the first time I feel like an admiring theatergoer as much as an indulgent father. Damon burrows into the text and makes the material his own.

It's not just my own biased view. A successful actress friend I've invited turns to me early on and says, "Bloody hell, he can teach *me* about acting Shakespeare!"

Partly, as always, it's the casting. Damon shares many traits with Mercutio and he plays all these qualities to the hilt, stealing every scene with his clever banter and ribaldry. And Shakespeare helps by giving him the best lines.

But Damon also displays growing artistry and maturation. While many of the performers race through their lines like a dutiful catechism, Damon takes his time and savors the words one by one, teasing out their full meaning and never shying away from the Bard's frank sexual innuendo: "If love be rough with you, be rough with love. Prick love for pricking, and you beat love down."

When the notorious showdown with Tybalt begins, I worry about Damon's ability to hold his own. The smallest person on that stage, he's been leaping about and verbally skewering everyone, but now the scene calls for direct physical confrontation. Damon's baseline energy is low and it's hard to see how his dandified, prattling Mercutio will *ever* fight.

But though a head shorter than the taunting Tybalt, Damon's Mercutio steps right up to the enemy Capulet and stares him down. The sight of true fearlessness can only arouse fear in those not so unburdened, and Damon's face is chillingly, defiantly *unafraid*. He draws his sword and forces Tybalt back with a powerful kick and parry, quickly gaining the upper hand.

"*Arrghh! Raahh!*" Damon's thrusts are accompanied by loud grunts, in case anyone missed that he's winning. But when Romeo tries to stop the fight, Tybalt, "under Romeo's arm, thrusts Mercutio in." It's an unfair attack, unwittingly abetted by Romeo, but it fatally wounds Mercutio and sends him to the ground.

As he confronts the horrific specter of his unjust, premature demise, Mercutio repeatedly curses both the Capulets and the Montagues. Damon underplays the scene—he sits slumped on the ground, pale, wounded, and caustic, his lolling head cradled by Romeo until detachment gives way to tragic recognition and bitter resentment at his galling fate:

"A plague o' both your houses! Zounds, a dog, a rat, a mouse, a cat, to scratch a man to death! . . . They have made worms' meat of me."

It's an unspeakable moment as Damon lies mortally wounded on the stage at the end of act 2.

"He can audition for us anytime!" my actress friend says, smiling, as we all applaud.

Chapter 35

I would just like to say that for having 2 days planning My Party
Rocked The Hizouse!!! Yes I said hizouse sue me! Yes yes it did there
was much sex (but none of it involving me . . . 😮 what a shocker
lol . . . ah self mockery where would I be with out it).

—*From Damon's blog, summer 2004*

Although Damon continues to socialize with his growing legion of friends
from theater and school throughout the summer—and to hold the biggest
and coolest sleepover parties at our house, aided by our easygoing attitude
(since we want him to have fun with the least exertion) and abetted by the
fact he's a chick magnet, on friendly if largely platonic terms with the most
beautiful girls, which draws all the guys too—Damon's summer is not all fun
and games.

This would-be eleventh grader has several classes and two New York
State Regents exams to make up. It's a tall order, but Damon has always kept
pace in school until this year, and he's determined to catch up. The fenestration seems to have given him a chance to regain lost ground and to rejoin his
cohort for the fall semester.

A tutor, Andre Lawe, comes to our house four days a week to work with
Damon. A Columbia University chemistry graduate preparing at twenty-
five to be a school principal, Andre is sensitive to Damon's medical ups and
downs. Tutor and tutee breeze through the work when Damon is up to it,
and when he's not, they set it aside for long heart-to-hearts.

"We chat about everything—life, music, relationships, movies, politics, books," Andre says in his mellow way. "Damon teaches me stuff every day."

Sometimes I come home from work and find Damon and Andre giggling and carrying on in the kitchen like two mischievous schoolboys. They are cooking up science experiments for Damon's chem lab and the whole place stinks. Shealagh has long since fled upstairs, after supplying the two principal investigators with pots and measuring cups, and I can see why. Having burned moth balls to demonstrate conversion principles, they seem to be cultivating mold in the sink and setting off a series of not-so-controlled explosions.

Damon gets through the Math Regents, the chem lab, and global history, leaving only the killer Chemistry Regents, which has a 50 percent fail rate. I plan to fly him to the *Deadwood* film set right after the test, as his reward and, hopefully, his incentive.

Damon is excited about the chance to appear on a major television show. He's been watching the critically acclaimed, X-rated western series on HBO in preparation, with special dispensation from his mother. Above his desk is a handwritten note from the show's creator and head writer, David Milch: "Dear Damon, I've written a part for a 16-year old red headed boy. Come out to Los Angeles and be on *Deadwood*."

It's a rare invitation but *Deadwood* is still a month away and New York is broiling in August, so we drive up to Martha's Vineyard, a summer tradition. Damon signs up for sailing lessons in Edgartown and makes impressive progress, learning technique, maneuvers, points of sail, how to read the water and dock.

"I can see he's serious about it," the instructor, a licensed captain who usually looks askance at his spoiled summer clientele, says approvingly.

Damon's health has worsened since last summer, and any physical activity now seems to stress his system. But he still manages to go clamming and fishing and to swim in the ocean with us, even if Sam challenges him on the Long Bridge and in other small ways. But on the Flying Horses and in the gaming arcade, Damon remains the reigning champion and undisputed leader.

Before leaving the Vineyard, Damon gets to do a solo sail in Edgartown harbor, demonstrating mastery of the basics at the end of class. The instructor rides with the other student but Damon, the star pupil, is allowed to skipper the boat by himself despite the busy harbor traffic.

He wears an orange life jacket and racy dark sunglasses and starts with a steady hand on the tiller. Everything appears smooth until he has to scramble and tack around a tight turn. The big boat wobbles and begins to stall—its wood groans and the sails fluff as if it's lost its headwind and might actually head *backward*—when Damon pushes the tiller toward the sail and heaves himself from the port to the starboard side with textbook timing.

The canvas fills again, and the boat resumes sailing in the right direction.

I watch from the dock as Damon steers the swift-moving vessel along the active harbor, a small, capable boy standing in the stern and piloting his large craft with impressive dexterity. He's checking a hundred details and making constant adjustments but keeping it all on a true course. As he glides past us, I spot the budding pride of a natural helmsman on his keen face.

"Yup, he's got the hang of it," the instructor says, nodding.

Chapter 36

Hey hey, it's Damon here giving you all a live update straight from Hollywood. lol. Yeah, so this is my second day here and I've already pulled almost an all nighter (my dad dragged me home) on the set of *Deadwood* which is an awesome set. The town is like life size and you can (and I did a couple of times) get lost. Oh for those of you who I forgot 2 tell (apologies) here is the deal: There is this show called *Deadwood* on HBO which is really cool. It's like this new style western complete with drinking gambling violence and whores lol. So my dad happens 2 be friends with the creator of the show who said he'd put me on. Which is awesome. And I just found out yesterday that I'm probably gonna get a speaking role which is very cool. Yeah.

—From Damon's blog, August 2004

Melody Ranch Studios, where the 1870s western series *Deadwood* is being shot, sits in Santa Clarita, California, in an arid canyon thirty-five miles northwest of Los Angeles. The location, site of such classic westerns as *High Noon*, was once a ranch owned by the singing cowboy Gene Autry. Now it's been converted by the best set designers and builders in Hollywood into one of the largest working sets, complete with a realistic mining town, a huge interior soundstage, a fifty-person crew with a hundred extras, plus twelve horses, five wagons, three buckboards, and one ox. Not to mention numerous offices, trailers, dining facilities, trucks, cranes, cameras, and all the standard backlot infrastructure.

When Damon and I first arrive—it's a forty-minute drive from Santa

Monica—we're amazed you can walk through this town as if it were real. It boasts authentic mining camp streets and period buildings with sides and rears, not just facades, so you can wind your way through the dangerous back alleys and shoot, stab, or fornicate with anyone you meet.

Sheriff Bullock's new house sits atop Main Street while farther down Main is the Gem Saloon, where the notorious Al Swearengen dispenses whiskey, whores, and his own justice. The murderously charismatic Swearengen is Bullock's chief antagonist and sometime ally, the pair embodying two sides of the same ambivalent need for order that underlies this complex drama and its devil's-bargain vision of American history. (Almost every character is based on a real person, not just Calamity Jane and Wild Bill Hickock.)

A hotel, doctor's office, and one-room newspaper offer temporary relief from more whorehouses, gambling dens, saloons, and shanties. These dwellings are interspersed with crude shops: a dry goods store, bakery, eatery, cooperage, boot maker, and butcher. Everything in this mining camp looks primitive and grubby, the naked sun beats down on the unpaved streets, and bloody animal skins hang everywhere.

David Milch, the man whose darkly moralistic vision has brought this world to life—the show's creator, head writer, and executive producer, as well as the famously profane Emmy-winning writer of such hits as *Hill Street Blues* and *NYPD Blue*—slouches tautly but amiably on a shaded part of Main Street when we first show up. Milch, bantering with the cinematographer James Glennon, stops to answer a question from set, receives fresh pages from a script supervisor, and finishes his story before walking over to give me a hug. He extends a very formal, courtly hand to Damon.

"It's an honor to finally meet you, Damon! Your dad's told me so much about you—only the good stuff is true, right?"

David wears his trademark faded black T-shirt and gold-rimmed glasses. He still looks lanky and oddly boyish as he nears sixty, an impressive, if largely genetic, feat, given the highly publicized abuse he's heaped on his body from decades of various addictions. A brilliant, twitchy, and complex guy, David has a big heart to go with his big talent and is a magnanimous host.

"Damon, that big camera you're staring at is for the day's first setup—can you believe this business? No one works until six P.M.!" David smiles. "But the desert sun is unforgiving, so you be careful, okay?" He sends a PA for sun cream and orders Damon watched. "Keep this boy out of the sun or I'll break your balls and chop 'em up!" David says with a grin.

David introduces Damon to his wife, Rita, and to the lead actor Ian McShane:

"Hey, Ian, say hello to Damon, he's also an actor. We're gonna write him a part . . . And, Damon, these lovely ladies are gonna dress you up."

As the wardrobe ladies fuss over Damon, I note it's in the nineties, even after five P.M., and the glaring sun, still high and raw, burns like a blowtorch. Damon's face is hot and flushed, even if he's too stimulated to notice.

"Rita, please take them to my trailer to cool down!" David hands us off to his wife, a painter and the mother of their three kids. "Damon, I'll see you later, pal."

Rita leads us to a posh "Rio Suite" from the production vehicle company Movie Movers. I make Damon take a water bottle from the well-stocked fridge. He sips, absorbing all around him, including David's notorious last-minute script "inserts." The room hums with air-conditioning.

"Wow, Damon, you do have amazing red hair!" Rita smiles. Damon's vivid locks have already sparked admiration from many quarters. Now Rita chats with Damon and catches up with me until we hear voices outside.

"That's Dave. He's here!" Rita winks.

David is escorted wherever he goes, and his movements on the lot are closely tracked by headset-wearing staff. But the trailer is private.

"Hi, Damon. Got all you need, pal?" David enters and shuts the door behind him.

"Yeah, it's nice and cool in here." Damon smiles on the sofa. "Very comfortable."

"Better be! Know what they *charge* for these suites . . . ?" David goes to the sink and swishes mouthwash. "So, Damon, you're in eleventh grade now?" David spits and grins. He taught at Yale and still has a touch of the assistant professor, but he's also the head writer and gently probes Damon about the kind of person, and actor, he is.

"I've mostly done Shakespeare and musicals, but also some comedy," Damon says.

"What, no television! And you're sixteen and call yourself an actor?" David deadpans.

"I'm still learning!" Damon retorts, and they share a laugh.

The PA knocks on the trailer door. "It's time, David! Crew call is for six!"

David turns to Damon. "I've been summoned. Want to ride over with me?"

"Sure," Damon says. They descend the trailer and step into a white golf cart.

David pushes the silent starter motor and sits back. "Okay, go ahead."

"But I've never driven anything but a bumper car before!" Damon protests.

"Well, this is the same—forward, reverse, accelerator—just don't bump anything."

Damon, nervous and excited, steps on reverse and almost crashes into a tractor.

"I warned you!" Damon laughs as David stiffens in the seat beside him.

"Try it again," David says calmly. Damon makes it across the road this time but oversteers, swinging in erratic loops and jolting them both in their seats.

"Sorry!" Damon giggles as David braces against the dash, ignoring his beeper.

A PA trots over with pointed urgency. "Everyone's waiting on set, David!"

David nods but stays put, displaying serene patience as he sits beside Damon. It's a side of David, who is notoriously fidgety and abrupt, I've rarely seen.

Damon finally masters the controls and proudly drops David off on set.

"Thank you, Damon." David salutes him before the waiting crew.

Main Street starts to fill with a colorful hubbub as the costumed cast trickles in for the six P.M. call. Production runs final checks, while the crew mans its stations.

A great sense of playful adventure hangs in the air, tempered only by the ticking of the five-million-dollars-an-episode money clock.

Damon stands rapt and watches as it takes the entire twelve-hour shift to complete a single scene. One actor keeps blowing his lines, and there are technical issues, like keeping all the torches lit and repeatedly hosing down the dusty road so it can reflect this light. Plus actor queries about why a character would do this or say that, followed by Milch's eloquent riffs on motivation and plot with a nod to history, psychology, philosophy, criminology, and modern culture.

It seems slow and drawn out but what Damon is witnessing from his perch near the director—a spiky-haired New Yorker, Ed Bianchi—is the nuts and bolts of filmmaking.

"It's so different from theater," Damon says. "The actors do it all in short takes!"

Damon loves all the rituals of being on set, including that "lunch" is always served six hours after crew call, even if it's midnight when we all go to the giant tented mess hall.

"Grab a tray and come with me, Damon," David instructs. The cast remains in period costume as we line up for hot food. We carry our trays to cafeteria-style tables filled by hordes of ravenous extras with filthy faces and bevies of statuesque, candy-eyed women in low-cut dresses. Damon is on cloud nine—he sits at David's table with several of the lead actors, talking shop in this carnival atmosphere—and he doesn't want to leave.

Outside time means little in this buzzing, brightly lit world.

The first night I let my mesmerized son linger on the set until four thirty A.M. before I drag him off to bed. In the next week, we go regularly to Melody Ranch though I try to get him back by midnight so he doesn't exhaust himself. I still rise by six A.M. and get in almost an entire day's work before I wake Damon up around one or two P.M. He rarely wakes by himself.

Sometimes when I watch Damon sleep, he looks so slight and retracted under the big covers, his pale body collapsing in on itself, that I start to worry again. But then I note his belly and face look less bloated, so we've made progress. And his improved appearance bodes well for his acting debut, assuming that happens, which is not a foregone conclusion.

"Will I really get my own part?" Damon asks after that first day, rightly uncertain.

"David assured me you'll have speaking lines, but he hasn't written them yet, and he's got a lot on his plate," I reply. "Plus, nothing is ever easy or certain in this town, no matter who you know . . . So we'll have to play it by ear, okay?"

"Sure, Dad. It's cool just being here."

"Why'd you let me sleep so late?" Damon asks the moment I wake him. But he knows.

"Don't forget your meds and your shot!" I remind him as goes into the bathroom. Damon now injects growth hormone daily, but he's grown an inch or two, so he's happy to do it.

After his regimen, Damon quickly brushes his teeth, dons shorts and a T-shirt, grabs his cell phone, and stands by the door, all in under five minutes.

"Okay, I'm ready!" he says.

I bring along his sun hat, which he always "forgets," but I let him eat breakfast in the car to save time.

We stick the latest CD in, put down the top, and take off. Damon enjoys my driving and leans forward in his seat as we zoom past one vehicle after another.

The wind picks up in the speeding convertible, blowing Damon's hair like wildfire in the snapping breeze. He's strapped in, but the propeller force of his flapping hair looks like it could catapult him into the sky. He grins at me and his blue eyes dance with the thrill of roaring power. I gun the engine and we rocket forward and experience the rush of pure velocity together. It's a scream!

The instant we reach Melody Ranch, the bond between Damon and me is broken and he can't wait to ditch me and join the cast. I take my laptop and go work in David's trailer.

I make occasional forays onto the set, but early on it's clear that even when Damon and I walk onto the same lot, we go through different doors. I'm oriented toward writing and writers, whereas for Damon, it's about actors and acting.

"You seem to fit right in," I say. "Is there a secret password or handshake?"

"No, Dad, we're just actors. But some of these guys are *really* good."

All the actors in the show welcome Damon. Ian McShane, who plays the fearsome Al Swearengen, reveals to Damon the gentlest disposition, along with a friendly Manchester accent, beneath that hard face and glaring eyes. "And how is young Master Damon today? You keeping that sweet peaches-and-cream out of this bloody awful sun?" McShane smiles and rubs Damon's back.

But it's Paula Malcomson, a gifted Irish firebrand and the show's blond poster whore, who adopts Damon from day one. "Let's get you out of this fuckin' heat, Damon! I got good AC in my trailer and a new copy of Yeats, the later poetry. No sane person should be walkin' out in this shit storm. They don't pay *that* well."

Paula and Damon hang out. They discuss literature, theater, life. They share confidences. One day I see them going into her trailer and realize they even *look* alike: Paula is petite and also has pale skin and luminous blue eyes, while her yellow-blond hair has the same intensity as Damon's coppery thatch.

"You could be brother and sister!" I tease them.

But the male crew members start a different rumor on set about all the time these two spend behind closed doors: "Hear what happened? Trixie got Damon!"

When Damon steps from Paula's trailer, he emerges with a new mystique. He blogs for his pals about it: "The cast is really cool especially the main whore aka Paula (Trixie). She was really nice and sorta showed me around and we also hung out in her trailer . . . NO! You people with your dirty minds you disgust me lol jk."

Another person who connects deeply with Damon is Gary Leffew, a stuntman and a world-champion bull rider. When Milch sought real-life cowboys to give him a flavor of that bygone world, all hands pointed to Gary Leffew, rodeo hall-of-famer and famous hell-raiser, as the nearest modern-day embodiment.

"Hey, amigos, when you only work for eight seconds a day, you got lots of free time for gettin' into mischief," Gary explains to Damon and me.

After we're friends, Gary tells me about the first day he met Damon.

"I seen this young boy standin' on the set in his own bright pool of light. It come off him like a glow!" Gary says. "He had a real powerful life force shinin' out—I tell ya, I never seen one that strong, it was just dazzling! I could watch it move with him whenever he moved . . . Man, I just had to go up and meet Damon!"

Gary takes Damon and me to the L.A. Equestrian Center, where he stables his horses for the cast to practice on. We mount and enter Griffith Park.

Damon and I are used to English riding and must adapt to the Western style. And Gary has no helmets for us. But it's Gary's wild, zippy horses that require the biggest adjustment. They don't just trot or canter but *gallop* up the twisting hillsides, nicking other riders and nearly plunging us over the ravine.

"Whoa! Stop!" we shout as they chase blindly after Gary's horse.

Gary is a great bull rider, the daredevil of rodeo, and can stay upright on any animal. But Damon and I are amateurs, and when not hanging on for dear life myself, I worry about Damon, who has a listing seat and little apparent strength or control. But Damon has good instincts, and when his horse gallops off unbidden, Damon bounces along in the saddle, tilting crookedly and riding it out like a rag doll until his horse slows down or one of us gives him a hand. Once I have to chase Damon down and grab his reins until his pony, throwing a fit, calms down.

Gary sits atop his horse with his perfect riding posture, chuckling. "Yeah, he'll do that every so often. He gets kinda feisty, but he don't mean nothin' by it."

It's a beautiful, rolling park with peaks and canyons and switchback trails.

A coyote appears and spooks Gary's horse, who rears and bolts, throwing Gary briefly off balance and sending Damon's horse and mine fleeing as well. There's a moment of pure panic until Gary manages to bring his horse back under control about a foot from the edge of a ravine, while I try to box in Damon's pony.

Fortunately, it's only a close call, but it makes me realize that although Gary is the best rider in the world, even he can't protect us. Damon and I must stay on full alert and fend for ourselves. Which may be one reason we wanted to come here with Gary—a paradox Gary, in his cowboy way, has grasped from the start.

As we climb, we see the modern sprawl, from downtown Los Angeles to Burbank with the Hollywood sign above. Yet we're enveloped by deep nature.

"Can we ride up to the sign?" Damon says with a cheeky smile.

"I never done it but I don't see why not," Gary says, impressed. "But we gotta hurry if we want to find our way back before dark."

We twist and wind our way up through the dense brush and watch the city drop away. It grows quiet and windy as we ascend the forested mountain, with steep escarpments and dramatic ravines. Even our horses fall silent as we round the last, dusty curve of the trail and come out over a high, narrow ridge.

There's just enough light as we overlook the valley. Across from us is a summit topped by a transmission tower, while a big range of mountains stretches on the horizon. Between lie sprawling urban centers with tiny, twinkling lights.

The cities of men look like a small thing from here, a glitch in the landscape.

We pat our horses' manes and stroke their damp flanks.

"Rockin' awesome!" Damon beams atop his golden pony, hatless and proud as all get-out.

Chapter 37

"It's my life! And I don't want to live forever . . . I just want to live my life!"

—Some song I can't remember at the moment

—From Damon's blog, August 2004

We return to the *Deadwood* set and it's still unclear whether Damon will get his part. Time is running out—Damon has to get back for school—but we still face several obstacles.

"You need a work permit," I explain to Damon. "An actor under eighteen must be an enrolled student with a C average but you had home tutoring the previous semester, so we don't have your report card."

"Maybe my tutor could send in my grades?" Damon says.

David Milch is also concerned about Damon's health. Like many people on the set, David has developed a real fondness for Damon. Unlike them, he knows about his illness.

"You sure he's up to this? We're in a record-setting, ball-shriveling heat wave and Damon's been looking a little pale to me. I don't want to push him—"

"Damon always looks pale," I counter, smiling. "And despite the heat, he can't wait to show his stuff. He really wants to do this, David!"

Finally, there is the business of a major studio production with a tight schedule and money riding on every shot. David has power, but it's not unlimited.

There's a day when it seems we won't make it. The production is behind schedule, and David isn't even on the lot. Our return flight is booked, and it feels like our window may have closed. Paula has no scenes today, so she's away, and Gary also has a day off.

"It's a hundred and one degrees!" the PA informs us at noon. Even the Gem Saloon, where "action" and "going again" echo all day, feels depleted. The snow-cone maker has melted.

At lunch we sit in the wilting mess hall with A. C. Lyles, a dapper eighty-six-year-old man who comes to the set every day dressed in a dark suit and tie, no matter how hot it is. Lyles, who's worked at Paramount for over sixty years and knew everyone, from John Barrymore and James Cagney to Ronald Reagan, is a living link with old Hollywood.

"Don't worry about your part; you're special, I can always tell!" Lyles says to Damon. "And David's a genius. He'll make it happen!"

Sure enough, by evening word comes that David has returned and he and his staff are working on Damon's lines. We know it's real because there's a ripple of excitement from wardrobe and makeup, big fans of Damon. We also hear from production and writing with more precise instructions.

Damon's status changes instantly. He becomes someone to watch.

His actor friends drag him to the popular Friday lottery, held under a big tree with all the cast and crew, from star to gofer, assembled.

The lottery is a weekly tradition, in which David hands out thousands of dollars from his own pocket in cash prizes, ranging from $100 to $500. It's a big, fun morale builder and a welcome weekend bonus to support staff and crew who earn modest scale wages.

"Five hundred dollars goes to—John Vitteli. John, get your ass up here!" David barks. The lottery is vintage Milch, because not only has David become rich from TV writing, but he's also wildly generous, carrying wads of cash and doling out hundred-dollar bills like candy to doormen, waiters, valets. He loves scattering chips from his winnings.

"One hundred dollars goes to"—David reaches into the hat—"Damon Weber!"

Blushing, a surprised Damon walks through the cheering throng to receive his prize.

"Man, some guys get all the luck!" David, who owns racehorses and gambles, grumbles affably as Damon comes up. He pats him warmly on the back.

Damon returns and shows me the $100 bill. "What do I do with this, Dad?"

"Whatever you want," I reply, but Damon isn't satisfied. "Okay, let's use it to buy David a thank-you present," I say. "Word is he wrote you a scene."

When we finally receive the script pages for Damon, we are very pleased.

"I got seven lines of dialogue with Sheriff Bullock's son!" Damon exclaims.

"Yes, it's a small, beautifully crafted scene—a brief idyll amid all that grimness," I remark. "Two young boys who glimpse the rare chance of friendship before it vanishes."

"My character is called *Damon*," Damon notes. "And my father, a gold prospector Gary plays, is called *Damon's Dad*. How do you like that, Dad?" Damon grins at me. "I got a real part . . ."

The next twenty-four hours are very exciting as we prepare for Damon's debut.

I feel like an aide entrusted with a young celebrity.

Damon himself is walking on air. He looks taller, more glamorous, more chosen.

He carries the script wherever he goes and studies it. Learning lines is something he knows, and seven lines is a piece of cake. I give him my scene notes and he nods politely.

We get several calls the night before from a diligent PA on the graveyard shift.

"Damon's first up on the call sheet, so we need him by eight thirty A.M.," he says.

"Fine," I reply.

Two hours later, he calls again. "Sorry, but can you bring him to set at seven A.M.?"

"Sure," I say, then hang up and turn to Damon. "That's a five thirty A.M. wake-up call for us!"

Still, it's flattering to be the focus of so much effort and attention. We can feel the gears turning on Damon's behalf as he becomes part of a powerful system.

All evening, I can see him mouthing words from the script and trying out different angles. He's rehearsing. A few times, I catch him grinning quietly to himself. He's happy and full of purpose, living in a world he cares about.

We go into the small outdoor pool before hitting the sack. Damon has been more active in the water on this trip, a good sign. He dives for plastic rings and swims between my legs. We toss a soggy foam football back and forth under the twinkling stars.

As we exit the pool, I notice how regal he looks in his big white terry bathrobe. When we ride the elevator, it seems other people also stare at Damon like he's someone whose name they should know.

As we get ready for bed, I stick my head out of the bathroom and catch him injecting himself. He's twisting across his trunk to insert the needle into his thigh, and his exposed torso looks very swollen and pasty.

Damon finishes and lets his pajama top cover his flank. Instantly, he's Damon again—the handsome boy they'll shoot. He flashes me a hard, furtive glance, as if to say this is one more insult, but he can manage it. And we agree, without a word, not to discuss it.

I lean over and kiss my star in the making good night.

"Sweet dreams, D-man."

Chapter 38

My dad's friend the executive producer/unofficial writer/unofficial
director (it's basically all his show) is also very interesting. He gets
around the set in a golf cart and changes the script last minute
which some actors aren't always thrilled about. lol.

—From Damon's blog, August 2004

We're on the freeway by six A.M. and it's blissfully free of traffic.

The sky is clear and the rugged San Gabriel Mountains glisten along the
Pacific Coast Range. I buy Damon fresh strawberries, which he loves, and
watch him nibble on the luscious fruit, smiling dreamily, as we zip out to
Santa Clarita in a red convertible for his screen debut. I don't know if it gets
much better than this.

We arrive on the lot at seven A.M. sharp. The PA, a stocky kid called
Kenny, greets us. "Thanks so much for coming on time! Can I get you any
food or drink? *Anything?*"

The day of deference has begun. Kenny leads us to a small day trailer
with a stepladder, part of a long Star Waggons unit. The name "Damon" is
on the door, which makes my son feel rightly special.

Next to Damon's trailer is a trailer with "Damon's Dad" on it. I smile but
don't go in. For today, it belongs to Gary Leffew.

Kenny leads us to Sheriff Bullock's new house, which sits on an elevated
site dominating Main Street. Damon's scene unfolds here.

The multi-gabled wood house is fronted by steep stairs that wind down
to street level. Halfway down the stairs is a dry "creek," which the crew is

filling from a hose. Various camera and lighting assistants position large filters and screens to deal with the anticipated glare. The air is still cool but the open desert sky is cloudless, and you can sense the gathering force of the rising sun.

The director Steve Shill has Damon walk through each shot to work out the markers.

David Milch arrives in his ever-present black T-shirt and five o'clock shadow, looking like he's slept on the lot. He's trailed by the usual retinue. David flips through the script pages. "Cut these lines on page six and add this!" David tells Shill. Damon has now been on set long enough to grasp that in television, unlike film or theater, the head writer/executive producer is top dog. David utters a few more instructions before loping over.

"Ready for your big day?" He gives Damon an affectionate pat but we can see he's distracted. There's much to do before shooting commences.

We go to the tent for breakfast and get ham and cheese omelets from the short-order cook. Everyone treats Damon like a VIP, which is what you turn into when you have a scene coming up. Kenny brings forms to sign from the Screen Actors Guild and Department of Justice.

Two women from wardrobe drape Damon in a burlap shirt, filthy blue overalls, and black lace-up boots, topped by a wool cap. The fashionistas have admired my son from day one and beam at his costume. "You rock, Damon!"

Next Damon is led around the corner to makeup, a long, narrow trailer fitted out like a chic hair salon. Four leather-and-chrome chairs swivel opposite four large mirrors, while wigs, brushes, and makeup kits line the counter. Tim Olyphant, the lanky leading man who plays Sheriff Seth Bullock, is sitting in the last chair, being fussed over by a team of makeup artists and enjoying it.

A trimly goateed man in a white shirt meticulously roughs up Damon's hair with his hands and fluffs it up with fine instruments. "You've got great hair—we don't have to do much!" Two female assistants smile and nod while a younger makeup guy in a *Scorpion King* T-shirt systematically begins applying a coat of dirt to Damon's face, his hands, and the back of his neck.

Damon steps out of the makeup trailer looking like a Norman Rockwell illustration from a Mark Twain novel. Tom Sawyer in South Dakota, circa 1870. A staff photographer takes a publicity shot of Damon standing beside a horse.

Main Street is busier now and the sun is already heating things up, though it's not yet nine A.M. Everyone sheds layers. The director, down to shirtsleeves, remarks, "Crikey, it's going to be a bloody scorcher!"

The big 35 millimeter Panavision camera has been mounted on a tripod on Bullock's front porch. The crew positions giant white, black, and silver panels around the camera to try to balance the streaming light. It's a tricky, moving target. They improvise, using ladders to hide auxiliary white lights under the burlap shade of an adjacent house.

Dozens of costumed extras flow through the town and begin to fill the street with the bustle of daily nineteenth-century life. Horses and wagons clop by while weary-looking men sit outside their tents with rifles slung across their laps and chopped wood at their feet.

Damon rehearses climbing into the wagon and Gary, playing Damon's father in a shabby gold-prospector outfit, gives him a practice ride up Main. "Gonna be a long hot day, son!" Gary says. "You best rest up 'fore we light out."

Josh Eriksson, who's playing William opposite Damon, arrives, though he's not in costume yet. His script dangles in one hand. The director introduces the two boys—they quickly size each other up while exchanging polite greetings—and then he rehearses them.

Damon already looks warm and stiff in his heavy costume—the experienced actors wisely wait until the last minute to suit up—and we all know it's going to get much worse.

The forecast is for triple digits, possibly the hottest day yet.

Paula Malcomson arrives and sits on the shaded saloon porch. Paula is not shooting today but has driven out to support Damon. Her hair is loose and she wears a casual pink top. "Hey, Damon!" She gives a dazzling wave.

"Hey." Damon blushes and smiles at his cheering section.

"D-man, drink!" I hand him a water bottle. His lips are dry and he's dehydrated. He obliges me with a perfunctory swig but he's got more important things on his mind.

The lighting crew continues juggling the angled screens by Bullock's house, trying to keep up with the blazing sun. "Put some Kinos down," the cinematographer, James Glennon, instructs. Glennon, a bulky, shambling figure, employs a first assistant to look through the viewfinder, a second to pull focus, and a third to move the camera on its tracks, but his keen eyes don't miss a mote of dust if it might show on-screen.

David Milch grins with delight at Damon's costume and makeup. "You look fantastic, Damon!" Then his scowl returns. "But it's over ninety degrees and not even ten A.M.! I want you to keep drinking and stay out of the sun as much as possible. I'll have a PA standing by with an umbrella for you at all times . . . Otherwise, just have a good time and try to enjoy yourself. You're a member of the guild now!" David notes.

"What does being a member of the Screen Actors Guild mean?" Damon asks.

"You get a minimum daily rate and health—" David starts explaining, then stops. "It means next year when you come out here, you'll have an agent and you'll shake me down for a lot more money!"

Hordes of extras now populate every inch of Main Street. A PA quickly tops off the creek. They want it brimming, but the sun keeps evaporating the water.

Damon and Josh get into position, Josh at the top of the stairs, where he's just emerged from Sheriff Bullock's house, and Damon facing him half-way down the stairs.

Steve Shill checks with David Milch and yells, "Action!" and the two boys, along with other actors, run through the whole scene once as the camera rolls:

Damon: You just move here?

William: Just yesterday.

Damon: I watched the sheriff build this house.

William: Mr. Bullock is my Pa's brother that married my Ma after my Pa
was killed, so now he's my Pa and my uncle.

Damon: Big trout lives in that deep part down there.

*Damon's Dad, a wiry gold prospector down at the ribbons drives up in a
buckboard.*

Damon's Dad: Damon!

Damon (over his shoulder, to his father): Comin'. *(to William)* My Pa and
me are going to Oregon to grow apples.

William: Are you coming back?

Damon: Pa says, we ain't never coming back. *Descends one step.* Keep
your eye on that rainbow. I call him Jumbo. *Damon climbs into the*

wagon beside his father and they begin to ride up Main Street and
out of Deadwood. William and Damon watch each other.
Bullock (coming out of his house): Mornin' William.
William: That boy is going to Oregon.

Close up on Damon looking back at William as his father drives them
away.

Although the scene will now be broken down into individual lines, and parts of lines, and shot many times from multiple angles, with many takes and retakes, a spreading murmur can be heard after this initial run-through. The precipitating cause is Damon.

The only person other than me who does not look completely surprised by his performance is Paula, who is already smiling and thinking of the notes she wants to give Damon. Otherwise, there are many open mouths on the set.

Until this moment, everyone, including David himself, had assumed the show-runner was doing a favor for a friend's kid and they'd have to get through this with the least amount of damage or embarrassment. It's not an unheard-of occurrence on a film set.

But now the air is charged.

Damon has them floored.

You can *feel* the buzz. Glennon, a renowned veteran, trudges over to me and says, "Congratulations! You can go into semi-retirement. That boy is really good—he's a natural!" He smiles in his dour way. "Tell your wife your kid will never be out of work in this business."

Glennon's assessment seems to be shared by other observers. They whisper excitedly among themselves. Several walk over to me and quietly express their admiration for this unexpectedly self-possessed young actor.

"He's been acting since he was five," I try to explain. "He knows what he's doing."

David Milch harbors a pensive, dawning half smile. He's been rooting for Damon, but he didn't expect this. I tried to tell him, but I'm the father. David had originally invited me to be on his show—"Come on out and we'll slap a pair of chaps on you and put you up on a horse"—when I suggested substituting my son, a real actor, and David wrote his note to Damon. Now it appears as if Milch knew what he was doing all along—giving a gifted young actor his first major break.

Once Damon's acting bona fides have been established and the pleasant surprise has worn off, there's still a big scene to shoot and lots of hard work to do. It will take a couple of hours, with the temperature rising steeply, in alarming increments, as we approach noon.

By ten thirty A.M. it's 95 degrees and by eleven it's 98 degrees. At eleven twenty we break into triple digits and by eleven forty-five a PA informs me that it's 104 degrees, the hottest day of the summer.

Everyone who's not in the scene or working runs for cover, mopping their brow and guzzling water. We are being cooked on the valley floor, with the mountains sealing in the heat. I wear shorts and a T-shirt but the toxic sweat drips off me, even in the shade.

Damon has to stand on the exposed steps and run through his scene in heavy costume and makeup as the sun reaches its zenith.

After each take, a PA steps up and holds a large blue umbrella over Damon, who looks like Little Lord Fauntleroy in dirty overalls, but the moment he hears "Action!" Damon steps back and replays his scene without flagging or complaining. He takes direction well, and he does not fluff his lines.

Early on, Paula Malcomson asks me if she can give Damon some notes. "Go for it," I reply.

Paula trots out to the blazing steps, pulling Damon aside to confer between takes. They form a classic tableau, the lithe, studious, blond-tressed actress huddling with her young actor friend, her arms crossed over her soft pink blouse while his capped head tilts down to listen. Two serious students of the craft, sharing and comparing.

After, Paula won't reveal what she said. "It's private but I'll tell you one fuckin' thing, I got as much to learn from him as he does from me!" She studies Damon on the monitor, donning brown eyeglasses and clapping on headphones to catch every nuance.

David Milch sits off to the side and studies the same monitor in a contemplative self-entwined pose. He's happy with what he sees but also worried about Damon, the heat, and existential issues.

David calls a time-out to give everyone a break from the sun. "Let's take five!"

Damon comes over and flops down in a brown canvas chair. He's hot and flushed but dripping with pride. He drinks from a water bottle with lordly gusto.

"How is it out there, Damon?" David checks in with his young actor.

"It's fun!" Damon says.

David nods with a dyspeptic smile. "You're doing great but I want you to take more time with your lines. Let yourself be awkward and try to fill the silences with more longing and disappointment," David says. "These two boys really wanted to be friends and are full of regret that it won't happen."

A makeup person dabs Damon's sweating face, and then David escorts Damon to his mark, walking beside his young actor and giving him more tips.

Under David's vigilant gaze, Damon pushes his part emotionally.

"Excellent!" David's face breaks into a small, appreciative smile.

The hardest part for Damon is the physical strain. It's bad enough to wear heavy overalls; a thick, rough shirt; and high leather boots for hours in the unrelenting heat. But what almost undoes him is the repeated action surrounding his last line of dialogue.

Damon must deliver the line in two parts: walking down the stairs after the first half ("Keep your eye on that rainbow") then stopping for the second part ("I call him Jumbo") before turning and hustling up into the waiting carriage with Gary. This last move demands a big effort as Damon grabs onto the seat rail, heaves himself up from street level, and clambers in. And it all has to look completely natural and fluid in the 104 degree blaze.

I know the enormous effort this seemingly routine action demands from Damon and how hard he's trying not to show it. I worry his cover could be blown if it goes on too long. So far no one, other than David, suspects a thing, but it's pushing Damon to the limit.

He's acting on more than one level.

I watch Damon as he turns and comes down the stairs with dogged determination each time, swiveling his hips, rolling his shoulders, and pumping his arms to gain enough momentum to propel his body into the carriage. I hold my breath every time.

Once, I spot Damon wincing and run up between takes. "You okay, D-man?"

"Yeah, I pulled a leg muscle but I'm fine now." Damon shrugs. He's so full of adrenaline, he doesn't feel a thing. It's 104 degrees and my son is in heaven.

And doesn't want me there, though he's grateful I'm near. I return to the sidelines.

They have to shoot this scene two dozen times. It demands coordination between Damon's and Josh's lines, Damon's descending the stairs and ascending the carriage, then Gary driving them up Main Street while Damon looks back at Josh and Josh looks at Damon. After each take, Gary must turn the carriage and ride it all the way back—even the horse is hot and tired!—and Damon must alight from the wagon and resume his position on the stairs. Meanwhile, fifty extras must take their posts and spring to life again.

Somehow, Damon hangs in until we hear the magic words: "That's a wrap."

David hands me a headset. "You need to see just how good he looks on-screen!" I know all about Damon's acting, of course, but when I view the monitor, I'm impressed by how the presence of other talented actors and *Deadwood*'s enhanced production values add depth and create a truly classical movie look.

David Milch high-fives Damon as he comes in and praises his fine work.

"That was serious acting! I pushed you and you dug deeper . . . I hope you realize how well you did. You gave an impressive, completely professional performance! Almost no one achieves that the first time."

David sends a PA to get his new star a snow cone. "Now you need to cool down and stay out of the sun the rest of the day. I mean it!"

Steve Shill tells Damon he's a real pro and it was a pleasure directing him.

I'm standing apart and watching as several other crew and cast members come up to congratulate Damon, when David Milch pats me on the shoulder.

"I understand." He nods darkly. "These guys think this is just a kid getting his first shot. But you and I, we know what else is going on. It's a fuckin' mysterious process . . ." David starts to leave. "You know, sometimes you do something nice for someone and it turns out well for everyone. That's a good outcome." David gives a beatific smile. "He's such a fantastic kid!"

He pats me again and walks off.

A sexy actress runs up and tells Damon how great he was and that she looks forward to working with him.

Damon blushes, tips back his handsome rapscallion cap, and thanks her. He looks tired but triumphant, a novice no more. He loosens his shirt and drapes one cavalier arm over the chair, grinning over a dripping snow cone.

Part IV

Chapter 39

So school begins tomorrow and I am in a strange way looking forward
to it but at the same time apprehensive. After all, it was only a few
months ago that I was missing so much school because of all my
medical crap that I dropped out and had to go on home instruction
which, although easier, is also very lonely. So the surgery has
definitely helped but the question is, is it enough? Although I have
been more or less fine over the summer, it is not the same. During
the summer, I could pretty much rest whenever I needed/wanted to.
But school, as we all know, is relentless. Do I really have enough
energy (protein) to get through it? And this is Junior Year, the one
that really counts . . . and I plan to direct a play and hopefully be in
model UN and actually have a life (way to pace yourself Damon!) In
truth, my numbers have not really improved that much, they've just
stopped going down, meaning I'm not in danger of wasting away or
being confined to my bed 24/7—whoopeee. And of course I have the
lovely infusions every 2 or so weeks now at my house, which is much
better but it's still going to be a bitch having to go home for those
especially when rehearsal starts. But really it's the same problem
it always is, which is very simply my energy. And I won't be able to
truly tell how much that's improved till school starts. At least I have
the comfort of knowing that my doctor is on the same page as me:
sending me back to school is an experiment that could very well fail.
Of course, I could always drop all the extra curricular shit, settle
for 70s and 80s, and call it me. I could also live someone else's
life but, surprise surprise, I don't want to. I suppose (at the risk of
being cliched) only time shall tell. So enough of me bitching, it's not

helping me and it's certainly not helping you. Sorry for those of you
who actually are reading this.

—*From Damon's blog, September 12, 2004*
(ten days after returning from Deadwood)

Despite a great summer and his early excitement about returning to school,
by October of his junior year, Damon starts to falter again.

"His albumin is down to two point one and he looks awfully pale and
weak. I don't think he can handle school," Shealagh says. "It's too much for
him!"

Damon is under attack all over, only this time, we've exhausted all of the
treatment options, except for a heart transplant.

Dr. Hellenbrand admits he has nothing more to offer us—"I'm really
sorry we couldn't do more for him with fenestration"—and no other doctor
or hospital has a better option.

Dr. Chin sends me a paper on "renovating the heart," the experimental
use of stem cells to repair injured hearts. But even Dr. Chin scribbles in the
margins, "I'm not sure if any of this really applies in Damon's case since his
heart has not been acutely injured."

My cousin Dr. Bar-Or still believes inflammation is the key to Damon's
illness but he has no ready solution. "I have some ideas," he says, "but they're
still in the experimental stage."

My friend Dr. Jeffrey Friedman thinks a mechanical assist device might
help but accepts that it's not feasible for now. "The market isn't there, so no
one's developing it."

Shealagh's best friend, Dr. Sonja Kassuba, has faith in alternative medicine but recognizes we need an "immediate intervention" to arrest Damon's
steep deterioration.

I do a final search for new papers and check in with doctors at a dozen
hospitals all over the world, until I've X-ed out every item but the last on my
faded master list.

Only the heart transplant remains. We have to accept it and explore it.

We start with Columbia, Damon's regular hospital and a pioneer in heart transplantation. Shealagh and I go to Dr. Hayes, Damon's longtime cardiologist, who has foreseen this day. "I know how difficult this must be for you, but you're making the right decision for Damon," she tells us.

Dr. Hayes leads us straight to the office of Dr. Amelia Mason,* the medical director of pediatric heart transplants at Columbia. Dr. Hayes's recommendations are invariably reliable and she speaks warmly of Dr. Mason. "Amelia knows all about Damon and is eager to meet you."

Dr. Mason smiles behind round glasses as she enthuses about the wonders of heart transplants at Columbia.

"It's almost routine now and people can live for twenty years or more with a first transplant," Dr. Mason says. "Many are still going strong in their third decade, and they can always get a second transplant, if they need it, and start the clock all over again."

"What quality of life can they expect?" I ask, noting her cheeriness.

"Oh, a very good one, just like normal. Transplant patients lead full, active lives. We have patients running marathons, skiing downhill, having babies . . ."

"That's good to hear," I say, encouraged but trying to square this with what I've read. "But doesn't Damon's PLE pose special problems for a heart transplant?"

"No." Dr. Mason doesn't skip a beat. "We've successfully transplanted many patients just like him. In fact, one of Damon's biggest problems post-transplant will likely be the risk of injury from all the excess energy he will have with a new working heart!"

"Are you serious?" I say as Shealagh and I exchange hopeful but skeptical glances.

"Yes! These kids can suddenly run and jump like normal children for the first time in their lives," Dr. Mason explains. "They're so excited, they often get hurt leaping around until they learn how to control their energetic new bodies. So you may actually have to *restrain* Damon at first and teach him to be careful."

"We can live with that!" Shealagh chuckles nervously. We're both very gratified to get such a positive overview from the presiding pediatric transplant expert at Columbia. But as Dr. Mason continues in this vein, I begin to feel uneasy.

---

*I have changed the names of "Dr. Mason" and her colleagues in the pediatric cardiology transplant team—Drs. "Davis," "Becker," and "Sanford." No other names have been changed.

"Forgive me, but what are you basing this on?" I ask. "Because this isn't what we've heard." I look at Shealagh. "I mean, if transplants are so great, why have we spent the past three years trying to *avoid* one? Have we been completely misled until now?"

"It really works, trust me! We have the experience and patients to prove it!"

"Okay"—I stare at her—"so how many heart transplants have you performed?" Then I fire off a series of questions: "How many were Fontans? And how many had PLE? For how many years had they had PLE? Did the PLE resolve? And how many years post-transplant did the patients live?"

Dr. Mason stiffens and for the first time, her fixed smile wavers.

She bristles. "I don't have it all at my fingertips!" She looks put out, as if I'm challenging her authority and spoiling the feel-good air.

I seek to reassure her. "Look, our only interest is Damon's well-being, but we've talked to many doctors and read many papers with a *different* view. What data do you have? We need hard numbers." Despite trying, I can't quite hide my exasperation.

"We have an outstanding pediatric transplant program, one of the best in the country," Dr. Mason declares. She either doesn't have the facts or won't discuss them with us. She looks to Shealagh for female solidarity—*Is he always like this?*—and keeps smiling at us with a beaming, content-free expression that says, "Trust me, it's all good."

But it's not all good. We can't get her to talk about any substantive details or any potential trouble spots.

I begin to worry we are getting a sales pitch. Dr. Mason wants to sell us a *product*. Her language is vague and imparts no real information. I must know a hundred doctors and scientists by now, including dozens of Nobel laureates and scores of world-class medical researchers and practitioners, several of them good friends—they form the core of my daily professional and personal life—and not one of them speaks, let alone thinks, in this way. Nor has any physician at Columbia ever addressed us in such a generic, unforthcoming manner.

"Look, I'm sorry, but that's just not good enough for us," I tell Dr. Mason while Shealagh nods. "We can't be the first parents to ask for real data. We're talking about our son's *life*, and we need more facts and more context to make the best decision for him."

I am polite but resolute and there is a long, uncomfortable stretch until

Dr. Mason, who has a determinedly bouncy air and has never stopped smiling, comes to recognize she can't close this deal without producing something concrete.

Suddenly she changes her tune and invites me into her confidence.

"So, although it's not published yet, our group at Columbia has a big paper in press that might interest you! It's a multi-decade, retrospective study that reviews, for the first time, all our patient outcomes for cardiac transplantation after the Fontan, including for PLE patients. And it documents all the case histories I referred to."

News of this instantly alters my frame of mind. I feel a ripple of hope and excitement.

"When's the paper coming out?" I ask. I know no such data has yet appeared—I've been searching for it myself—but if Columbia has peer-reviewed results, and if they're as good as Dr. Mason says, then we're in business. It would mean the outlook for Damon is much more favorable than we imagined and we're at exactly the right hospital.

"I can't recall the exact numbers but I can try and get you a preprint as a personal favor," Dr. Mason says. "It won't be published for three to four months."

"I would really appreciate that!" I reply, full of eager deference now.

"That would be so kind of you," Shealagh chimes in.

Dr. Mason, back in our good graces, smiles. "We could also handle the IVIG infusions for Damon, if you like. He now gets them at home under Mount Sinai's care, is that correct?" She fingers the stethoscope around her neck.

"Yes, but we thought Columbia didn't do IVIG. It's why we went to Sinai."

"Oh no, IVIG is part of our pre-transplant preparation program. We use it all the time to help fortify patients before the surgery," Dr. Mason says.

"Really?" I say, and share a secret smile with Shealagh, since we've long pushed IVIG for Damon but had to go it alone. I lower my voice. "It means we were right and Dudu was right, and we've been strengthening Damon all along!"

"Yes!" Shealagh says sotto voce. "But we should probably let Columbia take over now because it's better to have one place overseeing all his care."

We agree to consider having Columbia administer IVIG and set a meeting for Damon with Dr. Mason, parting from her on an up note. Heading home, Shealagh and I feel buoyed. Even if Dr. Mason is only half-right—I still have my doubts about her unqualified boosterism—we're still ahead of our expectations. Maybe a heart transplant really *is* the answer to our prayers.

Back home, I reach out to my brain trust, check in with several hospitals, and read up on transplants. But I don't dig in and burrow deep the way I did with PLE. Early on, Sonja, a strong physician ally and a support to the family, says to me, "This isn't like PLE, Doron, where they know so little and you had to become the expert and make every decision. They've been performing heart transplants for thirty years and have excellent systems and protocols in place. They know what they're doing, believe me! You don't need to take it all on yourself. You can relax a little and trust them on this."

I'm not relaxed but I am profoundly *exhausted*, so I'm relieved to hear we don't need to gather our own data, find our own experts, formulate our own medical plan, and second-guess every move that doesn't accord with the best current understanding and practice, or with our own instincts and common sense.

Passively relying on the medical establishment and trusting them to manage my son's care in his best interest is not, as Sonja rightly notes, a luxury I have allowed myself ever since I was jolted by Damon's diagnosis and the lack of appropriate treatment. So it's very tempting to indulge a little now and let them carry the ball for a while.

Even after Damon meets Dr. Mason, is examined by her, and reacts much as we did—"If you listen to Dr. Mason, transplants are so fantastic, *everyone* should have one, even healthy people!" Damon says dryly—I decide to trust the experts. Columbia has a world-class reputation and a seemingly outstanding track record with patients like Damon.

Chapter 40

Yankees slaughter Red Sox first three games but Red Sox come back to win four consecutive games make the world series and baseball history. Due partly to a player who happens to bear the name of Damon.

Which just goes to show you boys and girls: it ain't over till it's over.

It ain't over till its fuckin over.

—From Damon's blog, fall 2004

"I'm tired. I'll go to bed early and do my homework in the morning," Damon says.

Day to day, he continues to struggle. I can see the strain on his body and in his face. The surrounding atmosphere becomes less hospitable to him, the oxygen too thin. Every step takes something out of him.

"I'm out of breath! Where's my inhaler?" he cries.

As his energy wanes, Damon also becomes more moody and snappish. His siblings and his mother bear the brunt of it but occasionally, he's short-tempered with me as well.

It's more than male adolescence, though that's part of the mix. Because he needs me more than most teenage sons need their fathers, or because he needs me in a different way, it's trickier for Damon to vent his anger at me. But he does get around to it, especially when he needs to impress his peers.

One day Damon is hanging in his room with Kyle, Keith, and Keith's boyfriend. The rest of the family is at the front door, about to head to the local cinema, when Miranda says, "I have a stomachache. I don't want to go to the movies!" She marches back upstairs.

I pop into Damon's room, where he and his pals are sprawled on the carpet. "Hey, D-man, could you keep an eye on Miranda for us until we get back? We can't leave her alone in the house and Mom really wants to see this film." I pause. "Mom could use a break."

Although Damon need do nothing except stay where he is with his friends for a few more hours—they had no immediate plans to leave—he suddenly gets his back up.

"No, I don't want to babysit Miranda!" Damon protests. "I'm not doing it!"

"Look, if you don't cover for us, we can't go to the movies," I say.

"Well, that's too bad then!" Damon snarls while his pals look on.

"D-man, that's not very considerate," I remark, taken aback by his insolence. His friends watch to see just how far he will dare push his father.

"I don't care!" Damon taunts, emboldened. "I don't give a shit. It's your problem!"

Now he's crossed the line and I'm ready to discipline him when I spot a heartbreaking, exquisitely pained look on Kyle's face. She knows the score and she's bracing for what is about to happen to her friend. On the spot, I change my mind. I tuck my tail between my legs and walk silently out of the room. We can afford to miss the movie.

Another time Damon is having a late-night party when a bunch of guys and one girl decide to spend the night. Damon wants the girl to sleep in the living room but the rule is that girls need privacy with a closed door. Damon argues vehemently with me, and again I feel his strong need to defy me in front of his friends. But this time I won't cede. "She's sleeping alone in your room while you crash with the other guys, or else she's going home! It's your decision."

Damon challenges me with increasing sharpness, and I must find a middle ground between nurturing his fighting spirit and setting rules. But in private, when it's just the two of us, Damon remains his basic sweet self, albeit broodier. And while his life now revolves around his peers, he remains sensitive about his place in our family and in my affections.

"Hey, D-man, I want to try my first triathlon and there's a short intro race next week in New Jersey," I tell him one day. "It sounds from the website like I need someone to help me. You interested? We could hang out after."

Damon studies his middle-aged father, smiling. "No thanks, I got plans." As I foresaw, carrying my water is hardly his idea of a fun weekend. But I wanted to give him first dibs, as I always do, before going next door to Sam's room, where my prospects are better.

"Yeah, I wanna go!" Sam jumps at the idea of an overnight trip with his dad. For him, it's an adventure and a chance to get me to himself.

As Sam and I prepare to leave on Saturday—I wheel my bike by Sam's room while Sam eagerly grabs his canvas bag and joins me—Damon suddenly steps out of his room.

"Hey, what's up?" Damon rubs sleep from a puffy face. The bustle of activity has caught his attention, especially Sam's animation and high spirits.

"We're driving to that sprint triathlon in Jersey and then a little R and R," I reply.

"Huh?" Damon remains only half-awake and is distracted and irritated by Sam's giddiness. "Sam, could you pipe down please, I'm talking to Dad!"

"Remember that race I invited you to? But you weren't interested?" I prod.

"Oh yeah," Damon recalls. "*That* thing." He still has no real interest in going, but he registers, just as I do, that this is a break in tradition. Until today, this was the special kind of trip that Damon and I would make together, while the rest of the family looked on. But this time, it's Sam and me heading out, with Damon staying behind.

"I packed you guys sandwiches!" Shealagh now appears with Miranda, smiling.

"Does your hotel have a pool?" Miranda asks with keen interest.

"It's a motel, Miranda!" Sam corrects her. His lively face is full of pride at our impending voyage and his designated role as my race assistant.

"Well, good luck, Dad," Damon says, then goes back in his room and closes the door.

Shealagh picks up on Damon's vibe and takes me aside. "This is important for Sam. Damon can't get every outing with you. Look how excited Sam is. He deserves this!"

"I know, I even offered it to Damon first. And I want the time with Sam . . . Still, it feels like Damon is getting bypassed in so many ways now . . ."

"We can't hold the others back," Shealagh says, but I can see she's as upset as I am.

Damon starts to miss school every week, for one, sometimes two, days at a time. He sleeps late and complains of headaches and general weakness and fatigue. When he's not holed up in his overheated room, dozing, playing video games, or hanging out online with friends, he drags around the house with a blanket and wallows in the family room or in our bedroom.

"I'm just resting," he says constantly. I can see him cradling his chest and protecting it. He bends forward and leans on any nearby object—a counter, a chair, a table. As if he feels the heavy weight and mass of his heart, its enlarged physical pendency, and seeks to relieve this burden by transferring it to another, external support.

Occasionally, Damon shakes out his limbs and snaps his fingers with a sudden burst of bravado, as if trying to rouse himself from his torpor. "Yes!" He jumps to attention, as if a bugle call has just awakened him, and he's raring to go. He wants to be his old, active self, even if it takes a self-administered prod to jolt him to his previous state of alertness. But then, with his manufactured stimulus gone, he sinks back into lethargy.

There are small bursts of fun and excitement. Lachlann comes for a visit from the Isle of Skye and the two boys renew their friendship with parties and computer game rooms and boisterous mischief.

For Halloween, Damon summons his creative flair—with a big craft assist from his resourceful mother—and dresses up as a martini glass. He wears a silver bodysuit as the stem while Shealagh configures a pliable mesh frame from a waste-paper basket to serve as the glass bowl. They sheath the bottom in silver and crown Damon's head. Shealagh adds white foam to represent the liquid and a wedge of yellow for the lemon slice and Damon looks sublime and utterly drinkable.

In late fall, I invite Damon and the family to the Hamptons International Film Festival, where I sponsor a program similar to Sundance. I've gone out a few days early for my events, and one day I get a distressed call from Shealagh. She and Damon had spent an entire day at home sitting and waiting for his biweekly IVIG infusion—Damon even missed his rehearsals—but the nurse never came. Columbia, which had taken over his treatment, had canceled the appointment without notifying them.

Shealagh is distraught, close to tears, and Damon is very upset.

Promising to handle it, I call Dr. Mason's office—she's been seeing Damon—but I'm told she's not available. When I explain it's urgent and ask for a home number, I'm tartly informed Dr. Mason does not give out her home number but I can leave a message and she will call me back when she is available. I'm used to such screening methods from Hollywood but not from my son's cardiologists.

Two days later, I finally hear back from Dr. Mason. She professes not to know about the cancelation and says I should speak about it with Dr. Hellenbrand since he's still overseeing Damon's care. I call Dr. Hellenbrand, whose home number I do have because like Dr. Hayes and every *other* doctor who's cared for Damon at Columbia, he gave it to me on our first meeting. Dr. Hellenbrand, who's always been straight with me, swears he knows nothing about this snafu. By now I suspect what happened but it seems so at odds with customary medical behavior that I ask Shealagh to check with the home infusion people. Shealagh calls them and the company confirms it was Dr. Mason's office that canceled the treatments!

Indignant and dismayed, I call Dr. Mason for an explanation. But again, I get her answering service and again, I'm told to leave a message. It's hard to describe my state as I go about my business and wait for another full day until she calls me back.

The call comes as I'm driving, but since Dr. Mason is so elusive, I pull off to the side of the road and ask her to explain her behavior. She says nothing—no denial this time, just silence. Then she asks innocently why I'm upset since the IVIG treatment wasn't doing much good anyway. Irate, I tell her I'm upset because she has committed three major errors, each compounding the previous one.

"First," I tell her, "you made what we believe is a wrong medical decision about stopping IVIG! Not only do we feel IVIG has been helping Damon for over a year, but you professed to support this treatment. Second, even if that decision is medically debatable, you never discussed it with us but went behind our backs and unilaterally canceled a treatment that had become a regular part of our lives! Third, when I confronted you about what happened, you passed the buck and did not accept responsibility!"

I say all this with great heat, and it's clear from her tense silence that Dr. Mason is not used to being addressed in this way. It's also clear she has no defense.

"I don't know who in my office could have canceled the treatment," she says. Then she adds, "But at this point, we don't believe IVIG is helping Damon in a significant way, so I'm not sure what the benefit is anyway."

"Well, we think it's helping him and we're going to continue it!" I respond. I'm on a long flat stretch of Montauk Highway with power lines spooling in either direction and I feel a bitter sadness, even more than anger, that anyone can behave in this fashion. But although I'm appalled by Dr. Mason's conduct, I know to stop short of an irretrievable break because she is part of a powerful system and until or unless I find a better system, Damon's vulnerability may force me to deal with this one. I manage to end the call on a civil note.

Damon comes out to the festival and enjoys the films and the parties. He's now a member of the Screen Actors Guild with a bona fide credit to his name—*Deadwood* will resume broadcast in March, and we've learned he's in the third episode—and he has something to talk about with the other young actors, directors, and producers he meets.

But back home, it's clear Damon is slipping. He sleeps late and misses more days of school. He falls farther behind in his work. He's always trying to catch up and return to normal, but he never quite seems to get there anymore. It's increasingly about what the *next* day or week might bring, but not about the present, which is beset with obstacles.

One night, I come home with Shealagh from a big film premiere and after-party. Shealagh has become more withdrawn as a result of Damon's illness, but tonight my wife agreed to go with me, and despite herself, she had a good time and enjoyed the silly glitter.

As we're about to go up to bed, I notice that Damon's light is still on. I knock on his door and enter. "Hi, D-man. You're up late."

"Yeah, I'm just goofing around." Damon slouches on the low armchair in his overheated room, keyboard on lap, looking chalky pale and exhausted. Dirty cups, half-eaten food, and little balled-up white tissues litter his desk area. All of which I'm used to. What I'm not used to—what, in fact, I have never seen before—is the look of flickering fear and stealthy depression lurking beneath his haggard gaze. It darts across his face like a black cat and quickly hides behind the eyes, where he tries to keep it under wraps.

It tears at my heart and makes me realize how bad things have gotten.

Although I know he wants me to go, I decide I can't leave him alone in such a state. I must find a way to cheer him up, or at least to make that scared look disappear. I start blabbing about the evening's events, dropping names and chattering aimlessly. I don't care what I say, I need to banish the darkness that has settled over him.

Eventually I run out of chatter and exhaust his patience. I'm exhausted myself, and I'm dying to go to bed. I have no more excuses to linger. If I'm lucky, I've diverted him. More likely, I've just pissed him off. But I had to try. I say good night and exit his room.

Only now, I'm too riled myself to go to bed. I step out onto the front porch and look up at the late-fall sky. It's blue-black and chilly, with a pale moon over the park. A brisk wind brushes the tears in my eyes like shards of glass.

I realize tonight is my third and final warning in a dismal sequence. The first was Damon's falling asleep in the car after the Rangers game, and the second his premature exit from the Sundance party. Each episode was completely out of character and showed his illness starting to change him.

Damon is beginning to fall apart before my eyes and he's crying, silently, for help.

I cannot stand by and watch him decline further.

Chapter 41

"Guess I'll die another day, it's not my time to go!"
—*Die Another Day (From the latest James Bond movie)*

Hey what's up all, how are you?

I'm kinda in a weird place right now but that's life and this is most certainly not Wallgreens! I feel like the tapestry that is my life is unwinding and all the threads are blowing in different directions threatening to fly away completely. I want to reach out and grab them and secure them again but if I try for one thread, I am forced to loosen my grip on another and I may lose it entirely, so I just have to sit tight and watch the pieces flying off. And then of course there's that one thread whose color I desperately need to change, as it would make the tapestry much more beautiful and worthwhile. But then of course that thread might not be able to change colors and in trying I might turn it an ugly brown (like when you've mixed too many paints) and if that thread became brown, the entire tapestry would become ugly and not worth looking at, and maybe even not worth working on, I'm not sure. And *that* was my bad metaphor 4 the day.

Goin for a cath this Tuesday (that's like an operation thing where they knock you out, have a needle with a camera on it go through your body and take pictures). It was supposed to be short originally, but now it's not gonna be because other doctors who wanted other data got involved. Which means I'm not gonna make it to rehearsal tomorrow: sigh: damn, look at me letting people down. I should've known though, a medical procedure, me, short!, ahahaha shirley you jest! Well I guess that's all. Gonna go to sleep, sooo tired, but that never changes lately, sleep or no.

—From Damon's blog, fall 2004

"Hey, D-man, got a minute to talk?"

When, after consulting with Shealagh, I finally go into Damon's room to tell him it's time to consider a heart transplant—a decision I've been trying to avoid for three years and a moment I've been dreading for almost as long—he seems to take it better than I do.

"Sure, Dad, come in." Damon logs out of Warcraft, making room for me on the armchair footrest. He *wants* to have this talk. We both know it's not going well, and he looks to me, as always, for the game plan. I swallow hard.

"So, we're now looking at the heart transplant as our best shot. It has a lot going for it, more than I at first believed. It could be *the* solution." My eyes mist up. Damon has been counting on me, and I owe him an accounting. "I've tried everything. You know there's nothing I wouldn't do for you, D-man!" I tense my left hand and slice like a guillotine across my right arm.

Damon nods. He knows.

I clear my throat and run through the basics: that we haven't made a final decision on the hospital, but Columbia has very good outcomes with heart transplants for PLE patients like Damon. And while there will be new immune issues with a transplant, they're all manageable and consistent with a full and active life. "The operation carries some risk, but after, you'll have a new, fully functioning heart with new energy, D-man! And you'll be able to grow!"

Damon, absorbing every word, looks soberly relieved. He nods. "That makes sense, Dad." He knows he's in trouble and glad we have something new to try. He understands better than I do that the present situation cannot continue. "Be nice to put this whole thing behind me!" His face shows new hope and resolve.

We make an appointment with Dr. Mason's office and are assigned to her colleague Dr. Clarice Davis. The pediatric transplant group has four

cardiologists, all women, with Dr. Mason and Dr. Davis the senior members—though Dr. Davis, like the others, clearly defers to Dr. Mason, the
director.

"Damon, why don't you pull up your shirt so I can listen to your heart?"
Dr. Davis smiles in her correct, well-groomed manner. She examines Damon
and reviews his medical history, but the purpose of this visit is to go over the
heart transplant and what it entails. Heart transplants are big business—half a
million dollars a pop—and even the busiest places like Columbia handle only
about twenty pediatric cases a year, so each one matters to the bottom line.

"Do you feel tired even after you've slept? Is it hard just to do normal
stuff, like walking?" Dr. Davis runs through the standard questions about our
son's symptoms and quality of life, nodding each time. Suddenly she looks
up from her notes.

"You've tried everything, but sometimes your old heart just isn't up to it
anymore, is it?" she coos softly, as if his heart is a beloved, ailing pet on its
last legs.

Damon, our stoic, long-suffering son, looks disarmed. He nods. "Yeah."

"I know," Dr. Davis says. "But don't worry. We're going to get you a new
heart, and you'll be much better!"

I feel moved by the simplicity and directness of this statement, and by
Damon's frank response to it. I realize Dr. Davis has used this language
before—it's what she does for a living. Nevertheless, it's a sweet, touching
gesture that also shows a rather blunt, replace-the-battery optimism. Apparently, we've come to the right store.

Before getting listed for a transplant, Damon needs a catheterization to
confirm his pressures and other heart functions are good enough to make a
transplant workable. Donor hearts are in short supply, and Damon must pass
the test to get approval as a worthy candidate. Assuming he qualifies, we are
told Columbia's leading reputation, its regional primacy as a transplant center, and Damon's lifelong affiliation with the hospital will all help to ensure
he has priority and will get a heart within a reasonable time.

Dr. Hellenbrand will do the catheterization himself. Meanwhile, at our
request, he has reinstated the IVIG treatments and also doubled Damon's
diuretic, helping him shed five pounds. But despite short-term boosts from
the IVIG, Damon continues on a downward course. He misses entire weeks
of school and often sleeps well into the afternoon, going in only for play
rehearsals.

"Why don't we get Andre Lawe back to tutor you at home?" I suggest.

"If I take a leave, they might not let me enter the building to direct the school play!" Damon explains. He's been actively engaged with every aspect of *The Man Who Came to Dinner*, slated for mid-December. Auditions proved tricky because most of the actors were his friends but he's made the tough decisions and has the cast he wants. Now he must rehearse them every day and maintain his own energy.

When Damon arrives with his pals at my office for the annual Rhodes Scholarship filing, I'm struck by his scrunched, pallid appearance. He looks almost ghostly under the bright lights. And he moves in such slow motion that I simply discount his contribution to the folders. But he still manages to join in all the fun and after I buy everyone dinner, he pleads with me to take the remaining group to a midnight movie, *Team America: World Police*, a dirty-minded, howlingly transgressive satire that has the kids rolling in the aisles.

Damon goes in for his catheterization a week later. Inside the chilled operating theater, we must again watch our son laid out on the lone bed like a specimen while giant, C-shaped steel arms twist around his frail body and a half dozen masked faces peer at him with disembodied eyes. He succumbs fast to the anesthesia and then Shealagh and I must leave and go down the hall to wait, the loneliest walk in the world no matter how many times you make it.

My wife and I sit in the waiting room until Dr. Hellenbrand—his presence is the most reassuring thing about this day—comes out to tell us all went well and Damon is awake. He confirms that Damon has a good working fenestration so refenestration does not seem warranted, as Dr. Chin suggested, nor does pacing.

"All in all, Damon appears in better shape than many transplant candidates," Dr. Hellenbrand says with a workmanlike nod. "They'll need to take down his Fontan but his anatomical wiring is all in place and we found nothing problematic. He seems good to go!"

By Friday, Damon's results have been processed, and he's formally approved as a candidate for the transplant list.

Shealagh and I are pleased but we don't list Damon right away because we want to make sure we've given every nontransplant option a chance. And we're still not 100 percent convinced Columbia is the best hospital. Plus we want to wait until after Damon's play.

"It's three weeks away and rehearsals are the one thing that gets him out of bed. Otherwise, he's sleeping later and has even less energy," Shealagh says.

I send Dr. Chin Damon's cath results and he agrees they do not support a refenestration or pacing but he suggests we try digitalis. I talk to Dr. Warnes at the Mayo Clinic and she says we can try fractionated heparin. Even while preparing for a transplant, we explore every possible alternative.

Thanksgiving we spend quietly at home, just the five of us, since my parents and my sister have their own plans, and we're in a muted, defensive posture. Our old oven was on the fritz so we've just purchased a new one, and the big holiday turkey comes out looking golden and gleaming. Shealagh has prepared a handsome feast and everyone enjoys the good eating.

"Let's give thanks." I raise a cider glass. "To the family: Damon, Sam, Miranda, and Mom and Dad. And to Grandma and Granddad and Anat."

"And to Toby and Turpin and Julie and Granny," Damon says with a wink at me.

"And to Freddie!" Sam says as the nonperson in question licks his sly chops, sniffing the warm gravy. "How could you forget Freddie!"

"And to Rocky!" Miranda cries as her guinea pig squeaks in the next room.

"Yes, to all." Shealagh lifts a glass. "To health, prosperity, and happiness!"

"Cheers!" I say as we all clink and drink. I look at the assembled gathering.

"A special salute to Damon for directing his first play!" I smile at him.

"Here, here!" Shealagh chimes. "And to Sam, for winning first place in the debate competition!" She shows off Sam's fancy gold medal, a recent triumph. If either Damon or Miranda had won such a trophy, we'd have been pleased, but coming from tight-lipped Sam, it's close to astonishing, a reminder our middle son is full of surprises and trying to pick up the slack in his own way.

"And to Miranda for advancing to the next level in Irish dance!" I add.

"Thank you, Dad!" Miranda beams at me and sticks her tongue out at Sam.

We play Trivial Pursuit after, with sharp sibling bickering and one-upmanship, and then Damon screens the 1930s movie version of *The Man Who Came to Dinner*. We review and analyze it in great detail.

"At least the actors all know their lines," Damon observes.

While the family watches TV, I slip off to my study. Traditionally, I try to do something civic-minded with Damon on this holiday, like helping in soup kitchens, but his current state precludes such activity. So instead, I decide to pick a charity and send a contribution in Damon's name. Part tradition, part superstition, since I'm trying to align all the universe's forces on our side. And I know, despite our unrelieved sense of crisis, that we're not the only ones who are suffering.

Surfing the Net, Have a Heart: Adopt a Soldier catches my attention for obvious reasons. It's an effort to provide our forces fighting in Iraq with personal items to ease their overseas tour. Although the war is unpopular, I've reminded Damon that regardless of one's politics, there are young men and women still fighting and shedding their blood for us every day, just as during Vietnam, and we can't forget them. Damon will be seventeen on his next birthday, the same age as some of these troops, and I've always thought of him as a soldier in his own war.

So now I write a check and follow instructions, which includes sending a photo of Damon, first name only, with a short message. I scroll quickly through my digital camera—Shealagh thinks I'm sneaking off to check e-mail and is yelling for me to come back—when I find a good picture of Damon, standing in front of a horse, with a glorious smile on his face. It's from that memorable day we rode with Gary to the top of Griffith Park. I'm struck now, glancing backward, by how unwell Damon looks in most of the recent photos, but in this shot, I got lucky and caught him in a blessed moment, when the light was just right and fell lovingly across his red hair and radiant smile.

I print out the photo, and on the blank side, in my own hand, I tell my adopted soldier about Damon's long, hard campaign, and how I pray that by next Thanksgiving, the two of them will be back home, safe and sound.

Chapter 42

"But there's no need for turning back 'cause all roads lead to where I stand, and I believe I've walked them all no matter what I may have planned."

—Don McLean (Crossroads)

—From Damon's blog, December 2004

In seeking the best hospital for Damon's heart transplant operation, New York-Presbyterian/Columbia University Medical Center remains the place to beat. Not so much because of its reputation or because Damon has been a patient there all his life and will thus get priority—though these factors do carry weight—but primarily due to Columbia's unparalleled experience with post-Fontan PLE transplants—with patients just like Damon.

When Dr. Mason first hands me the raw, pre-publication statistics from her study—she presents them proudly, as if they vindicate her claims—I am jolted by the numbers.

"Hold on. If I add all this up, it means forty percent of patients who received new hearts died during the operation, or shortly thereafter?" I stare at Dr. Mason with a sick feeling in my stomach. "That doesn't sound like a great cure rate to me!"

"Yes, but look at the dates!" Dr. Mason explains that almost all the deaths occurred in the 1970s and early '80s, when patients were much sicker than Damon before they ever went in for their transplant. Several were on ventilators and could no longer function on their own. Columbia's recent outcomes for post-Fontan PLEs are vastly improved. Virtually all are successful. "We've learned how to do this today and solved the earlier problems!" She smiles.

I look more closely at the numbers and see that Dr. Mason is right. For the earlier and more debilitated patients who died, all the fatalities occurred within twenty-four hours of the transplant or soon after. But for the more recent patients who survived to discharge from the hospital—average length of stay, four weeks—the five-year survival rate was 96 percent and the ten-year survival rate was 92 percent, astonishingly good figures, especially when one considers that Damon generally *beats* the spread.

"And it looks like *all* the PLE patients who made it to discharge saw their PLE resolve *completely*," I say excitedly because this issue had concerned me.

"Yes, and long-term, these patients even do moderately *better* than general transplant patients, perhaps because they're more compliant about their meds."

"This is great news!" I declare, ready to hug Dr. Mason. "It means our biggest challenge will be to get Damon through the operation and past the monthlong recovery period so he can come home. Based on these numbers, once he's discharged from the hospital post-transplant, Damon's prognosis looks *excellent*."

"Yes, though the first year is also important," Dr. Mason says. "He has to comply with all his meds and we have to keep a close watch over him."

"Sure"—I nod—"but Damon is a model patient, well schooled in compliance from his years of PLE . . . And Shealagh and I are scrupulous and seasoned patient parents . . . Plus, you guys have a *whole team* that specializes in post-transplant care!"

"Oh yes, we're nationally ranked." Dr. Mason nods. "In the top three."

"Great!" I say. Despite the well-documented dangers, this sounds better than I'd dared hope. Dr. Mason's study—I notice Dr. Davis and Dr. Q are coauthors—will become my key document. I parse every line and pore over every statistic. Since it's not yet in print, I relay its data, with permission, to cardiologists at other hospitals and ask how their numbers and their success rates stack up.

Comparing outcomes and judging relative performance would seem like an obvious basis for making an informed decision about a matter of life and death for our son. Since every hospital I've talked to has volunteered to perform Damon's transplant—the half-million-dollar fee again!—I want to know how well they've done with similar patients and similar operations in the past. A no-brainer, one might assume.

But apparently not, I explain in frustration to my wife.

"No one can answer my most basic questions because there's no central database or any systematic method for tracking the number of operations with these types of patients, nor is there any obligation to report outcomes and success rates to patients and their families. And no hospital wants to divulge its numbers because it's a competitive game, and a rival hospital could have *better* numbers."

"They want to filter the information and have it all their way," Shealagh says, as frustrated as I am. "It's not right."

"No. They're effectively asking us to fly *blind,* and to rely on subjective terms such as 'good name' and 'reputation' and unreliable methods such as self-reporting or 'best hospitals' lists . . . To be fair, Columbia normally would not release its numbers and it's only because they happen to be doing a retrospective study—a study that shows them in a positive light and will be good for their bottom line—that they've agreed, after my badgering, to share their data with me."

"Still, at least we have *something* from them," Shealagh says.

"Yes! We can use it as a yardstick with the other top institutions." I nod.

I call up Dr. Michael Freed at Boston Children's Hospital, a cardiologist who's reviewed Damon's case for me. Like everyone, Dr. Freed cautions there are many factors in choosing the right place and raw numbers don't tell the full story.

"Statistics can be read in many ways; the devil is in the details," he warns me.

"True, and the number and success rate of PLE transplants won't be our sole criterion, but it's *one* hard measure, and without it we're missing key data."

After more debate, Dr. Freed allows he has not seen Columbia's study. "But if these numbers are right, I don't think Boston Children's can match them."

I phone Dr. Warnes at the Mayo Clinic. She is surprised both by the number of post-Fontan PLE transplants Columbia has done and by their success rate. Because I admire the Mayo Clinic's approach to patient care, I invite Dr. Warnes to tell me why I should take Damon to Minnesota for his heart transplant. But Dr. Warnes, who assumed the Mayo Clinic had the largest transplant population for every category—she poses a number of astute questions about Columbia's data—is scrupulous and balanced, as always.

"I cannot, in good conscience, claim that Mayo has greater experience or greater success with this specific patient subgroup than what Columbia is reporting," she tells me.

Finally, I call up Dr. Chin, who's been as involved in our case and as helpful as anyone. Yet even Dr. Chin, despite his proven commitment to us, cannot assist us here. He sends us to the surgeon Dr. Spray, who sends us to the transplant program medical director, Dr. Chrisant. Dr. Chrisant once worked at Columbia and is, in fact, a coauthor on the Mason study—it's a tiny, rarefied world and they all know each other, as I've discovered. But Dr. Chrisant, after trying to recruit us as patients, is unforthcoming. "We don't have aggregate data on our Fontan patients I can send you," she says.

Even at Dr. Chin's institution, I cannot get hard data! Dr. Chrisant's reticence leads me to conclude that CHOP's experience must lag Columbia's.

I continue talking to everyone I can. Perhaps no expert better sums up the reasons for staying with Columbia than Dr. Bruce Gelb, a cardiologist at Mount Sinai. I consulted with Bruce fifteen years earlier, shortly after Damon's birth, when he was starting out and I knew his father. Bruce is my cohort, and he's on the ball, so we quickly plug back in.

Bruce sympathizes with my inability to get good comparative data for Damon's operation and admits each hospital is a fiefdom, a world unto itself in a Balkanized system.

"As for choosing the right hospital, I know Tom Spray and he's one of the best, but at the end of the day, the transplant surgery, even in Damon's case, is not that complex. You and I couldn't do it, but for the top cardiothoracic surgeons, it's just another operation. Any of the leading guys at the major institutions can handle Damon's transplant, including ours, which has a world-class team, in case you're interested . . ."

Bruce smiles when he says this, and we both understand he's just doing his job.

"But with transplants, the aftercare is as important as the surgery, so a hospital's proximity is critical," Bruce says. "You'll have to come in often during the first year after transplant. If Damon is showing any signs of rejection or infection, the two most common problems, you'll need to bring him in right away, night or day. So driving two hours to Philly to check on every sniffle may not be very convenient. Whereas Columbia, much closer to your home, and accessible via subway or car, sounds more practical for you."

"I don't mind the inconvenience if it will give Damon a better chance," I say.

"Sure. But look, I know Amelia Mason and her team, and they're fine, as capable as any of the other groups, so it probably makes sense to stay there. Columbia has been treating Damon all his life and they will have his full medical records as well as a long institutional memory and a sense that he's their patient, which can also help."

Bruce makes a persuasive case, especially when I consider the Mason study shows that if Damon makes it home from his transplant, he has a 100 percent chance of surviving the difficult first year with Columbia. Those are odds *no one* can beat, and even if I don't expect it to be easy, this is Columbia's specialty, and they're apparently very good at it.

Dr. Mason may not have started as my favorite physician but if she can help ensure a good outcome for my son, I'll be her best friend and number one fan. In fact, my highly plastic brain already is embarked on a makeover for the now-essential Mason.

The clincher is Damon. "I want to stay at Columbia for my transplant," he states.

It's not any individual doctor that wins Damon over. In fact, he seems to share our concerns now that the straightforward Dr. Hellenbrand has handed us over to the more nebulous "pediatric transplant group." But Damon does harbor a sense of loyalty and faith in the institution that's treated him from birth. Or perhaps it's just a need for reassurance, a feeling of greater comfort with a place he's known all his life. Whatever it is, I've learned to listen closely to Damon and to trust his instincts and try to honor them when I can.

If I had good evidence to the contrary—for example, if another hospital had a markedly higher success rate—I might have to reconsider. But in the absence of such counterevidence, I work on the assumption that Damon knows things we don't or can't know, and if he feels better, or more secure, he'll do better.

And the data is so strong. It's nice to think we've been at the right place all along.

Chapter 43

You see I can't seem to sleep
But fear not it's not cause I weep
I'm tired as hell
but see there's a bell
incessantly ringing
do you know what to do?
can you stop the dingdinging?
a bell in your head?
No no no, you misread
more like a thousand all goin off in my mind
and no matter what I can't stop, pause or rewind
these thoughts that are flowing
Where the hell am I going?

—From *Damon's blog, December 2004*

Damon sleeps longer and longer now that he's on home tutoring again. Some days it looks like he'd go on sleeping into the next night if we didn't wake him up, as he's asked us to, for after-school rehearsals. The Tech fall production, only two weeks away, has become the focus of his remaining energy and drive.

"I can't miss one rehearsal!" Damon says. "We still have a long way to go!"

He rises around one P.M., instantly alert, and knows exactly what he must do. He showers, dresses, and composes the daily cast sheet, printing copies.

Then he jabs a heparin injection into his bruised flesh. "I hardly feel it anymore," he says.

Damon pads down to the family room. "Freddie boy!" he greets the pooch, who rushes excitedly at him. Using an old towel, Damon begins to spin his dog through the air. Freddie's gleeful teeth grab on to the ropy cotton as he swings in a low arc about Damon's rotating trunk, almost *willing* himself off the ground and into orbital compliance as he sails prettily about his paling Svengali. Even now, no one quite possesses Damon's showmanship. But like everything else, this trick is becoming harder for Damon to pull off, and he soon tires.

Damon heads to the kitchen and gathers his stockpile from the cabinet and fridge. "Here we go!" He perches on the high stool and begins to slog through his pills, vitamins, supplements, and oils. The more recalcitrant ingestibles he coats with applesauce.

"Let's see what's playing." He remotely clicks on the small TV above the counter and gloms onto any diversion while swigging, swallowing, and gagging his way through his daily stations of the oral cross.

It's a quick fifteen-minute car ride to school, and Shealagh is eager to drive Damon and spare his diminishing strength. She tries to coax him to eat something solid, an apple or other fruit at home and, if he's up to it, an Egg McMuffin ("hold the cheese") at the drive-through on the way to Tech. Damon usually arrives just as school is letting out, around three P.M., and heads into the South Elliott Place entrance. A resolute, pint-sized figure, he braves the giddy stampede of a thousand bodies pouring from the building, high-fives a few friends, and makes his way inside. He's popular with the security guards at the sign-in desk, which helps, since technically he's no longer enrolled at the school.

"Just gonna rehearse." Damon smiles. He heads for the big auditorium and enters a cavernous, semi-desolate space with a sunken orchestra pit below a vast, remote stage. A scattering of students hang off the railing while factions loiter in wayward aisles and shadowy corners. But Damon's arrival, like the sheriff hitting town, presages the dawn of order and coherence.

"Hey, everyone, Damon's here! Time to get started!"

The director in every sense, Damon knows his audience and comes prepared. "Okay, listen up, here's your daily sheet!" He hands out a typed list with the day's scenes and activities laid out. Damon can count on a few allies: the drama mentor, Mr. Wasserstein; Alexandra, a talented actress and president of the drama club; Josh, the reliable stage manager; and Damon's good buddy Max, his right-hand man. But teen discipline and attention span can still be erratic, so Damon introduces new routines.

"I got a new tape with some great chill-out music!" Grinning, Damon pops the latest New Age tracks into the player and the ambient music instantly alters the mood. He leads the class in exercises, focusing them before they start rehearsing.

But new problems arise, starting with the issue of a life-sized wooden sarcophagus into which a scheming character is enticed. Lifting the tall box with a live body inside is tricky, while the lid keeps sticking, raising claustrophobic alarms and wild banging from within: "Get me outta here!"

Damon also must deal with the anxiety of a young actress worried she won't be able to kiss a fellow actor, as the scene demands, because of his unromantic appearance.

"I know it's hard," Damon says. "Just close your eyes and pretend he's Brad Pitt."

More ominously, Damon loses his lead at the eleventh hour, jeopardizing the entire show. The director must scramble to keep the production from imploding.

"Okay, I need someone who can learn all of Sheridan Whiteside's lines and carry the play with less than two weeks to go!" Damon sighs.

As if things aren't bad enough, the drama club needs extra money for the production. Shealagh and I underwrite some costs, and Damon hawks knickknacks with his friends at school lunch to raise more funds.

For props and costumes, Damon's biggest asset is his mother. When he needs an antique 1930s suitcase, eagle-eyed Shealagh spots a canvas case with leather handles out on the sidewalk. For an old-fashioned feather duster, Shealagh finds a good bamboo-handled facsimile in Chinatown. For period dresses, Shealagh rummages through the racks at the Salvation Army. When she can't improvise, Shealagh drives Damon and the costume designer, Vlada, to the big costume warehouse in midtown and buys them the right outfits.

It's hard to believe Damon is overseeing every facet of this sprawling production and rehearsing his actors—including the new lead, who doesn't yet know his lines—in the midst of his deteriorating health and the ticking transplant clock. But he is.

We've agreed that right after the play, I'll take Damon to L.A. to see his

Deadwood pals before we list him for a transplant. Once listed, Damon can't travel, nor will any of us dare to leave home base, until he gets his new heart. The offer could come at any hour—usually from a car accident or sudden trauma—and we have to be ready to move fast.

"They estimate the average wait is three to six months, but I think it could happen sooner given your size, blood type, status, hospital, and other preferential circumstances," I tell Damon. "But we can't count on that, and no one can promise us anything. So we have to prepare to put our lives on hold and be on call around the clock, for an indefinite period."

Given this imminent lockdown, I make a quick business trip to Paris just before Damon's play. During a free afternoon, I take off like a cooped-up kangaroo and hop for miles through the city where I once lived and studied, turned twenty-one, and had one of the great love affairs of my youth. I cover half the metropolis on foot, striding at breakneck speed. Finally, I circle back to Trocadéro, where the old cinematheque served as my second home; shoot past Balzac's house; and descend the rue Raynouard, where the cops would stop and hassle me for driving my girlfriend on the back of my Mobylette.

I'm pleased to find the apartment building where I rented a tiny *chambre de bonne* is still there, with its narrow attic window overlooking the Eiffel Tower. But what most strikes me on my swift walkabout, other than my blistering feet, is how *altered* my life now is. I search in vain for the ambitious, romantic young man who hungered after every intimation of beauty and truth this magical city seemed to offer, and who threw himself headlong into love and art—the two seemed inextricable—believing no higher goal or nobler purpose existed. The notion of marriage and kids never entered *his* consciousness.

Yet now I live for my wife and my children, and Damon has become the center of my existence. It occurs to me *he* is my romance now, or some platonic version thereof, and I love him and fight for him with the same ardor I once reserved for the love of beautiful women and the pursuit of artistic inspiration.

I'm still pondering this back home in Brooklyn, sitting in the kitchen with Damon on Saturday afternoon. Shealagh has taken Sam and Miranda ice-skating in Prospect Park, so it's just the two of us. Damon is downing his pills, slowly, which is how he does everything now, when he turns to me. "So how was Paris, Dad?"

I can't tell whether he's really interested or just passing the time while taking his meds, but soon he's probing boldly and has me saying more than I intended. Under deft interrogation, I tell Damon about falling madly in love the summer of my freshman year in college and cohabiting with a wild spirit.

"Where did you meet her?" Damon asks.

"On the beach in St. Tropez. We were lovers before I knew her name—or how many other guys she was still seeing." I glance at my son, realizing I've passed the point of no return. "She was eighteen and hard to resist. I was nineteen."

"Cool." Damon nods as if I'm showing him a bootleg film, with his unrecognizable father in an unfamiliar role. "Then what happened?"

"She led me on a mad chase, I followed her halfway across France, persevered, but refused to let it be a summer fling. I came back the next year, and we lived together in Paris while I went to university, or tried to . . . It was an exciting roller coaster, but then the ride ended. It's hard to be free of any social rules and live only on the edge of each moment. She was bolder and more out-there than me, but a little unstable too, and it got worse."

"How?" Damon tries to sound casual and downplay his avid interest.

"Well, there were lots of things . . ." I sigh. "I guess the short version is, sometime after me, she spent six years in prison for accidentally killing her lover."

Now I have Damon's complete attention in a different way.

"She didn't intend to," I quickly explain. "I think she wanted to settle down with this guy. But the knife slipped."

"What was she doing with a *knife*?" Damon screws up his features.

"It's complicated . . . She was a purely spontaneous person, always true to her impulses. That can be dangerous but also very alluring, especially when the transgressing person happens to be beautiful. I fell hard for her. I was young."

Damon's lips drift into a secret smile as he processes this information.

"Probably better if we don't let your mother know we discussed this." I wink at him. "And of course, not a word to Sam or Miranda."

"Of course." Damon nods. "Thanks for telling me, Dad."

"Yeah, no problem. You asked, I answered. I don't regret any of it, though we both got hurt. She once asked me, years later, if it was possible to love too much . . . The moral, in my view, is *go for it*—whatever 'it' turns out to be for you."

Damon raises an earnest, pale ginger eyebrow. "How will I know?"

"You'll know, believe me!" I chuckle but Damon isn't satisfied.

"It's easy for you, Dad, because you always got what you wanted."

I laugh, flattered he'd think so. "Not always, D-man, not always! No one ever does. Not if you're playing for real."

Damon studies me, taking this in. "I'm still not sure how I'll be able to tell."

"If you want to break it down," I reply, "when you're willing to lose everything and make any sacrifice, including giving up fiercely held notions of yourself, you'll know."

Damon looks like he's still trying to get a handle on this. I smile.

"You have wonderful surprises and undreamed-of delights in store, but you'll know what's true when it appears. I have total confidence in your abilities."

"If you say so, Dad." Damon gives me a skeptical but intrigued look.

That evening we all go to see *Finding Neverland*. The film explores the life of J. M. Barrie, the author of *Peter Pan*, and reveals that Barrie lost his older brother as a child and created the figure of Peter Pan and the notion of Neverland, a place where no one grows old or dies, in part to try to console his shattered mother.

I thought I was taking my family to a nice holiday movie but I leave the theater feeling as if we've all been ambushed in the dark and forced to confront a taboo subject. It seems there's no escaping our predicament. But as we drink hot chocolate and unwind after, everyone says they liked the film and no one seems upset.

I don't share my feelings with anyone—I don't wish to think about them myself—but the next day, after working at my desk all morning, Damon approaches me in the kitchen. He's been notably warmer since I shared my past.

"How's your novel going, Dad?" He fixes his sparkling eyes on me.

"Okay." In truth, I haven't been able to write for months due to his situation but I continue to jot notes on my plot and characters. So now I mention a major shift given fresh impetus by the film we just saw. "I'm moving away from *Romeo and Juliet* and toward *The Tempest*."

I'm using literary shorthand, but Damon instantly gets what I'm saying. Soon, I'm telling him as much about my novel as I've told anyone, and he's not only nodding as if he understands, he's asking me astute, penetrating questions.

It's an epiphany for me. I'm simply floored that this young man sitting across from me, whose education and development I've helped guide at every stage, is now providing *me* with enlightened feedback on my own creative work.

There aren't more than three or four people in the world I can usefully talk to about my writing—who know enough, and care enough—and suddenly I realize my son has become one of them!

It's like waking up to find an amazing gift under my pillow or a priceless gold coin in my backyard.

The universe has just become that much less vast-seeming and solitary for me.

Chapter 44

Damon Weber (Director, Vice President of the Drama Club): *The Man Who Came to Dinner* is a simple comedy about not so simple people. So was the process that led to the production you are about to see. Like Mr. Stanley, I was not the same person by the end. The play before you is the result of two months hard work by a wonderful, charismatic cast and a dedicated and committed crew whom I've been lucky to work with. Although we had our fair share of octopuses, large bills and the occasional cockroach, we somehow managed to pull through. I would like to thank my parents, especially my mom for her much needed assistance with props and costumes. Lastly, I would like to thank everyone who came here tonight because the audience is what brings a play to life.

> —From the playbill to the Brooklyn Technical High School
> production of *The Man Who Came to Dinner*,
> December 2004

We sit on the floor along the proscenium of the stage with our winter coats on our laps, and a profusion of hats, scarves, Kleenex, and cough drops scattered at our feet. Almost everyone has come to support a friend or relative.

This overstuffed drawing room farce by George S. Kaufman and Moss Hart is a somewhat dated screwball romp, and most of the time Damon has his hands full just keeping the sprawling twenty-nine-person ensemble on their marks and on cue. But the dialogue and action keep flowing at a good pace with no showstopping snafus—the lead relies on youthful cockiness and sheer exuberance when his actual lines elude him—and there are myriad comic turns and hilarious caricatures. Even the upright mummy case is effective.

When it's over, the audience applauds and gathers around the cast but I remain seated, still mulling the subtle shaping intelligence of Damon's direction.

"Did you just see what I saw?" I turn to Krista, a theater teacher.

"Nice job. He improved on the film version in a couple places," she says with a smile.

"Damon, Damon!" The cast clamors for the director to join them onstage.

Damon jogs up and takes a quick, deep bow at the waist, the suave young director in his glory. For the first time, I realize the true depth of his artistry.

Afterward, our proud family congratulates him. "Damon, did you get that girl out of the mummy case yet?" Miranda looks concerned. Then we all wait as he wanders through the auditorium and makes his good-byes one by one.

"Think he has any idea how good he is?" I ask Shealagh.

"It's hard to tell but I think he's just happy he managed to get out of bed and stand here tonight!" Shealagh says with a mix of welling pride and relief.

I continue pondering Damon's craft as we meander up chilly DeKalb Avenue and troop into Applebee's with his pals. It's crowded and noisy on a Saturday night, and we have to wait for several tables so we can all sit together.

Damon is several seats away from me, ensconced with Kyle and his other buddies, so I cup my hands above the din to get his attention.

"Amazing job, D-man! You really showed me something new tonight!"

The play is already old news and Damon is eager to keep up with his friends and their latest preoccupation, but he still manages a quick, grateful smile my way. "Thanks, Dad."

I try not to think about how pale he looks. For tonight, his accomplishment imbues him with a shining luster, and as I sit back in my molded plastic chair in this packed, voluble, and stupefyingly ordinary chain restaurant, I'm proud to salute an emerging young artist and to place an honorary crown on his head.

With the countdown to transplant ticking loudly, Damon and I fly to L.A. and visit the *Deadwood* set. It's as if outside time has stood still in that remote canyon. We see all our buddies and the cast members as they troop into the dining tent in their 1870s frontier garb and makeup after several hours of shooting.

David Milch tells Damon that every person who's watched his performance was knocked out by it and asks Damon to take a first pass at writing his own expanded part for next season.

"Wow, thanks, that sounds like a cool opportunity," Damon says.

"You bet your ass it is." David grins. "But I know you have good ideas."

The rodeo star Gary Leffew, who didn't know of Damon's illness, is shocked by the news and amazed he still rode with us. "So it's showdown time? He's gonna do great, I ain't seen no man tough as Damon . . . I'll be pullin' for him with all I got! For you too, my friend! Stay strong. Ain't nothin' harder than this."

Although we planned to stay on set till nighttime, Damon runs out of energy—I'm struck by his deteriorations since the summer—and we must leave early. As we make our somber farewells, David Milch approaches Damon very gingerly and asks if he can give him a kiss.

Damon pauses to consider, then slowly nods.

The actress Paula Malcomson meets us for tea the next day and shares the same easy rapport with Damon. "They finished editing your scene and it looks fuckin' great, Damon . . . So how was directing your first play? Aren't actors a pain in the ass?"

Later Damon and I are sitting poolside when his friend Max calls from New York, frantic because he couldn't reach Damon and feared he'd gone in for his transplant.

After Damon calms Max down, we wade into the pool and toss a rubber ball back and forth. I notice Damon, a tad wobbly, still catches my throw each time. I recall when we spent hours practicing to improve his motor skills but now he can handle anything that comes his way. We toss the ball, ten, twenty, thirty times . . . We pass fifty, then a hundred throws, hooked in the back-and-forth. I watch Damon in red swim trunks as he zeroes in on the flying orb and nabs it with perfect hand-eye coordination each time. How can a boy so ill be this proficient? Can I really let them *rip out and replace* the heart of such a flawless performer?

Our last night, I take Damon to the premiere of *Meet the Fockers* and he has a good giggle over this star-studded comedy. Then we head to the gala reception under a huge tent, where I introduce him to various film people I know.

We spot the actor Dustin Hoffman, surrounded by security and a crush of fans. I sponsored a panel with Hoffman two years earlier, and after I prod him, he recalls the event, claims to remember me, and lets me introduce him to my son.

"So what kind of acting have you done?" Hoffman asks. He wears makeup above his powder blue shirt and actually listens and responds to Damon.

Damon's face lights up as they talk, and not just because Hoffman is a major star, a genuine talent, and an intelligent conversationalist. What also hits Damon—right between the eyes, as it were—is that Hoffman is not much taller than he is!

I watch my son rise on the balls of his feet and lift up his head as he discusses their shared love of the craft with the renowned actor and registers that *this could be him*. It's involuntary and owes as much to other similarities he can sense close-up, but the size is a leveler exposing a deeper truth: *Hey, maybe I could do this.*

Damon is far too modest to utter such a thought, but I see the flash of recognition in his face as he stands and holds his own beside Hoffman.

As I watch the two dapper figures, their heads bent close, bright-eyed and smiling, I'm struck that despite the fifty-year age difference, they have something important in common. And I grasp that if Damon continues on his current path, and if he keeps getting the right breaks, Hoffman represents one kind of actor route, or a plausible acting context, for such a career direction. It's a heady thought, but I don't feel grand or prideful about it. It's just one possible window into Damon's future, and Damon might not even choose that path, nor am I sure it's the best path for him. And of course he might fail, if he did choose it. But it's a preview of, and a highly privileged glimpse into, where, theoretically, Damon could fit in, if that were the path he followed.

Chapter 45

It's a bird, it's a plane, no it's Damon updating! Lol Hey everyone,
I'm back. What tis up? So lots has happened but you get none of it.
So anyone know a good place to have a New Year's party cause I feel
like relaxing this new year aka not hosting the group's New Year's
party lol. I still love you all, some more than others . . . Yeah so, if
anyone's got an idea 4 a New Years' party that doesn't involve the
words "amish country" or "Damon's house" please share . . . Been
playin massive amounts of World of Warcraft and it's been much fun.
Btw why is everyone saying bueno? Well that's all 4 now, later dudes
and dudets.

—From Damon's blog, winter 2004

Having made the General Decision for a heart transplant for Damon, and
having selected our return from L.A. as the Decision Period for getting his
name on the wait list, we now face the Decision Moment—that precise instant when we make The Listing Call.

That triggering act will unleash a cascade of events culminating, if all
goes well, in the surgical removal of Damon's original heart from his chest
cavity and its replacement with the fully functioning heart of another, freshly
deceased individual.

It's a huge step—a leap of faith, as well as science.

"We've consulted *every* medical expert and exhausted *all* known therapeutic options," I tell my wife. "Not a single practical treatment of any kind remains on my list!" I make a show of crumpling the now-useless piece of yellow paper in front of her and trashing it.

We've had to accept not only that transplantation is the sole remaining option but also that we must act soon if we hope to successfully avail ourselves of it.

"He's getting chills and looking more listless and enervated," Sonja notes on her latest visit. "I wouldn't wait much longer."

We see the warning signs and know she's right. From the start, we've understood there was a fine balance between trying to avoid a transplant altogether and not completely closing off the transplant window, so that this procedure remained a viable alternative if none other could be found. Now the balance has tipped. While Damon's latest tests show he's still in relatively decent shape for this operation, time is running out.

Yet now, with the day of reckoning at hand, it becomes challenging to pinpoint the optimal moment for listing Damon. The hospital has provided little guidance. "You can list him whenever you're ready but we don't need to see him for two months," they tell us. Shealagh and I feel it's far more urgent—a matter of weeks or even days, not months—but my wife leaves the exact timing to me. It's a complex, monumental decision, the biggest I've had to make, and I run every scenario to get it right while grappling with powerful, conflicting emotions.

"It could take six months or longer to find him a new heart and he could decline fast before we do, which is one reason to list him now," I tell Shealagh. "But it could also take twenty-four hours to find him a donor heart, which means we must be ready to let him go into the operating room from the minute we list him!"

Every extra day with Damon is precious now. He sleeps late and hangs around the house, playing computer games and blogging and IM-ing his pals. He takes his pills and his shots. He watches a lot of TV, wrapped in a sweatshirt and blankets in the family room.

I catch him when I can, especially around the television set. *Scrubs, Family Guy, What's My Line?* and *Sex and the City* are his current favorites, though he also tunes in to endless reruns and just about anything on Comedy Central. "What you watching, D-man?" I sit beside him no matter what's on and share wry commentary or a wordless communion.

I'm so eager to be near Damon I request a tutorial on World of Warcraft, his most consuming pastime, and spend hours battling monsters and undertaking quests in the trippy kingdom of Kalimdor.

We go to my parents' house in Queens for the first night of Hanukkah, a family tradition. Many relatives and friends are there and all are aware of our situation—Damon looks small and hunched in his *Deadwood* sweatshirt and his bowl-cut hair frames a chalky face—but we try to pretend it's just another holiday.

We lay out our presents by the teak cabinet and gather to light the menorah. The silver candelabrum stands on a cloth that Damon painted in kindergarten: it's filled with his bold, brash colors, all unified by a glorious overarching rainbow, once his signature motif. My wife and I share a wistful pang at this pictorial memento of our firstborn's sunny childhood.

Shealagh has cut her hair short and wears an embroidered purple blouse. She puts on a brave front, but the suffering is etched into her face. Sam and Miranda, both vivid in colorful T-shirts, provide a stark contrast with their subdued older brother. Their careless bouncing energy underscores his sluggishness and increasing marginalization.

As my mother prepares to light the first candle on the antique, finely wrought silver candelabrum, she turns to Damon.

"This menorah is from my home in Leipzig. It belonged to my parents and is one of the few things I had from them before they were killed with all my relatives . . . When the time comes, I'm going to give it to *you* to keep in the family!"

My mother's voice trembles and Damon, who's heard this before, bows his head, humbly acknowledging the firstborn honor. "Thanks, Grandma."

My father hands my mother a prayer book from her home in Germany and takes one from his parents' home in Glasgow. My mother recites the blessing and lights the candles on two menorahs and we sing "Rock of Ages." Damon joins in the rousing victory song. He looks pasty by the glow of the hanging lamp, and his oversized sweatshirt swallows his doughy body, but he's determined to participate in the celebration and adds his conscientious notes to our motley warbling.

"Sammy, what are we celebrating today?" My father dives into his catechism mode as we sit down to eat at the long, resplendent table.

Sam looks at Damon, who shrugs and looks right back at Sam with steely silence. Damon's patience with his siblings has suffered, along with everything else, during this period, even if Sam's veneration of Damon is undiminished.

"The miracle of the oil," Sam pipes up, after seeing he's on his own.

"What kind of oil, like at the petrol pump?" My father keeps a poker face.

"Daddy, spare us the history lesson till later, okay?" my sister cuts in, ostensibly on our guests' behalf. "It's a Jewish holiday, they're all the same. They tried to kill us, we survived, now let's eat!" She grins with tart charm.

"Everyone can sit down. I'll put on the first latkes," my mother says.

I bring out my camcorder and start to pan across the table, noting each attendee. But when I get to Damon, he shifts sideways, out of frame. I wait but he uses his glass of hot cider with cinnamon stick to keep my view obstructed. He's become very resistant to being filmed.

"Come on, D-man, I'm shooting everyone. It's a record of the event."

"No," Damon says. I can't determine if it's because he's more self-conscious about his appearance or if he sees my effort to record him as a tacit admission of uncertainty about the future. Or perhaps it's simply because he's a teenager and I'm his father.

But Damon now regards me and my camera as an intrusion, and I must catch him off guard if I want a clean shot. It's a big change because ever since I filmed Damon as a four-year-old sitting on the doorstep of our Adirondacks cabin—a young boy bathed in sunshine and surrounded by green blades of grass, smiling at a slow summer day—my son and I have had a special rapport through the camera and Damon has always *encouraged* me to record his unfolding glory.

Yet now, even after I respect his wishes and put down my camcorder, Damon remains an elusive figure. He eats sparingly, like a bird, and flits off several times, darting to the bathroom or roaming about the house.

"Is Damon okay?" my mother asks once. "He seems to have disappeared."

"I'll get him," I say, and put down my fork. I search the house and find him upstairs in my old room, lying down on my old bed in the dark. I can't see him at first and it's very quiet, but I feel a faint presence enfolded in the gloom.

"That you, D-man?"

"Yeah, I just came up to phone my friends, and I must've drifted off."

I wait for him to wash his face, and we go back downstairs together.

Later, after the orgy of gift-opening and shredded wrapping paper, Sonja walks over to me, her back to Damon. "You know I'm really very impressed by everything you've done for him. No medical expert in the world could have done more than you have for your son, and you should feel good knowing that."

My sister leans over and says, "I couldn't agree more. You're amazing parents!"

These comments, which I hear from several quarters lately, only increase my anxiety, although I know people mean well. If I'm such a good father, why is my son so sick, and why haven't I been able to make him better? And if the transplant really offers hope, why does everyone sound like they're trying to console me *before* the operation?

My mother walks around and hands out big jelly donuts, pressing the traditional sweets on every guest. Damon politely accepts a donut but lays it aside on the glass table, leans back against a beaded cushion, and closes his eyes. Everyone sees how out-of-it he is.

We wait for a seemly interval and depart, earlier than usual.

We're very close now and it's only a matter of days before we make The Call. Winter break has started and school's out for everyone, not just Damon.

Each morning, we wake up wondering if today is the day, and each evening we find something worth cherishing and holding on to: a small affirmation of what we still have, be it Damon's brief outing to the library or a friend's sleepover, Damon cackling on the phone or plotting a New Year's Eve party. It's surprising what comprises an acceptable quality of life when the alternative is unknown. Never has the status quo looked more appealing and worth hanging on to.

Why give him up, or risk losing him, any sooner than we have to?

There may be some denial and wishful thinking behind our delay. If we just wrap Damon up in our deepest embrace and hunker down, enveloped in the safe cocoon of a love-filled home and its daily routines, surely this will pass?

But there's also a pragmatic, selfish reason for waiting: we don't want to let Damon go one nanosecond before we must, and we feel so connected to him that we trust our own independent monitoring system to signal us when it's time.

The new Columbia study has made us much more optimistic about the risk/benefit ratio for transplants. And there is a strong likelihood of a life-altering *improvement* for Damon. But it's still a dire step.

So we prefer to wait. But I check Damon almost hourly.

One evening, I return to his room to continue our conversation—I left to answer the doorbell—when I find him laid out on the carpet, completely immobile. He's fallen asleep, as if in midsentence, his mouth gaping like a fish's. It's only five P.M. but already dark beyond the curtains. The air inside his overheated room is insufferably close. Sticky spoons and open medicines and white balled-up little tissues litter the ground. I can see the life force ebbing out of my son.

If we wait any longer, we're sealing his fate.

I go upstairs and find Shealagh. "It's time, baby. We gotta do it!"

"I know." She sighs deeply.

I call up Columbia and get Damon listed. It's three days before Christmas.

Chapter 46

Anyway, a belated Happy New Year's to all . . . Went 2 Max's for New Year's twas fun. It's ironic all the days over the break where I was just bumming around (except 4 Max's thing) were the most fun and the days when I had plans wound up sucking . . . Oh if I forgot to mention it, which I think I did, there are whispers of putting me in the hospital . . . coincidentally around the same time, there are also whispers that Damon has started carrying his Turkish knife around: . . . hmm . . . . . . coincidence, I think not. Note 2 self: must sharpen that thing. (what Damon you have a Turkish knife! Uh, where? How come none of us has ever seen it or know where it is?? Think about that question 4 a minute and see if you can't answer it yourself lol.) Thank gosh 4 Krista (my neighbor) 4 rescuing me Friday. I went over 2 her house and watched Jaws (which I'm ashamed to admit I had not seen till tonight, it was awesome) If I am going 2 die I hope its cause someone shoves a big pressurized gas can in my mouth and then shoots it. What a way 2 go lol. Though I don't suppose that's the kind of medical malpractice or mistakes 1 usually hears about: lol. (Oh btw, Krista is 23 so don't get any ideas lol I know how your minds work)Thanx Nicole and Nef 4 your comments. Ok goodnight all.

—From Damon's blog, January 2005

From the start, getting Damon listed for a heart transplant is a flawed process.

When the time finally comes, I take a deep breath and call Dr. Davis at Columbia. It's been a long, painful journey, but now that we're there, I'm hoping for a little orientation and support. I expect she'll be very responsive, since we've accepted their assurances that a heart transplant is the right way to go and they are the right people for the job.

However, despite the excruciating struggle that precedes this momentous decision, it turns into a big anticlimax because Dr. Davis is not at the hospital when I call. Nor is Dr. Mason on the premises. And no one can tell me how to reach either of them.

I've phoned to announce our readiness, at long last, to hand over our son into the care of the pediatric cardiac transplant unit at Columbia—the single most agonizing choice we've ever made—but there's no one on the other end to receive the news! Nor is anyone on hand to tell us about next steps or to provide the standard set of instructions.

I'm left hanging on the phone with the solitary, beating echo of my own heart. It's especially frustrating because neither doctor has given me her contact information, so I have no way of getting through to them.

I leave a message for Dr. Davis, saying I need to talk to her about Damon *right away*.

"We've never been shut out like this by physicians managing Damon's care! Not at Columbia, nor at any other hospital!" I complain to my wife, who is equally perturbed.

"And he's never been this sick before! How can they just ignore us?" Shealagh says, fuming.

I wait all day but Dr. Davis does not return my call.

"I don't get it," I tell Shealagh the next night. "Even Columbia, one of the biggest centers in the country, only does about twenty pediatric transplants a year, so *each one* is a big deal, with a whole team assigned to every case. Our call is supposed to initiate an entire protocol, so it's very odd no one has bothered to phone us back."

"I guess it's the Christmas period," Shealagh says. "Harder to find people."

"We're still several days pre-Christmas . . . And patients can be *ignored* if it's inconvenient?" I frown. "They should be prepared for us and on top of this!"

That night, before going to bed, I send Dr. Davis an e-mail saying I fear we're running out of time and I need to talk to her about next steps. I leave more voice messages with her answering service, underscoring the sensitivity of this matter.

The next morning, I check my e-mail but still no response. Nor a voice mail. I phone the hospital again. I feel we're ready to make the biggest leap of our lives, a concession wrung out of us after years of resistance, only no one seems to care. On the third day, increasingly worried about this lack of response, not to mention the lack of responsibility, I call the transplant unit, determined to get through or raise hell.

Dr. Davis and Dr. Mason are still nowhere to be found, but after refusing to leave another message, I am transferred to a Dr. Thea Becker at New York Hospital. Dr. Becker explains that she is one of the four cardiologists on Columbia's team, the other three being Dr. Mason, Dr. Davis, and a Dr. Sanford. Although Dr. Becker is clearly the junior member—we haven't heard of her until now, she is part-time at Columbia, and her voice has the stiff, by-the-book callowness of a graduate fellow—Dr. Becker assures me that all four cardiologists in the pediatric transplant unit are "interchangeable."

"We pool all our information, so anything you say to one of us is shared with the others . . . So you see, even though I've never met Damon or examined him, I know all about his case and I can help you as well as any of our other cardiologists," Dr. Becker says.

"With all due respect, that's an absurd concept!" I tell Dr. Becker. "Whatever happened to continuity of care and direct, firsthand observation of the patient?"

Although I'm appalled by this notion—it sounds like a fancy excuse for no-shows and lax supervision by senior doctors—and although I don't intend to let a raw novice like Dr. Becker, who's never even taken Damon's blood pressure or listened to his heartbeat, manage my son's transplant care, it occurs to me she might serve as well as anyone for our immediate needs. Getting Damon's name on the national transplant registry is a technicality in a largely bureaucratic process, and no personal knowledge of Damon is required. If Dr. Becker can help us speed up this protocol, we could save valuable time. And the junior Dr. Becker seems eager to prove her utility. At least she's *there*.

"So what do I need to do to get Damon listed?" I ask, softening my tone.

"If his transplant evaluations are completed, you don't need to do anything."

"You sure? That sounds too easy," I say with a laugh.

"That's it, but I can check on his status just to be certain," Dr. Becker says.

Two hours later, Dr. Becker calls back to say Damon has been placed on the transplant wait list. She mentions this so casually it takes a minute to sink in.

"He's listed?"

"Yes. He's on the national registry. His evaluations were all in order."

"Great . . . So from here on, the offer could come at any moment?"

"That's technically correct, yes. Though it usually takes several months."

Dr. Becker sounds very offhand, almost cavalier, which bothers me.

"But it could happen *tomorrow*, right? You can't predict! . . . So what should we do?"

"Haven't you read the booklet?" Dr. Becker asks.

"I skimmed it and my wife's read it about twenty times," I explain. "And I'll memorize it now that I know it's real. But can you please just give me a quick recap?"

Dr. Becker sighs. "The main thing is to have an overnight bag packed and ready to go to the hospital . . . You'll also want someone to look after your other children if both you and your wife plan to stay with Damon . . . He will need to wear a beeper and we'll want a list of all your phone numbers—home, office, cell—so we can reach you the minute we find a donor match . . . The transplant coordinator will contact you with further details."

It takes a moment after I hang up to accept what we've done. I relay these developments to Shealagh, then go and share the news with Damon.

"Cool," he says. "It'll be nice if we can fix my problem for good."

He seems relieved a search is under way and pleased at the possibility of success. Even as we speak, his face and belly are puffy and he exudes a muted, Buddha-like air as he calmly awaits release from his imperfect body.

I run through the broad outlines of the process for him. "Do you understand what's involved, D-man? You have any questions for me, or anything else you'd like to know?"

"I think I got it and if I need to know more, I can always go online," Damon says with a shrug.

I'm surprised he seems to be downplaying this. Then I realize how sensible he is. He trusts me to handle the details, he'll rally when he needs to, but otherwise he just wants to get on with his regular life. What else is there to do? It's a wise strategy and I don't mess with it.

Shealagh and I discuss what to tell Sam and Miranda.

"They know Damon is in trouble and that we're talking to doctors," I say. "And like all kids, they know more than their parents think . . . But now we need to fill in the blanks."

"Yes, I agree. Why don't you go first?" Shealagh says. "I'll give them the soft version after." My wife smiles.

It's not easy to explain to one's children that their brother's failing heart must be replaced with a stranger's heart—a freshly deceased stranger, whose size, age, and blood type must roughly match. But the kids, in their way, grasp the concept about as well as us.

Miranda accepts my words at face value and goes to brood in private— she's either sparing her feelings or mine, probably both—while Sam assails me with questions.

"Why does he have to stay in the hospital so long?" Sam demands.

"A month isn't that long. His body has to heal," I reply.

"But why does he have to keep taking all those medications?" Sam's still upset.

"So he doesn't reject his heart, and so he doesn't get an infection," I explain. "Since it's not his original heart, his body will attack it unless we keep his defense system down. But if his defenses are down, he could catch an infection, so we have to protect against that too."

"But why does he have to take all those medications *for the rest of his life*? It's not fair!" Sam cries as if it is all subject to my control and I could change it.

"Look, Sam," I finally say. "Damon will have more energy, and he can grow with his new heart, and those are *two* great things we can't afford to pass up!"

We talk to my parents, who respond with customary stalwartness.

"We're on standby and ready for duty," my father says. "Once Damon enters the hospital, we'll move into your house and camp there for the duration."

"Thanks, you guys! Only one parent is permitted to sleep in Damon's room but both Shealagh and I intend to be on the case twenty-four/seven."

"Call for you, Dad!" Miranda says, and my heart skips a beat. Every time the phone rings, we hold our breath because it could be The Offer. At work, I alert my assistant to my whereabouts constantly, though she still doesn't know why, and I check my cell phone compulsively. Shealagh and I speak several times a day and get nervous if too many hours have elapsed without an update.

Damon continues to have large groups of friends over to our house during the Christmas vacation. I still come downstairs and find teenage flirting, petting, and strutting around, but I notice the kids leave earlier and fewer spend the night. When I remark on this to Damon, he says with an enigmatic sigh, "Well, it's different now."

"I can't tell if it's different because the kids all talk about college and moving on while he's fallen behind," I tell Shealagh, "or because he can't keep up physically with them. Or is it because they feel funny knowing he's waiting for a heart transplant?"

When an old friend, Daniel, visits, the boys spend all their time on the computer. After Daniel leaves, I ask Damon what Daniel had to say about his upcoming surgery.

"We didn't really talk about it," Damon replies.

"Any reason?" I ask, trying to mask my surprise.

"No, it just didn't come up," Damon says with an ambiguous shrug.

But for our family, it comes up, as text or subtext, in *everything*. For New Year's, Damon has a party at Max's while the rest of us are going to a bash in Manhattan. We'd love to celebrate with Damon but we're happy he has his own plans. Damon promises to keep his cell on and we can get to Max's in no time if The Offer comes.

As we start to drive off, I realize I never wished Damon a happy New Year. He's still in our house with friends, and I won't see him again until 2005! To Shealagh's consternation, I shift into reverse and speed backward along our one-way street before leaping out of the vehicle, charging into the house, and embracing my son—"Have a happy and healthy 2005, D-man!"—before I jump back into the car and tear off again. Shealagh is upset with my driving and we fight all the way into the city until the big party diffuses the tension.

At midnight, as the colorful fireworks explode over Central Park and the glass windowpanes shudder, Shealagh calls Damon on his cell. She speaks to her darling boy from the window seat, then hands him to Sam and Miranda, who eventually pass him over to me.

Damon sounds champagne giddy, with lively party noises in the background. He's riding high. I can still hear a tremulous catch in his larynx but his merry, resonant voice soars with impish delight, reassuring me that our world remains intact for a little longer.

A week later, after returning to work, I become increasingly concerned about the continuing lack of communication from Columbia Presbyterian Hospital.

Dr. Davis still has not answered my e-mail, nor has she or Dr. Mason called me back. Absent my one talk with Dr. Becker—she's never around, and no one seems to know her—it's as if nothing has happened, nothing has changed.

We've had no instructions about the transplant preparations, nor does anyone seem even mildly interested in Damon's condition. Dr. Hayes, our longtime cardiologist, is off the case, and Dr. Hellenbrand, who temporarily took over, has handed us on to the transplant unit. Both Dr. Hayes and Dr. Hellenbrand were highly attentive physicians and responsive caregivers, but neither Dr. Davis nor her boss, Dr. Mason, whom Dr. Hayes entrusted us to, seems to have taken the most basic responsibility for our case.

"No one's examining Damon. They're not even giving us his weekly lab results, which we always got before, so *we* can tell how he's doing," Shealagh says.

"And they're not tracking changes from his new meds or calling to check on him," I add. "They're not even returning our calls. It's as if we've been dropped!"

I decide to send a stronger message to Dr. Davis. This time, I don't just describe my frustrations but I title my e-mail, "Who's in Charge of Damon Weber?"

I've noted Dr. Mason's marketing mind-set pervades her entire team, and I surmise Dr. Davis will not want such a telling question visible in her inbox.

Sure enough, within three hours, Dr. Davis calls back and agrees to meet us.

Shealagh, Damon, and I go in to Columbia. Dr. Davis, smilingly polite, examines Damon and asks how he's doing. She reviews the transplant procedure and preparations, walking Damon through all the steps and describing each stage. She has a bright, cheerful manner and is very thorough and professional.

"How long will it take you to find me a new heart?" Damon asks.

Dr. Davis explains that transplant patients are classified under three categories: status 1A, for those in the most urgent need; status 1B, for those with the second-highest priority; and status 2, for all other "active" patients on the wait list.

"Damon, since you are classified a two, the lowest priority, you'll have a six-to-twelve-month wait, though it could be sooner—being under eighteen years of age may work in your favor—or alternatively, even later. No one can predict." Dr. Davis smiles.

As I hear this, something nags at me. I recall that Dr. Bruce Gelb, in one of his asides, had mentioned Damon could qualify as a 1B due to his small size, under the criterion "failure to thrive." I hadn't fully understood what Bruce meant at the time, but his words come back to me now, and I ask Dr. Davis about them.

"No, that's not true. Damon is a two," Dr. Davis says. "You're mistaken."

"I'm sure you're right," I reply, "but I'm surprised a leading cardiologist like Bruce Gelb, who's a pretty sharp guy, would make such an error."

"I can't answer for him but I know transplants, which is my specialty!"

"Of course." I let it drop. I don't want to risk further antagonizing Dr. Davis after my e-mail, and it's possible I'm the one who made the error or misremembers.

Dr. Davis continues to instruct Damon about his big day in a clear, cogent manner, but she seems beset by second thoughts and turns to her assistant.

"Erica, could you go get me the big manual on heart transplantation?"

Moments later, Erica returns with a tome. Dr. Davis tears it open and races through the pages, searching with her index finger like an avid medical student.

"I'm not sure"—Dr. Davis finally looks up from the manual—"but you *may* have a point about Damon's status. I'll research it more and get back to you."

I'd already given Dr. Davis the benefit of the doubt, so this fumbling uncertainty unnerves me. We leave feeling uneasy about what's going on, obviously hopeful for a status revision in our favor but also worried about what such a revision might signify.

The next day we get a fax from Columbia informing us that Damon's wait-list status has been officially changed from a 2 to a 1B.

It's the difference between being high priority and low priority, between waiting for a few weeks or up to a year. It could also mean the difference between life and death.

We're naturally pleased Damon has moved up the ranks and now stands a better chance of receiving a new heart in a timely manner. But it also confirms that for the past two and a half weeks, Damon has been erroneously listed.

It's unsettling. My sense that no one was taking charge of our case proved truer than I suspected. Had we not challenged Columbia, Damon could have missed a lifesaving opportunity. And it was only by a fluke, a stray remark from a more knowledgeable physician, that I had any inkling about this snafu.

Around this time, Dr. Chin e-mails to ask me how it's going. I describe the listing error and other flaws, venturing that the transplant surgeons at Columbia may be first-rate, but the transplant cardiologists seem to verge on incompetence.

"Have I made a mistake?" I ask Dr. Chin, giving him a chance to set me straight and also to criticize a rival institution.

"You probably wouldn't do much better at CHOP, since half the cardiologists there were trained at Columbia!" Dr. Chin writes back.

I take it he shares my general view of the cardiologists but does not consider Columbia's listing error as startling or as unusual as I do. It could be my standards are too high and exacting, an occasional weakness of mine.

Eleven days after we correct Damon's listing classification, we get The Offer that a donor heart has been found for him.

Chapter 47

"Have you heard it's in the stars, next July we collide with Mars!"

—Some Cole Porter song

—From Damon's blog, January 2005

One snowy afternoon in the final days leading up to his transplant—it must have been a weekend but for the life of me, I can't recall exactly when— Damon is hanging out with his friends by the front of our house. I am sitting out on the green metal porch chair in my bulky winter coat, having brushed the fresh white powder off the seat. It's cold but the sun is shining. I'm watching the boys throw snowballs.

Damon is on the top step and he doesn't have much energy but he enjoys flinging down a few loose blobs at his pals on the pavement below or absorbing a shot or two with a soft white splatter on the meat of his coat.

Splat! He opens his arms and twists his torso so the snowball lands smack against his flank. He grins as if he scored the direct hit himself.

While his friends continue pelting each other down at street level, Damon shuffles over to me in my porch chair and innocently, as if it were the most casual act in the world, deposits himself in my lap. He perches chirpily on my knees, like a bird alighting on a statue.

The move catches me completely off guard. It's so at odds with Damon's customary teen behavior—especially when his friends are around!

At first, I assume he's stealing a breather, and I play it cool, so as not to embarrass him. But instead of pulling away and dismissing it as a gag,

Damon stays put, showing clear intention. He snuggles up to me and gets more comfortable in my lap. It's a touching overture, as well as a very willful and conscious regression. Damon deliberately makes himself into a child again—into *my* child—and cleaves to me with endearing filial adoration.

I'm totally disarmed, and my heart melts faster than the snow dissolving in the bright sun. Damon doesn't say a word as he sticks to me and ignores his friends, but he doesn't need to. He's aware of everything and is making a clear statement.

It's the most beautiful gesture and the most eloquent tribute I have ever received. Damon salutes our unique history and our deep bond while acknowledging, without any conditions or inhibitions, his great love for me.

I wrap my arms around my son and try to balance him on my knees—even with his illness, he's much bigger and heavier now—and I hungrily respond to his show of affection. I strive to maintain decorum for both our sakes, since we're sitting out on the porch and everyone can see us from the street. But we're not really a part of the world anymore, at least not in the same way.

I hold Damon tight and register his weight and his warmth and his spirit. He leans against me with his baggy coat while I press my face against his neck and shaggy head. We clasp hands. It's the deepest conversation we've ever had, or will have, about what's happening in our lives and how we feel about one another.

Yet not a word passes our lips.

I can't remember how many years it's been since we sat entwined like this, embracing openly. And I can't believe it's my acerbic sixteen-year-old son who has initiated this intimate exchange—despite the full-daylight company of his friends. He doesn't seem to care, as if he's taking time out to deal with more important matters.

We hold this position for a blessed interval and I am filled with gratitude. Damon is not only showing me his love but allowing me to reciprocate without restraint or censure.

My cup runneth over, and I never want this moment to end.

Chapter 48

Hell, I wouldn't mind a date lol. Well this is the first time I've been home alone on a Friday since forever and it sucks. I'm so lonely. There's nothing to do or at least nothing I can do. Been trying 2 amuse myself by bouncing my empty medicine capsules off the cork board in my room. For those of you who have never tried it (all of you) DON'T! I've also tried 2 use my syringes as darts. Doesn't work too well cause they're too light and if you try throwing them with any force there's a risk of them bouncing back and hitting you in the eye. In fact they've done a lot of interesting things except 4 stick in the cork.

It doesn't help that I've gotten even worse. I have no energy anymore. I often find myself sitting there in this lethargic state doing nothing and I keep falling asleep on my floor. I could right now if I let myself. My brother had to wake me at 3:30 pm today. I'm fast becoming the one thing I've fought not 2 be: a homeridden weakling. And no, I don't care that many kids who have a single ventricle system and never even got PLE have been on homeschooling their whole lives. I'm not many kids.

But what can I do at this point, just fuckin wait? I can't fuckin stand waiting and I don't know how I'd last more months of this. World of Warcraft is fun but it's not a supplement 4 life . . . Wow that's the most pathetic statement I've ever written. (hehe "wow" anyone see the irony?)

I'm not sure what 2 do with myself. I can't make new friends like I used to cause I'm just too out of it 2 be myself. The only people I can still enjoy hanging out with are my old friends like in small groups or individually. But I'm worried my life is slowly slipping away from me and there's nothing I can do but sit back and watch. And wait.

Well I guess all I can say is I need something . . . and it better fuckin b a heart!

—*From Damon's blog, January 14, 2005*

Shealagh is folding laundry in the family room around lunchtime when the phone rings and Columbia informs her they have an offer of a heart for Damon.

We've been warned to expect false alarms but since we can't know for sure until we get to the hospital—presumably a donor-organ-harvesting team from Columbia is on its way to the donor site—we must move quickly.

Shealagh wakes Damon, who sleeps late into the afternoon now, and breaks the news in a wavering voice. Damon nods and begins to get dressed, remaining calmer than his mother.

Then Shealagh phones me at the office. I'm in a meeting and have to step out.

My wife tells me about the heart offer. We review our plan and coordinate schedules. Shealagh sounds extremely tense, so I remind her not to panic. This is what we wanted.

I grab my coat and tell my assistant I'm out for the rest of the day on private business. I call my parents and a few friends en route.

Shealagh loads two bags into the car and meets me at Sam's school with Damon and Miranda. She asks me to drive. Damon sits in the back in a sweatshirt and baggy jeans, looking deceptively composed, like a boxer before a championship bout. I ask him how he's doing and he says fine, he was fast asleep but is coming around. He listens to his iPod.

I try to look at him through the rearview mirror or steal a glance over my shoulder. He's so vibrant and alive it's hard to imagine anything bad could befall him. He's just a sweet teenage kid who needs a new heart, like the Tin Man in *The Wizard of Oz*, a film Damon watched so many times as a toddler he wore out the videotape (although he loved the Cowardly Lion most). Now we're going to the Emerald City to get Damon *his* new heart.

We arrive at the hospital quickly, earlier than expected, and they must scramble to accommodate us. We're shown to a lounge-like preadmission room. A TV screen displays a "Hello Damon" crawl. It impresses Sam and Miranda more than Damon.

Dr. Becker, whom we've never met, comes to greet us. She's a young, sober Indian woman, correct and a little stiff, exactly like her voice. She checks Damon's vitals and takes blood but lets him keep his regular clothes. We're so early, having reached Columbia well in advance of the organ procurement team, that the situation remains in flux.

I try to imagine the donor heart being removed, examined, carefully packed in a cold fluid, and loaded onto a helicopter. The logistics have always been fuzzy, and I once upset Damon by joking we had to wait for the right person to croak before he could get his new heart. The idea of anyone suffering for his benefit is intolerable to my son. Now we must remain on standby and stay in the hospital, possibly for hours, until the heart gets here, further tests are conducted, and a final determination is made regarding its viability as a donor organ for Damon.

Dr. Becker reviews the basics and brings us forms to sign. "I do not have specifics, but we must assume it's a go until we are otherwise notified," she says.

It's clear Dr. Becker does not have much experience or authority and is acting as a go-between. When I indicate we'll withhold our final consent until we get more information, she promises the surgeon will come speak to us before anything happens.

"Who's the surgeon today?" I ask. There's Dr. Q, the superstar called in for special cases, and Dr. Mosca, the distinguished head of transplant with the most operations.

"Dr. Jonathan Chen." Dr. Becker mentions the youngest member of the surgical team. "He's brilliant, a rising star recruited after a national search," she says, trying to reassure us.

It's a lottery system, and we've drawn the least familiar card. I console myself they must not consider Damon an especially difficult case.

My parents arrive and swell our group to party size, though the mood is anything but jolly. Sam fiddles in the corner, eyeing his brother and biting his lip; Miranda sticks close to Damon and clings to his every move; Shealagh packs and repacks the overnight bags, trying to keep it together; and I pace and harangue the medical staff with endless queries and commands. Nor can my parents help much. My father, an affable extrovert, is discomfited by stillness and uncertainty, and my mother, a resilient survivor, carries her own historical baggage.

But everyone is there because they love Damon. And this collective warmth and solidarity, the family turnout, does signify. Like the dockside send-off to a perilous solo voyage, our group presence provides the human context and the basic orientation for Damon's journey. We are both the start and the finish line, and Damon knows he just has to get back to us in order to be safe.

Damon slouches in an armchair with a book on his lap, a play called *Kimberly Akimbo*. It's a mordant comedy about a sixteen-year-old girl with an illness that makes her age at four times the normal rate. I'd gotten Damon and my mother tickets and now my mother prevails upon Damon to read aloud from the play.

It's a shrewd distraction because Damon loves to perform, but I'm too focused on unfolding events to heed him. Will the donor heart get here in time, or will we go home empty-handed? I recall reading the human heart can survive only four hours outside the body before it loses the ability to function post-transplant.

But at some point Damon's rich, lively, and dramatic voice, an inexhaustible spigot of words and storytelling verve, reaches me too. My son declaims with relish from the slender volume in his pale hands, and he has his audience, as usual, rapt. The writing is sharp and funny, with a wry, outcast irony. Even the medical staff stops to listen, arrested by this uncommon use of the facilities. And it strikes me, watching my son weave his familiar spell, how Damon is always at home in the realm of art, even in the hospital before a life-threatening operation.

Two physicians in white coats appear, one of them Dr. Chen, who informs us that the donor heart is in good order, and we are moving forward.

My system instantly switches to high alert. So this is *not* a run-through.

Dr. Chen appears a capable sort, youthful and still aspiring, but with enough experience under his belt, and I decide I like him. Not that I have much choice. (I could refuse the offer if he didn't seem up to the task, but it would leave us waiting indefinitely.)

Dr. Chen reviews the procedure, answers our questions—displaying a firm, supple intelligence when I press him—and departs with a confident, provisionally reassuring smile.

Now everything turns more breathless and accelerates.

My parents gather Sam and Miranda, and after heartrending hugs, they go. Damon changes into a gown and slippers. He's wearing a red ribbon from Kyle for good luck. The nurse lets him keep the ribbon on his left ankle but below, she tags him with a white plastic snap-on bearing his name, date of birth, hospital ID number, and admitting cardiologist. She attaches an identical white plastic tag to his right ankle.

They place Damon on a gurney, put in an IV line, and recheck his vitals.

The anesthesiologists come by and ask their questions. They leave.

Dr. Becker scurries up the hall to tell us they're almost ready in the OR.

Shealagh and I hover near Damon, finding any excuse for physical contact and any premise for small talk. Anything to avoid confronting what's about to happen.

"That soldier we adopted in Iraq wrote back. Her name is Dana," I tell Damon.

"Cool," Damon says, though he looks surprised. "I didn't realize you sent in my picture, Dad . . . I'll write back when I get out of the hospital."

"When can we see that new portrait of you and Max?" Shealagh asks. Only yesterday, Damon posed with Max for a painter friend of Max's parents who became enamored of Damon's "look" when she met him New Year's Eve.

"Ask Max's mom. It's her friend," Damon says. "She has a gallery."

"Think we can buy the painting from her?" I inquire.

"You might want to see it first, Dad!"

A transplant nurse in a moon suit, her face obscured by a mask, traipses over in elastic overshoes. She has come to take Damon to the operating room.

We glance down the long, empty corridor and stiffen. It's time.

Damon, who's sitting upright on his gurney, asks if he can walk to the OR instead of being wheeled in. The nurse, surprised, admits there's no medical reason he can't, if he really wants to and if he feels up to it.

Damon immediately slides off the bed and stands. Even at this stage of his illness, he's proud. And not without capability. He's going to walk in unassisted.

Shealagh and I exchange proud smiles. It's such a Damonesque move, so unintimidated and full of his signature spirit, that it buoys us. Maybe we really *can* beat this thing and turn it into just another station on our journey.

I stroll beside Damon in his blue gown and help push his IV pole. Shealagh walks on Damon's other side, holding his hand while drying her eyes.

The nurse follows behind us, steering the wide, empty gurney down the hall in our wake. *Clickety-clack*. I remind Damon that by the time he wakes up, the worst will be behind him, and he'll already be on the road to recovery. Damon scans my face closely, like a child probing with his fingers, and gives a faint nod.

We've reached the end of the corridor. It's time to hand Damon off to the surgical team with its scalpels and stainless steel wires and massive, circulating heart-lung machine.

I look at my son. There's so much to say but I decide it's better to keep things as normal as possible, since that's how we want them to end up. He knows what's at stake—we all know—but hasn't he been here before?

There's a positive outcome to this operation, a known path to success, and Damon just has to come out on the right side of it. But we need him to go in with the same confidence and sense of security that's sustained him thus far, and he needs to know we share that confidence.

I recall the first time I had to leave two-year-old Damon alone at preschool. He wouldn't stop clinging to me as he bawled his eyes out on the threshold. I thought my heart would break, but I knew I had to leave him, and I knew it would turn out okay.

Only this time, the outcome is far less clear, and it's not Damon crying.

Shealagh chokes up as she hugs Damon and walks off sobbing.

Then it's my turn. I embrace Damon with open arms, tasting his soft hair. He hews stiffly to me for an instant, but I let him know this is not farewell and we will have time after. I pat his back like a coach before the big game.

"Okay, D-man. This is it, but remember, you know how to do this! You're the toughest person I ever met . . . I want you to go in strong, with good thoughts, and I'll see you in a few hours . . . Love you, big guy!"

As I let go, all too soon, of Damon, I try not to think that I might never hold my son again or get to talk to him and tell him how I feel. Those are just abstract concepts, dark, flitting ghosts, and I simply banish them.

The nurse leads Damon toward the steel doors of the OR, where the faceless surgical squad eagerly awaits him. We watch Damon shuffle forward, a little shaky but still advancing on his own two feet, a small, pale, incredibly brave sixteen-year-old boy with a lion's heart they can never take away, no matter what instruments or drugs they deploy.

The doors swing shut after him.

Chapter 49

"I fear no death nor pain."
"What do you fear?"
"A cage."

—The Lord of the Rings

—From Damon's blog, winter 2004–2005

Shealagh and I sit and wait in the lounge of the Cardiothoracic Intensive Care Unit.

This is where Damon will be sent post-transplant.

It's the longest wait in the world.

And the most desolate.

All my research has shown that Damon's time in surgery—the six to eight hours when he lies on the table under anesthesia, his bladder drained by a catheter, his breastbone cut and parted, with a heart-lung machine circulating his blood, until the surgeon removes his original heart from its connection to the great arteries, sews the donor heart into place, and initiates activity so that the new heart can begin to function, unrejected, on its own, enabling Damon to be untethered from the heart-lung machine—constitutes the single most dangerous period in the entire process.

Damon either comes out alive, or he doesn't.

End of story.

And hopefully, a new beginning.

Though no one wants to give me, or any family member regarding any operation, an actual risk assessment, I piece together my own by combining multiple variables, cofactors, medical history, hospital records, and meta-analyses. Then I take my estimate and get it indirectly confirmed by physicians who tweak it. Doctors can't resist correcting you and showing how much they know, especially if you're on their turf, and I can't tolerate not knowing. So we back into agreement on a ballpark number, even though the doctors would never volunteer or publicly acknowledge an average mortality rate, because it would expose the illusion that they can manage everything.

Numbers tell only part of the story, of course, and I give Columbia the benefit of every doubt concerning their long experience and their improving, self-reported results. But even when I factor all this in, Damon still has, conservatively, a one in three chance of dying in surgery. It's higher if I look at the raw unscrubbed numbers over time.

One in three is still better than the odds of PLE, except PLE plays out over many years and this will be over in six hours. The verdict will come in very swiftly, and there is no further recourse or court of appeal for us.

In my own heart, I feel that if Damon can make it off the operating table and return to us with his recognizable, fighting self intact, we will persevere. But he has to get out of that room *alive*.

So now we continue to sit and wait in the gray airless lounge. A wall-mounted television flickers with remote, meaningless images, pale reminders of an outside world that once mattered.

A nurse emerges every couple of hours to give us a progress report. We scrutinize her face, her gait, her body language, for any "tells" as she marches across the floor toward us. It's all I can do to stop from running up and shaking the information out of her.

The nurse finally reaches us and starts to speak. The minute she resumes the narrative, I know the story hasn't ended, and I relax. The nurse describes various minor developments and turns in the procedure, all of which I glom on to and store. But there's only one real question I care about, and the answer seems to be "So far, so good."

I pump my fists and yell like a fan after the first quarter. "Yeah, D-man, go, D-man, go!"

Shealagh disapproves of such naked cheerleading, not to mention premature celebration, but I'm a believer in positively focused energy and momentum.

Or I'm trying to be.

The long day turns into night. I call my friend David in Seattle, the only person I can talk to at a time like this. Shealagh speaks to my parents, who are staying at our house. They report that Sam and Miranda had a nice, big dinner—they both wanted seconds—and went to bed without a peep. All is quiet on the home front.

We get a second positive update but the same letdown ensues once the nurse leaves.

We're getting to the meat of the operation, and there's more to worry about now.

The hospital vigil drags on. And on.

We drift, suspended in a no-man's-land between terror and hope.

We cross the midnight threshold, and then we're into the wee, dark hours.

Time loses definition and grows amorphous. We float in the void, trying not to disappear down any black holes.

The elevator pings and footsteps approach. My stomach craters and I realize it might be better not to know, because in uncertainty, I can still hang on to faith. I brace myself but in this instance, it's a false alarm. The footsteps aren't for us.

There is comfort in open-endedness but also a point of no return, and as the black hour-hand scythes across the grim clock face, we fast are nearing it.

Damon's operation is taking too long!

Delay can't be good, and Shealagh and I both grow tense. We know the old heart is out and they're trying to put the new one in. But what if the new heart *won't start up?* Damon cannot stay on the heart-lung machine indefinitely. His original heart is toast, and he has no backup if they can't make the new heart work.

As more time passes without a sign, we become even more agitated. What's going on? If Damon isn't out by now, there must be a problem. It's been almost eight hours. Based on their last update, we should have gotten the all-clear over *one hour ago*.

I start paging the transplant nurse when the figure of Dr. Chen suddenly appears in the lounge, and a ghostly chill passes over us.

He wouldn't show up himself unless he had cause.

I try to avoid despair as I zero in on Dr. Chen from across the lounge. You can tell Damon's surgeon has been through a major battle. He's wearing scrubs like fatigues and resembles a commander returning from the bloody field.

I look him straight in the eye as he reaches us, knowing his first few words will determine the future course of our lives.

"Everything is fine." Dr. Chen cuts to the chase. Neither of us moves. "We put the new heart in and it's functioning well," the surgeon reports from the front lines with evident satisfaction. "Damon did great. They're closing him up and moving him from the OR into the ICU. You'll be able to go in and see him shortly."

It's impossible to describe the impact of his words, unless you've heard angels sing.

We thank Dr. Chen and heap praise upon his magnificent feat. We're so grateful to him! This means everything to us! He's awesome and amazing!

Dr. Chen smiles, sharing our joy and basking in a successful night's work. He looks mightily pleased and lingers to chat, unwinding like an athlete after a great performance.

"Damon's donor was a very sizable adult with a big heart, so we had to squish things around in order to fit the new heart inside Damon's chest cavity," Dr. Chen says. "It might be a little tight in there until Damon's system adjusts, but it all worked out and I don't anticipate any problems. Damon now has a big, strong heart he can grow into!"

Dr. Chen is also pleased they managed to get supplementary tissue from the donor lungs, because he needed extra pulmonary arteries and veins for his reconstruction.

"I had to fashion a wider connection for the vein between Damon's neck and heart—we refused two previous donors because they didn't have enough extra tissue—but I'm very pleased with the result, and I think you will be too."

Dr. Chen describes several other features of Damon's new anatomy. As I learned from managing Damon's PLE, the structural details of an underlying surgery can have long-term consequences, and it's in our interest to learn all we can. But right now it's the middle of the night and Dr. Chen is exhausted, while we want to go in and see our son. We agree that in a few weeks, we can review all this more calmly if I come by his office for a primer.

When we finally get to see Damon—it always takes longer than they say—it's a shock. But a necessary shock, once we adjust to it, not a grim one.

He lies on his back in the ICU bed, his inert, traumatized body supported by an array of bubbling, suspiring machines and flashing, beeping monitors.

Damon's eyes are puffy and closed, with goop on the stressed lids to keep them from chafing. His trademark red mane bobs above the white hospital pillow, one of his few unchanged features, though it highlights the adjacent deformations. Damon's mouth and nose are mashed by bifurcating respirator tubes taped in harsh X's across his face, while a central IV line enters the right side of his neck in a bloody, Frankenstein-like tangle.

Encumbered with a thicket of inflowing and outflowing ventilator hoses, three chest drainage lines, a urine catheter, IV tubes, pacing wires with silver foil, a green arm board, a black pressure cuff, blue EKG sensors, and a red pulsing probe—all exposed under extra-bright lights—Damon's supine figure is lit up and wired like a Christmas tree!

But perhaps what's most striking, amid all this damage, is how *good* Damon's color already looks. His skin, perfused as never before, *glows* with a warm, rosy sheen. He's flush with pulsing blood, while all traces of blueness, from his face down to his extremities, have been erased.

We've never seen Damon with such a ruddy, healthy-looking circulation!

The source of all this pumping vitality and excitement, the fantastic, throbbing object in question, is visible on the left side of Damon's chest. We can see it moving just below the surface, a creature in its own right, alive and hopping like a jackrabbit. It jitters and flutters and jerks, creating a big stir underneath its translucent envelope of skin. This new, beating *thing* is so large and so frantically active, it looks like it could escape its fragile subdermal lair and leap straight from Damon's chest onto the bed.

Shealagh and I stand in awe before this marvel of human engineering. Damon has a big new heart transplanted into his old body. We can feel its raw, surging power, like an outsized new engine revving up inside a compact car.

Meanwhile, Damon remains in critical care and many of his functions still require intensive support. His body must make its peace with the donor heart while each of his systems recuperates. Any failure anywhere could lead to massive breakdown everywhere.

Even before Damon wakes up that first day, we have things to worry about.

His blood pressure is too low, as is the urine output from the kidneys.

His CO_2 level is too high, which means he's not breathing enough. The giant ventilator that breathes for him by pneumatically compressing air several times a minute—it emits a deep, steady suspiration, as if the whole room were inhaling and exhaling—has to have its rate adjusted.

And while Damon needs diuretics to chase out excess fluid, he also needs more blood volume because he lost blood during the operation. Even now, he continues to bleed sporadically through three long, spotty drainage lines that exit his body into a clearly marked collection chamber. So the doctors must push more albumin into his body—it comes in big, clear fluid sacs—to increase his blood volume.

By early afternoon, Damon's eyes open and he comes to. Shealagh and I stand on either side of our son, holding his hands, stroking his hair, and trying to comfort him. We fill him in on what's happened and congratulate him effusively.

"You made it with flying colors! Everything's going to be okay!"

Damon nods, his eyes rheumy and bloodshot. He's very weak but cognizant. We watch him check his surroundings and register his new state of mute captivity. He seems most discomfited by the choking respirator tube. The fentanyl and morphine help with the pain, the dobutamine and epinephrine keep his heart pumping strong, but nothing can deflect the apparatus jammed down his mouth, nose, and throat. It forces oxygen into his lungs every ten seconds. He's like a fish who can only stay in the water—who can only stay alive—if it keeps the hook in its mouth. Reluctantly, Damon swallows and accepts his fate.

Shealagh cools Damon's brow with a white towel while I dab the one available corner of his parched lips with wet foam on a stick. We keep him apprised of how well he's doing and what still needs to be done. We can't tell how much he's absorbing, but we can feel him finding a new equilibrium. The fresh incision line where they split his chest looks as if it's already healed, and his whole body radiates with a glowing new epidermis. We even spot Kyle's flimsy red ribbon clinging to his ankle, a small bright emblem of inextinguishable love.

All the surgeons, Dr. Davis admits, say the transplant went "better than expected."

Shealagh and I beam. We knew if they gave Damon a chance, he'd beat the spread.

Chapter 50

"Guess who's back
Back again
Damon's back
Tell a friend"

Yes, it's really me and as I'm sure you've all heard already from numerous sources, I'm alive and well. Still in the hospital but out of the ICU and that's all 2 be expected. Hopefully be comin home sometime next week but it's still up in the air.

Soooo what is up everybody?! How did you survive without me? lol. I heard Irena managed 2 get the group together 4 a party which is mucho cool. Sorry I couldn't make it dear, I was slightly preoccupied but perhaps next time.

Twill probably be a while before I can have the group at my house en masse (just because of all the immune suppressant medication I'm on and I don't particularly feel like hangin out with you guys with a mask on the entire time (nothing personal) lol And no Jano, Zak it's not a monster or Zorro mask or anything like that so don't get excited lol jk. But I will figure out a way 2 see all of you as soon as I can and in the meantime I'm sure the group is resourceful enough 2 find a new base for a while.

My room's pretty cool. It's spacious and there's a bed where 1 of my parents can sleep and a tv, a phone and a computer which I'm updating from now. Unfortunately though you have 2 be an admissions user 2 install anything which means no games (and the computer in the "learning center" has a grand total of OMB of space, now I don't know much about computers but that's not a lot of space so no Warcraft or anything else 4 me). I have internet access (obviously) so if anyone knows some good online games or coolsites or anything, please let me know. In other words people, *entertain me,* I don't care how. Tell me what's been going on with you, what's been happening at Tech, a joke, no matter how bad I assure you it will be better than a blood test. I'm bored as hell in this hospital and there's nothing 2 do but read and pop pills . . . and not the fun kind.

Btw thanx 2 the group and everyone 4 all your support during this. You guys have been awesome! Damn this entry took me a really long time proving that I'm not yet 100% but I knew that, well later all.
—*From Damon's blog, February 10, 2005*

Damon makes good progress in the hospital following his heart transplant operation but a hail of errors, gaffes, and setbacks threaten to undo all the benefits of his surgery.

Hospitals turn out, paradoxically, to be very dangerous places, and the longer one stays on the premises, the more dangerous they seem to grow.

Even when the doctors and nurses are first-rate, as scores are, the system often conspires against them. And when they are less than first-rate, as far too many turn out to be, they can pose a threat to the patient, which must be defended against at all times.

For the first days following his transplant, Damon shows steady, even remarkable improvement. By day two, he's fully aware and communicating with us via pen and paper, using his left hand because the right is immobilized with the IV line and the arm board. He's weak and sore and very thirsty but he doesn't complain. He even has his sense of humor. When Shealagh and I bicker over who stays overnight, he scribbles *stop arguing!*

Dr. Davis comes by and reiterates the prevailing sense of satisfaction with Damon's operation. But now that the surgeons have done their job, she explains in her mellifluous hierarchical manner, the pediatric transplant group will take over.

"So Dr. Mason is *in charge*," Dr. Davis trills, needling me ever-so-subtly for my earlier e-mail ("Who's in Charge of Damon Weber?"), which she obviously hasn't forgotten.

But I just smile back and beam at her. Damon is doing well, and I'm ready to hug them all. If Dr. Mason, a stocky woman who bustles into our ICU room with an unmistakable air of self-importance and her own entourage, wants to claim ownership for a successful patient, then God bless her. I just want to get my son home, and I'll help elect her president of the AMA if it will assist in that process.

We bond now, Dr. Mason and I, in the aftermath of a good transplant, and reach a happy accommodation of mutually shared goals. I find new, unseen virtues in her and she's happy to play the wise, experienced overseer, which sits squarely in her comfort zone.

Dr. Mason confers with the surgeons and consults with the specialists, coordinating the various expert inputs, before she presents the daily plan of action.

"We want to try and extubate Damon today!" she announces early on.

It's only the second day, but Damon's blood pressure has reached its target, his urine output has improved, and they don't want his body growing dependent on the ventilator, which can occur after traumatic surgery. Also, Damon's X-ray shows extra fluid around the lungs, which is easier to resolve once he's using his own muscles to breathe.

Weaning an ICU patient off the respirator is always a critical step toward recovery. Can the postoperative patient breathe on his or her own without mechanical assistance? But it's especially significant for Damon because following his first open-heart surgery as an infant, Damon required a full month to come off the respirator. Many attempts were made to wean him, and all ended in failure because he was too weak. Neither Shealagh nor I has ever forgotten that nightmarish month in the ICU, which felt like years, when our son was held captive to a machine and it looked like he'd never come off it.

We know what a big deal this is, and we're apprehensive about it.

Damon also seems worried and shows uncharacteristic anxiety when they ask us to leave the room before extubating him. He starts to cry, the first time we've seen panic from our son during the whole transplant process. It's like having his umbilical cord cut, and he's frightened about losing the external support and being able to make it on his own.

The pulmonologist, familiar with this reaction, tells Damon he can have one parent stay in the room if it will make him feel better. Damon calms down, glances about, and points straight to me. Since he has only two parents and I'm more assertive, it's hardly a surprise pick. Nevertheless, I feel strangely touched that Damon would need *me* in this way, because I've become so accustomed to thinking of *him* as strong and self-sufficient.

It's so easy to forget he's just a kid!

Watching Damon being weaned off the respirator—Shealagh peeks in too, from behind the curtain—is like watching our son be reborn. I stand beside Damon and urge him on while Shealagh roots silently from the ICU corridor. Damon gags and chokes and sputters, and his floundering body jerks and flails as they pull out the endotracheal tube. Ejected into a harsh new environment, he claws and scrabbles forward until he emerges among us, a fledgling, wobbly, self-breathing young creature. *Ecce homo.*

"Bravo, D-man, bravo!" I cheer lustily.

Now we wait to see if Damon can *maintain* this independent state. His chest heaves and all his monitors flash. He shivers and gasps and blinks. It looks like we may have to hook him back up . . . But slowly, he manages to take in oxygen and expel carbon dioxide, and his body finds a precarious new balance.

Like a newborn infant one minute after birth, Damon passes his first Apgar. He's ready to meet the world and breathe on his own.

It's a tremendous milestone, and a cause for great relief and celebration.

Damon runs into his first setback on the Saturday after surgery. I have weekend duty, giving Shealagh a much-deserved rest, and I find Damon with his upper arms and face dramatically swollen. "How you feeling, D-man?" I frown.

"I'm a little uncomfortable and my arm is pretty tender," Damon admits.

Alarmed—my son is taking on the puffy air of the Pillsbury Doughboy!—I look for a doctor. But it's the weekend shift and no physician or nurse is around. I page the ICU attending and wait over an hour until he shows up.

The doctor says Damon could have inflammation in the neck caused by a clot that must be dissolved right away. They prescribed a drug for it earlier.

"What time did he get it?" I ask, surprised at the absence of any effect.

He checks the chart. "Looks like he didn't get it yet. But I'm sure he will."

"What's the holdup?" I snap. "Didn't *you* just tell me it was urgent?"

I wait with Damon for several more hours, then page the ICU resident, a high-strung young woman with the air of a somnolent undergraduate. I show her that Damon's face is still swelling up. "We need to do something *now!*"

"Yes. Timeliness is key. I'm on it," she says before she runs off.

After lunch—it's now five hours since the order!—I page the resident but she does not respond. No one knows where she is. I head down the ICU corridor and check every room, but she's not there. I start getting desperate when I spot her immured in a small alcove, lost in a pile of reference books. She jumps up guiltily.

"Where have you been?" I cry. "My son is *still* waiting for his medication!"

"I-I'm sorry," she stammers, her face reddening. "I was going to do it."

I storm out, buttonhole the new ICU attending, and read her the riot act. She stays calm, and within twenty minutes, Damon gets his medication.

I watch the drug go in and pray it's not too late. Damon is so bloated he looks like he's ready to *explode,* and I'm not far behind. The new ICU attending tries to mollify me. "We're one of the fastest ICUs in the country," she says.

I stare at her, openmouthed. "You had this order since eight this morning!"

She pauses. "You're right. I don't know why this wasn't done earlier."

I'm struck by her honesty—I'm used to a policy of constant denial—but I remain worried. Damon resembles a blimp. I sit by him, hoping the drug works.

A new resident arrives. "Hi, I'm Jim, I'm here to help in any way."

I explain what's happened, but Jim doesn't react. He just lingers. So I ask a series of medical questions, but Jim offers nothing but the blandest platitudes.

It's clear Jim knows very little and has no medical task to perform.

"I'm here if you need anything," he keeps saying, although the only thing we now need is for him to go away. "I'll be here all night if you need me."

I'm trying not to be rude when Jim finally goes. As he exits, I hear a small, wry voice pipe up from the bed with perfect timing: "Well *that* was pointless!"

I smile, greatly relieved that Damon, who seemed so out of it, remains alert. It's the best indicator I get that despite his puffiness, he's not slipping away.

That night, as I curl up on the cramped armchair-cot beside Damon's ICU bed, a thin sheet covering my T-shirt-clad body, I feel like an exhausted bodyguard unable to switch to off-duty. I worry about Damon's swelling and about every flashing screen and pinging indicator.

Fluid tends to pool overnight, so I'm on the alert for that. Damon's heart rate is down to 100—they've weaned him off the epinephrine and dobutamine—which is okay if it holds, but not if it drops. But his oxygen saturation, whose fluctuations send my own heart fluttering, sporadically dips to the mid-80s while he sleeps. Since a higher saturation is better for wound healing, and for just about everything else, I prompt the night nurse—a big improvement over the day nurse—to place an oxygen cannula by Damon's nose.

I monitor all the machines plus the stream of doctors, nurses, and staff who flow in and out of this dimly lit circle. Nothing gets past me. Occasionally, I open one eye to check on Damon's saturation, or the arterial or venous pressure, or the nutrient IV bags, or a new technician. Mostly, I can track them with my eyes shut. Eventually, I drop off for a spell.

Sometime in the dead of night, I am awakened by a shattering sound and terrible screams, followed by frantic footsteps. Once I verify that it doesn't concern Damon, I recall that earlier in the lounge, I saw a group of Hasidic Jews praying. One man has a very sick baby in the ICU, and I heard a nurse say the infant was unlikely to survive. Now, based on the shrieking lamentation and the mournful chanting that fills the halls, the baby has apparently died.

It is a tragedy, and although I don't know any of the parties, I register the loss of a human life in my dim, sleep-fogged brain. But then, as I console myself that Damon, *my* charge, is safe, a dastardly thought glints: if the angel of death was sent to take one life on this ward, then let this anonymous stranger be that sacrifice, and let my son be left alone!

By morning, things look better. Damon has begun to reverse the fluid overload in his upper arms, neck, and face. He's still swollen, but the Pillsbury Doughboy is deflating.

Damon also gets a great nurse, Angela, who removes his mattress pad since the new beds don't require pads, a fact seemingly unknown to several previous ICU nurses that has resulted in a bedsore. Angela changes all Damon's sheets, gives him a clean new diaper, and refreshes all his dressings, IV lines, and tubes, bringing order and harmony to a sorry mess. She's a godsend, like her name.

Damon's X-ray still shows a hazy wet patch on his lungs, so it's imperative we keep him sitting upright and moving about to help the fluid disperse.

"We gotta get you out of bed, champ!" I unclip his chest sensors and gather his central and peripheral IV lines in my hand. Then I carefully shift him to the edge of the mattress and let his feet find the floor before I help him stand.

"That's it, good!" I say. Damon leans his light, frail body against mine. I lay a sheet and pillow on the armchair, ease him into it, then cover him with a blanket and drape his IV lines and tubes over it. I turn on the TV.

"There you go, all the comforts of home!"

Damon remains sitting semi-upright for several hours, an excellent development. I divert him, and intermittently, I even coax my son to eat in his bird-like way. He consumes two crackers, half a chicken nugget, about ten French fries, a couple of Fritos, part of my Twix chocolate bar, and one orange segment. He also takes applesauce with his pills and drinks water and lemonade.

I have Sunday football on and Damon, not a fan, starts to take an interest, the first time he's engaged with the TV. Once he stretches and yawns luxuriously, and I feel he's *almost* himself. Problems persist but they seem more manageable.

"My back's sore," Damon complains several times.

"It may be displaced pressure from your big new heart," I say. "Here, let me give you a massage." I work around his tender neck, shifting the filigree of IV lines. His scapula feels bony and frail and I have to be very gentle. But the massage seems to help, at least while I'm giving it, because soon as I finish, he asks apologetically for "more, please!"

We unwind and chat. Damon jolts me when he reveals that he awoke during the last part of his heart transplant operation.

"I could hear the nurses gossiping and trying to move me. They turned me right on my *eye*, which was open against this cold metal slab! My brain wanted to speak, but I couldn't move my mouth . . . I had to wait while they shoved me around until they finally got my body into position. Then it felt like they were sewing up my chest with stitches!"

I grit my teeth and silently curse the anesthesiologists—this is the second time it appeared that they failed to properly sedate my son!—but I let Damon talk it out because it was clearly a traumatic experience whose enormity he's still trying to comprehend.

Damon drifts off, dozing, with good numbers. I make calls. Shealagh and Sam ask me a thousand questions, while my parents are happy to hear Damon is improving. My friend and mentor Art Singer offers to call up Nobelist Eric Kandel, a Columbia star, and have him put in a word for Damon.

Sunday night, Shealagh comes in to relieve me and brings a Big Mac with her. The doctors have warned Damon to consume more calories or they'll have to force-feed him.

"Here, sweetie, I got you something you like!" Shealagh says. Damon sits up in his bed and tries to take on the overstuffed burger. At first, it seems too much, but he manages a small bite and then another, and soon, as his digestive system cranks up, he displays flashes of real appetite, with juicy dribblings down his chin and a fortified gleam in his eye.

"It's good!" Damon nods as if he's just discovered eating. Shealagh and I smile. Damon doesn't finish the burger—he's still a ways from that—but things are looking up.

After ten days, Damon leaves the ICU and goes down to the sixth floor. He still has several more weeks in the hospital under a best-case scenario, but he's judged to be out of immediate danger. It's another major milestone.

Damon's recovery room is spacious, with a TV, telephone, computer, and guest bed. It's like a halfway house, and it puts us one step closer to our dream of returning home.

Everyone now feels sanguine about Damon's prospects. Dr. Hayes visits, beaming with palpable joy and relief. She's known Damon since he was three days old and couldn't be happier for us, especially after all we've been through.

"He looks so good!" she says with a grin.

Dr. Chen, the surgeon, stops by to check in on his patient. He's very pleased with Damon's progress and seems fond of our son. They banter. A *Deadwood* fan, he discusses Damon's upcoming debut. "I can't wait to see your episode, Damon!"

One day, Dr. Chen brings Dr. Eric Rose, the illustrious chief of cardiology renowned for performing the first pediatric heart transplant in the country. Dr. Rose visits us at the behest of Eric Kandel, and his arrival sets tongues wagging.

"Now you're going to meet a real VIP!" Dr. Chen grins at Damon and Shealagh. I'm at work so I miss the walk-through, but Dr. Mason, among others, is all agog about what drew the august figure to Damon's bedside. "How do you know him?" she asks.

Dr. Rose chats with Damon and Shealagh. He describes his first transplant patient, just celebrating his twenty-second anniversary. That patient had to be retransplanted, always an option, but today they know so much more about the immune issues—"they have it under control now"—that Damon is in a far better position.

Although Damon continues to recover, he hits several snags along the way. He gets a first biopsy revealing no sign of rejection, which is wonderful news, but the cath also shows a narrowing between his old SVC—his superior vena cava—and the donor veins, which will need to be widened with a balloon or a stent.

"I'd wait about six weeks till he's stronger to fix it," Dr. Hellenbrand advises.

Damon also continues to have issues such as high pressures and low saturation, requiring daily monitoring. As he heals, he's weaned off medications and faces new imbalances, such as low potassium. His chest X-ray still shows too much wetness around the lungs. And his chest drainage tube, the last major support system, continues to collect too much blood and pus, delaying its removal.

But Damon's biggest problem, we learn, is that once out of the ICU, he's no longer a priority and we must be even more active in managing his recovery. We do all the obvious things, like pushing him to stand and then walk inside the room. He leans on us and totters forward. Later we get him to take his first tentative steps out in the hallway. He dons a mask and pads slowly as we help wheel his IV pole. He's very weak and doddery and must take frequent breaks, but it's still very exciting for us.

"You're walking on your own, champ!" I cheer. We practice with him daily.

Unfortunately, Damon still has serious medical issues that we can't manage and that no one is attending to. We track all his medications and monitor all his readings and we report all his symptoms. But no one seems to be monitoring *us*. The doctors are unreliable or absent, and the nursing is erratic.

Two weeks after Damon's transplant, we seem to have fallen through the cracks.

Dr. Mason makes fewer visits and is harder to reach. Often she doesn't appear until the evening, when it's too late to do anything, and sometimes she doesn't appear for *several days* despite repeated paging. I refrain from any criticism—I cling to my honeymoon with Dr. Mason—and I ignore her prolonged absences so long as Damon's overall trajectory remains positive. But my wife grows increasingly dissatisfied. One night, after paging Dr. Mason for the third day without a callback—Shealagh is told she's away—my wife spots Damon's missing doctor on TV, standing in the very hospital we're at and smiling for all she's worth in the background of a well-publicized case!

Shealagh is furious and ready to file a complaint. "Damon has serious issues and Dr. Mason *still* hasn't seen him!" she cries.

Dr. Sanford, the third cardiologist on Dr. Mason's team, is supposedly helping to care for Damon. But Dr. Sanford does not make regular appearances. At one point we don't see her, or any doctor, for *four days*. I protest loudly and threaten to report this dereliction of duty until Dr. Sanford finally appears.

"No one's been in to examine Damon for four days!" I thunder.

"Well, we try to limit his exposure to other people," Dr. Sanford replies.

"To *doctors*?" I cry. "Isn't that why he's in the hospital—*to see doctors*?"

"It's not like no one has seen him," Dr. Sanford says defensively. "We have doctors and nurses who watch him when he walks out in the hallway."

"Please! You're doing *drive-by exams* now?" I can't believe my ears. "This is your idea of *world-class* care?"

"And Damon wears a *mask* in the hallway, so how much can you really *see*?" Shealagh points out, more measured than me but equally indignant.

Dr. Sanford, a big, stately, and somewhat academic young woman, gives a tight sigh, realizing we're not buying any of it. "Look, it's been pretty busy around here. I'm pulling double duty. I'm the transplant cardiologist but I'm also the attending doctor on the floor. So I may have been a little overextended."

I'm mortified by such a pathetic excuse but I try to focus on results, not recriminations. "Well, our son needs *a doctor* to look in on him *daily*. He's a heart transplant patient, remember? If you can't do it, we'll request a replacement."

"I can do it."

But even when Dr. Sanford comes to see Damon, her physical examination leaves much to be desired. First, like an increasing number of hospital doctors, she seems as interested in looking at the computer as in examining the patient. Second, her observational skills are poor. When Shealagh warns her about an incipient white growth in Damon's throat, Dr. Sanford examines him and says, "It's nothing." Now, several days later, Damon has a case of oral thrush, a well-known fungal infection that requires immediate attention.

We ask Dr. Sanford how she could miss such a common complication after we'd pointed it out to her. She replies that it was too *dark* in the room to see properly.

After three roller-coaster weeks, as we begin to focus on leaving the hospital, Damon's chest drainage tube becomes a big issue. He continues to put out too much fluid, a mixture of air, pus, and blood, and we can't remove the tube, and all its appurtenances, until the discharge has abated. We check his output every day and wait for it to subside.

One morning Dr. Sanford enters, glances at the computer, the chart, and my son, and says Damon's drainage is low enough to pull the tube. She leaves.

Shealagh, Damon, and I are thrilled. We've all been waiting to liberate Damon from the chest drainage paraphernalia, which emits an incessant aquarium-like bubbling and gurgling. The noisy contraption follows him everywhere, like an underwater ball and chain.

As we wait, I start to fret about Dr. Sanford's numbers because they sound too low. I bend down to the floor and inspect the collection chamber. I do a double take, because I see *three times* her estimate in the cylinders. And that's just for the overnight drainage, since the chamber was emptied the previous evening.

It's the difference between a safe and a dangerous environment for pulling the tube.

I can't believe it. If Dr. Sanford had bothered to bend down and look with her own eyes, she'd have known her assessment was an impossible number!

Riled up, I complain to the nurse and have her check the computer. Sure enough, the data is wrong. But she just enters the new figures onto the old ones, as if they never existed. Outraged, I tell her she has no right to cover this up.

Just as unsettling, this mistake means we must wait for Damon's chest drainage to *truly* subside, and we can't even *think* about going home until his outflow has abated.

Three days later, I'm on weekend duty again, and Damon and I go on an extended stroll. It's his longest walk yet. As we near our ward on the return, I hear a sudden whistling sound emanating from Damon.

I look down and see his chest tube has separated from its insertion point, and air coming from a tiny exposed hole in his pleural space is hissing like a kettle. It sounds bad, so we flag a nurse, who quickly covers the hole and summons a doctor.

The doctor, a prim-looking woman with glasses, removes the chest tube.

"We need to prepare for an emergency reimplantation in the ICU," she says, and orders a chest X-ray. While we wait, I talk to her and see she's on the ball, a genuine, thinking physician. When the X-ray arrives, she studies it and says, "We could reimplant the tube or try leaving it out and see what happens."

"That sounds interesting," I say. "What do you mean exactly?"

"It's a calculated gamble," she explains. "Worst case, the fluid migrates behind the lungs, making it a little harder to extract. But his body also might adjust to the change and find its own equilibrium *without* the chest drainage tube."

"Go for it!" I tell her, knowing we might not get another chance like this.

Damon lets me convince him because he *hates* the gurgling tube and would do anything to ditch it.

It takes a few days—with one bad night when it looks like we might have to reinsert the tube—but Damon does finally find his own tube-free equilibrium. I silently bless this fine young doctor.

New issues crop up at the last minute. "I'm having a little trouble with words when I read," Damon says one day. Doctors give him a visual field test and note he has difficulty with one section of it. When we ask how serious this is, the senior neurologist replies, "It usually resolves, but sometimes they go blind. It's hard to predict."

Shealagh and I try not to think about this dire specter or the cavalier way it's conveyed. Fortunately, we are assigned a neurology fellow who works with Damon every day and helps him get a handle on this problem. She's just starting out but already has the gift. Once again, a young, talented, and motivated woman doctor does her job and helps Damon over a potentially debilitating hurdle.

We're biding our time now and praying that no more mishaps occur. One morning, the nurse brings Damon a 1,200 mg pill of ibuprofen instead of magnesium—after everyone has warned him that he must *not* take any ibuprofen. This time it's Damon, more alert now, who catches the mix-up and sends the toxic pill back. He talks to me about it repeatedly.

"Dad, she gave me the wrong pill! If I hadn't noticed, I'd have been in big trouble . . . We have to watch *everything*, it's just like you said!" He's shocked and looks at me with new understanding. I'm known as the barking dog by my family, and God knows what else by the hospital staff, and now Damon sees firsthand how critical our vigilance is.

As Damon improves, he seeks diversion and focuses more on the future. He chats on the phone, blogs on the computer, and listens to his iPod. Shealagh orders films for him to screen on our DVD player and reads aloud to him. They devour Laurence Olivier's *Confessions of an Actor*. Damon works out with a physiotherapist and starts to train his body. And he has his mother get an application for his learner's permit. He plans to get his driver's license on his seventeenth birthday and buy a secondhand school bus with his friends for a cross-country trek.

Now that he's better, Damon also receives more visitors in the hospital. Sam and Miranda and my parents and my sister come, and so do several of Damon's friends. Kyle visits several times. Once when I drive her home from the hospital, Kyle turns to me and says, "I have to admit, he looked much better than I expected!"

Trekking up to a big hospital to visit a sick friend who's just had a heart transplant is a brave act for teenagers, and everyone who makes the effort impresses us.

Near the end of Damon's ordeal, my own body starts to recoil against the hospital. For a whole month, all my days and nights have either started or ended in this grim location, often both, and my life has narrowed to one tiny repetitive loop.

I'm sick of the dank 168th Street subway station, of every greasy fast food joint and takeout place in the area, of the guarded entrance with the string of ambulances outside, of the vendor with his stale peanuts, of the twenty-four-hour crush of desperate people in various stages of distress, of the security guards and the endless winding corridors and tiled floors and fluorescent walls, the insipid cafeteria, the slow elevators, the hollow vending machines, more endless corridors, and then the dusty floor and the weary, white-coated nurses and doctors and technicians and cleaning staff, and the inescapable sour hospital room itself with its tired bed and musty monitors and limp equipment, and my bag of dirty clothes and bare toiletries waiting in a forlorn corner between the cot and the sink.

We finally get the word on a Friday afternoon when my mother and Sam are visiting. Shealagh and I are both in the hospital room with Damon.

Dr. Mason comes by to say that Damon will be discharged tomorrow.

Although we've been anticipating this, it's still an astonishing moment of liberation.

We all cheer and applaud. It's hard to believe. We've been here thirty-two days!

I go over and give Damon a big hug, then offer a formal handshake to my hero. Everyone pays equally heartfelt and personal tribute.

Damon sits on his hospital bed, quietly glowing.

Chapter 51

"I'm Free! . . . I'm Free! . . . and freeedom tastes of reality!"

—I'm Free, The Who

That's right, I am. After 4 weeks and 4 days I am finally out of the hospital and back at home. What a frickin relief. The computer in my room at the hospital broke down so I couldn't update every other day like I'd figured I would, apologies. Got back on Saturday and have just been recovering and discovering what I've been missing all these years.

Went to play some WC3. I love you guys. I'm not sure how I would have got through all this without you. Thanx to Will, Zak and Max.

—From Damon's blog, February 22, 2005

I can't believe it.

We're back home.

With Damon.

Who has a strong new heart and is doing really well!

He's back in his room, sleeping in his own bed, and eating meals with us.

He's back on his own computer, blogging and IM-ing and Warcrafting.

He's back on the phone with his pals, lolling on his chair and gabbing for hours.

He's back in the family room, building things with Sam and Miranda and playing board games and watching TV and hanging out with all of us.

Damon is also back with his beloved Freddie. He takes the mini-pin for short walks around the block. The energetic dog does not leap at the front door, as usual, but meekly offers up his long neck as Damon slips his red collar on and snaps the buckle. Freddie lingers patiently inside until Damon, still weak, has donned his winter coat and white face mask and signaled it's time to go.

"Come on, Fred." The two companions step outside. Damon holds the leash and pauses to survey things from the porch, once again master of his dominion. He smiles softly. Freddie has enough play on the sixteen-foot lead to run ahead and explore. When the dog gets too frisky, Damon yanks on the Flexi leash and Freddie looks up guiltily, recalibrating his pace so as not to strain Damon.

They return, invigorated, and cuddle together on the sofa.

On his first day back from the hospital, Damon sits down at the piano. He hasn't touched it for years but now he picks out the popular spiritual "He's Got the Whole World in His Hands" and begins to play. He's a little rusty and the piano is a little out of tune, but soon the uplifting gospel strains fill the house.

It's an extraordinary new situation we find ourselves in back home.

The worst is behind us, and while we must continue to monitor the situation closely, the odds now favor us for the first time in a very long time.

It seems too good to be true, so I hunt for flaws and weaknesses. On Damon's last day in the hospital, for his last blood test before discharge, I ask the nurse to check his albumin and total protein, even though it isn't indicated on the order. In all our anxiety about Damon's recovery, I have not forgotten that the underlying reason for the transplant—the cause for such a radical operation in the first place—was Damon's PLE. And I need to see how we're doing on that score, even if the doctors insist it's too early to tell and the test won't mean anything at this stage. But I remain haunted by studies showing PLE may not resolve, *even after a heart transplant*, and I need to verify we've avoided that particularly vicious fate. So I cajole the nurse to check the appropriate box on the blood test form.

That night, after Damon has jettisoned his ID tags and exchanged his hospital gown and slippers like prison garb for his own clothes, and after he's marched out of the hospital on a sunny but cold February afternoon with a cautiously triumphant smile beneath his white face mask, and after he has arrived home to a Winnie-the-Pooh-style hero party with a welcome banner, ribbons, and balloons, and after my kind parents, living in our house and minding our kids for a month, have left with our boundless thanks and everyone else has retreated upstairs, I get a call from Dr. Mason's office. Her nurse informs us, with breathless pride—I note they're always prompter with good news than bad, per the marketing mentality—that Damon's albumin has jumped to a PLE-busting 3.0!

It's not just icing on the cake, it's the whole cake!

Even the pediatric cardiology transplant team, which was opposed to measuring the protein so soon, concedes this is very exciting news.

I thank them for telling us and I hang up, profoundly grateful and relieved.

Now it's definitive, and I can really believe it myself and celebrate wholeheartedly.

A week later, our joy runneth over, as Damon's albumin hits 3.5, which is like mine and yours and that of everyone else who's is healthy, normal, and fully functional.

Damon has an efficient new heart and a brand-new lease on life!

Nevertheless, for many days, even weeks, following Damon's triumphant return, I cannot completely process this information. For the past nearly four years, my entire existence has been dominated by this battle for survival and the ceaseless deployment of all available resources toward one overriding goal. And now that the goal has been attained—Damon's illness is cured, and he's recovering—I don't quite know how to let my guard back down or what to do with myself in the freed-up space.

I begin by thanking all the doctors who helped us, from Columbia and from all the other hospitals, including my dedicated private brain trust. But because old habits die hard, and because I don't wish to be lulled into complacency—even if we've bought Damon fifteen to twenty years, what happens *after that?*—I prod my advisers about future therapies. I'm interested in artificial hearts, xenotransplantation, and stem cell therapy.

Everyone tells me they expect a new era of advances, but I should just kick back and enjoy Damon's success for now.

"I'm very optimistic about Damon's outlook," Dr. Rose e-mails me after I thank him for his help. And everyone seems to share this confidence. So I start to let go and relax. I accept that the nightmare is over, that Damon has been released from his captivity, and that I, too, am liberated.

I'm six weeks from my fiftieth birthday and aware of diverted plans and unmet goals—though it all seems worth it now that Damon is home, safe and sound.

I draw up a list of new goals and plans, including expanding my professional opportunities. I accept several travel and speaking invitations I'd deferred. I apply to a college writing program that requires only a short summer residency. I also register for my first Olympic triathlon. It's only six months away and I've done no training, but it's a spur to both action and imagination.

After the initial euphoria of Damon's homecoming, there is the day-to-day reality of recovery. Yet albeit slower and shakier, that reality is in many ways even *more* thrilling, because now it's all about Damon adjusting and growing into his new capabilities and learning to do things he could never do before.

Damon remains weak from his surgery, with much ground to make up, but even the nature of his weakness has changed for the better. Now when he climbs the stairs from the family room to his bedroom on the main floor, or from his room to our second-story bedroom, he doesn't get out of breath as he used to. His big, new heart keeps his blood pumping vigorously. Instead, it's his muscles that feel the strain, lagging behind his new cardiovascular prowess. "My legs feel sore," Damon says with a wondrous half smile.

But building up his muscles is a workable proposition, and Damon now embarks on a daily exercise program. He stretches and does calisthenics. He performs modified sit-ups, squats, and push-ups. He takes bracing walks with Freddie. And he works out with hand weights, lifting small dumbbells and relentlessly toning his body around the clock.

Now that he's lost all his excess fluid from the PLE—except in the face, where the steroids puff him up—Damon is down to eighty-six pounds. His arms, in particular, look thin. But his appetite is back, and he's diligent about his regimen, eating regularly and exercising several times a day with fierce concentration. He makes steady, impressive progress.

"If you keep this up, we'll be able to run triathlons together!" I tell Damon, and knowing his disciplined determination, it's not as farfetched as it sounds.

It's not just his body but also Damon's mental attitude that bounces back strong. He's full of schemes and plans, and none takes any post-transplant limitation into account. He will catch up on his course work over the summer and apply to college with everyone else during the fall semester of his senior year.

"You may want to stick close to New York for the first year or two, when hospital visits are the norm," I suggest during one college discussion.

Damon bristles. "No! Why would I do that?"

"Hey, New York's not a backwater. You got Columbia, NYU, many goo—"

"No!" Damon repeats. He gives me the baleful teenage eye for daring to hem him in or daring even to *contemplate* such a possibility.

This reaction is mild, however, compared to the resentment I elicit during another discussion of Damon's future. Though he still plans to return to *Deadwood* over the summer, he worries that acting, which he loves, is not serious or public-spirited enough for a full-time career. He's long been interested in diplomacy, and we've talked about the State Department after college. Although such a decision is years away, I incur Damon's wrath when I suggest he might wish to reconsider such a path in light of his heart transplant.

"In the State Department, you must take any assignment they give you," I say. "And most new recruits get sent to the Third World. Now you'll be on immune suppressants your whole life, making you that much more vulnerable to any infection but especially to rare or exotic pathogens, so I'm just saying *maybe* this is not the *ideal career* for you."

"No, I don't agree!" Damon cries. "There's no reason I can't do it."

"True, though your medical history is part of the application . . . But why take the *added* risk? I have friends with normal immune systems who picked up nasty bugs in Asia and Africa . . . There's so many *other* things you can do, D-man."

"But not if this is what I want!" He's so adamant and irate, I decide to let it go. Why have a major dust-up over such a distant possibility? And I don't want to crush Damon's dreams, or even more importantly, to crush his *spirit*.

He even convinces his mother, who then prevails upon me, to let him go to Tech and meet the Group for a first post-transplant get-together. They congregate after school by the park, and Damon promises to wear his mask and to exclude anyone with a cold if we'll let him go. We're supposed to limit his contact with other people but Dr. Mason thinks it's okay if he doesn't overdo it and Shealagh promises to supervise.

The outing is a big success with a large, spirited turnout.

"What happened to your original heart, Damon?" Max asks in his high-spirited, analytic way. "Don't throw it out. You should keep it in a jar and give it to the woman you marry!"

"I don't know, Max." Damon grins behind his mask. "Maybe a little ghoulish?"

"No, it would be so cool and so romantic!" Max insists. "You should do it!"

"Hey, Damon, you ever get your donor's dreams and memories?" Zak asks.

"Hmmm, not as far as I can recall, Zak." Damon smiles.

Damon has checkups at Columbia several times a week. I'm back at work, so Shealagh handles the visits, which take place in Dr. Mason's office. All seems good but Shealagh wants to know about a stubborn, thrush-like growth in Damon's mouth.

"He needs to do a better job of swishing with his disinfectant," Dr. Mason says.

"But he rinses meticulously and very thoroughly, several times a day as directed, and I watch him, so I know!" Damon's vigilant mother replies.

Dr. Mason shrugs. "If he keeps using the disinfectant, it will all work out."

Shealagh still finds Dr. Mason a touch high-handed and too dismissive of her concerns. "She's so bloody sure about everything—'It's *all routine*'— even when she doesn't seem to have a clue!"

But Shealagh is a worrier, Dr. Mason has treated many transplant patients, and Damon is doing well, so we're not about to complain.

Damon quickly resumes his independent teenage existence. Beyond daily pills and regular doctor's visits, there are only minor nods to his physical recovery.

Every few days, I must help with his DuoDERM skin dressing. His pressure sore has still not healed, and it's in a sensitive spot near his tush, so I must bend down and find the tiny target. "Okay, you're good, D-man," I say as I stand back up. It's like a last vestige of intimacy, a throwback to all the time we spent together in the hospital.

Otherwise Damon has only a few minor scars near the incision line, and his skin tone is magnificent, with rosy face and pink body.

"I think you're actually growing!" I remark.

Damon tries to repay me with his usual sweetness. On Oscar night, the family is sitting around the TV when he comes up and starts to rub my shoulders. I relish Damon's massages but am worried about the strain on him post-surgery. But Damon digs in with both hands, and using his whole body as leverage, he manages to exert surprising force. He stops after about ten minutes.

"Sorry, Dad, I'll do better next time. I'm still not a hundred percent."

"You kidding? That was great, D-man. Thanks!"

Shealagh and Miranda go up to bed at the halfway mark but the boys and I wait until midnight to see Clint Eastwood's *Million Dollar Baby* win the Oscar. The next day Damon asks me if we can go see the movie. The small theater in our multiplex is almost empty—the film's been playing for months—so Damon doesn't even have to keep his face mask on. It's a thrill to buy popcorn and soda and sit in reclining seats in a dark theater with my son after all he's been through.

When the film's over, we hit a local joint for dinner. Damon was more moved than me by this Hollywood film about a female boxer who's para-lyzed after an unfair fight.

"I liked that the main character decided life wasn't worth living on a respirator," he says. "Her dreams were crushed and she wanted to go with dignity. And I liked how her trainer, who loved her, still decided to give her what she wanted by helping her die."

It's a charged subject for Damon, who's just come out of the hospital after a long ordeal, including total maintenance on life support. He's okay now, but he must have experienced many dark, desperate moments. It dawns on me he knows this material far better than I do, and I listen closely to what he says.

It's a great evening for the two of us. We're doing all these routine things together—going to a neighborhood movie, eating dinner at a local restau-rant, having a real talk—that we could only dream of doing while Damon was so sick.

Damon polishes off his food in record time, then glances up at me with a mixture of blushing pride and sheepish apology.

"I'm still hungry, Dad. Could I have another burger?"

I grin at my embarrassed teenage son. "D-man, you can have ten bur-gers—a hundred burgers—have *anything* you want!"

I call the waiter over and order another burger and fries. I've never seen Damon eat like this, and it's exhilarating to watch. He has that sleek, raven-ous look in the eye, as if he needs to make up for all those years of frugal eating and meager calories. As if he intends to *consume* his way back to full strength and health.

Chapter 52

—*From Damon's blog, March 9, 2005*

Sometime in early March, I notice Damon's albumin level has dropped to 3.3. A reading of 3.3 is within the margin of error of 3.5, Damon's previous level, but I still don't like the direction. When the next reading comes in at 3.0, I start to grow concerned. I note also that Damon has a slight cough and that he looks droopier. But maybe I'm just being overzealous and have unrealistic expectations for a magical transformation.

I query Dr. Mason about this trend, but as expected, she brushes it off.

"These values jump all over the place in the first months, you shouldn't even be *looking* at them!" she tells me. I e-mail Dr. Chin and Dr. Rose, inquiring from each, "Is this drop within the normal range of fluctuation for a post-transplant patient?"

Dr. Chin replies we'd need to graph more values and study the overall pattern; Dr. Rose suggests I ask Damon's cardiologists, because anything he says would be pure conjecture.

These responses do not allay my concerns, but neither do they induce panic. I just heighten my alert level and watch Damon more closely.

The next day, a Friday, Shealagh takes Damon to see Dr. Mason for his regular visit—he goes three times a week—and Dr. Mason continues with her breezy dismissal of any concerns. She says our son is doing well and there's nothing to worry about. But that same night, around eleven P.M., when we're at home, Damon comes up to our bedroom.

"I just got this kinda *shivery* feeling," he reports, frowning. His breathing is shallow and rapid, he has the chills, and he looks pale. Our son is no hypochondriac, so we take his temperature. It's 100.8, indicating fever, a warning sign of possible rejection or infection.

"All the manuals state that the slightest indication of fever in an immune-compromised patient is significant and should be followed up," Shealagh says.

We don't like this at all and quickly call the hospital, reaching Dr. Davis. We assume we must bring Damon in right away but Dr. Davis says she doesn't think it's necessary.

"A temperature of a hundred is borderline. You can keep an eye on him and call back in the morning. If he doesn't get worse, you could wait until Monday for his regular biopsy."

Shealagh and I are surprised—we've been told that transplant patients must come in immediately for any hint of a symptom—but we're not looking to make extra hospital trips, and Dr. Davis has more experience than us, so we accept her advice and stay home.

By Saturday, Damon's fever is under 100 and he seems calmer. But he still doesn't look quite right to us, though we can't tell if this is normal for the post-transplant period.

We take him in Monday morning but the hospital is slow and doesn't process his biopsy order for an entire day. We will have to wait until Tuesday for the test. We're upset about this but the doctors say they want to keep him in the hospital regardless, so they can start him on a three-day anti-rejection course.

"Isn't that premature, since you haven't even tested for rejection yet?" I ask.

But Dr. Becker—neither Dr. Mason nor Dr. Davis is there to see us—says no. "It's most likely rejection—I heard a gallop when I listened to his heart. Even if the biopsy is negative, it could still be rejection in a different part of the heart."

I scowl. "Doesn't that render the test effectively *meaningless,* since you've prejudged the outcome regardless of the test result?"

Shealagh nods with me, equally confused by this tortured-seeming logic.

"No, this is standard procedure for a patient in Damon's situation," Dr. Becker says. "I assume you don't want to risk a major rejection episode, do you?"

Shealagh and I huddle. We're upset that Dr. Mason is not there and that no biopsy was done all day. Shealagh points out that the junior Dr. Becker has never listened to Damon's heart before, so she has no baseline for diagnosing a "gallop." But we both feel we can't risk *not* giving the course, just in case she's right.

Once we've convinced ourselves, we still have to convince Damon.

"No, why should I take all this new medication *before* we do the test?" Damon protests. "I don't have rejection, believe me! I know my own body."

Shealagh and I feel like shills as we explain the hospital's convoluted rationale to our son. "Sometimes we just have to trust their expertise," we tell him with a deep sigh.

Damon begins the anti-rejection course that evening, and the next morning he goes for his biopsy. The result comes back in the afternoon, and it's negative—there is *absolutely no sign* of rejection. Damon registers 0 on a scale of 4.0!

Damon flashes a sharp "I told you so" look. Shealagh and I feel greatly relieved but remain wary given the conflicting information we're getting.

The doctors not only maintain they did the right thing by *starting* Damon on the anti-rejection course, they now want him to *finish* it too. Dr. Mason shows up the next day, self-assured as ever, and confirms this is her recommendation.

"A biopsy is taken from only one section of the heart, so Damon could test negative and *still* have rejection in a *different* part of his heart." She smiles. "We've seen it before!"

Shealagh and I shake our heads but we don't have enough knowledge or experience to risk ignoring this advice. We're unhappy but at loose ends.

"Why don't you go back to the office? I'll take it from here," Shealagh offers. "It's just waiting around at this point. At least Damon will be home soon. This is our lot now."

Damon stays in the hospital for several days and blogs to his friends about it:

Yep I'm back at the hospital. Just for 3 days though so I should be leaving tomorrow morning. Actually pretty standard especially in the first 3 months they all warned me that this was something that frequently happens but it's annoying none the less. Came in Monday 4 the usual check-up and the biopsy (that's when they go in with a needle and take out a small piece of your heart). Hadn't been great the past few days I thought it was a cold, *they* thought it was rejection. So they decided they were gonna keep me for the 3 days to give me the IV steroids (standard rejection treatment). I said how bout waiting 4 the biopsy results cause everyone I asked including the doc who said it was rejection said that a cold or other mild infection aka flu fever could and would cause the same symptoms. But better safe than sorry and all that jazz so Monday finds me in a hospital bed. Tuesday afternoon finds the biopsy results. Guess what boys and girls—no rejection. 😲 But of course they'd already started the steroids and its possible so might as well finish the job so I'm here till tomorrow morning. Yippee 😊.

Realized and been realizing many things. Can't possibly explain them all don't quite understand them all myself yet. But one thing I'm slowly beginning 2 understand is just how weak I really was before (the heart transplant for those who are confused). Honestly I'll never understand how I got through the last 3 years as well as I did. And now when I think of what I might have been able to do with those 3 years had it not been for PLE it makes me kinda sad. I guess I never really accepted it or admitted it before but now it's suddenly sort of hit me; I had a disease and a bad one, one that could and did kill people and one that no one really knew anything definitive about and who could blame them. About 10,000 people in America have had my operation (the original 1) and 10% of those get PLE that's not exactly much of a data base. And one that could have eventually killed me and was weakening me day by day.

Strange I never really thought of myself that way until now looking back on it all. But it's not quite over. When I first got out of the hospital I felt great and I still do but the past week and especially being brought back 2 the hospital has made me realize that recovery will not be quick or easy. It's going 2 take time and work and patience. I only mind the time. How much more time is this all gonna take/waste and what am I going 2 lose or miss in the process? But as long as I am moving forward though minor setbacks are inevitable life is very good and I've got a lot of make up 2 do. ☺ ☺ ☺ ☺

After three days, Damon leaves the hospital and returns home. He seems okay and there are no more acute episodes. We're all relieved. But he still has a cough and a peckish aspect. And the steroids have given him a distorted moon face and a swollen neck, which, when he first appears in my study in the morning, makes me start. It's painful to see my beautiful boy with such grotesque features.

We go downstairs, where I help him take his morning meds and make him breakfast. We sit and talk, but everything feels off-kilter. Damon looks like he's wearing a troll mask. He describes strange hallucinations in ghoulish detail.

"This fiendish figure was standing behind the door, ready to attack me!"

I ask Dr. Mason about these visions. "Oh, that's not unusual with the strong doses he's on, it'll stop once he tapers off," she replies.

Shealagh also is unhappy with Damon's condition but relieved he's coming off the steroids. She keeps taking Damon to Columbia and reporting various cold-like symptoms: headaches, sniffles, fatigue, swollen glands, breathing problems, and stomach pain. She is especially concerned about the fact that Damon is losing weight—he should be gaining—and that he's experiencing mental confusion. But Dr. Mason says the confusion is typical as patients adjust to cyclosporine, the weight loss is from ascites decrease, and the puffiness is from the anti-rejection course. "There is nothing to worry about," she tells Shealagh.

Shealagh takes Damon to Columbia on a Friday afternoon and despite the all-clear, the next morning he gets the chills and a fever again. This time his temperature is 101 but we're less panicked about it. We call up the hospital and Dr. Sanford, who's on duty, says to bring him in to the emergency room and she'll meet us there. Since it's a Saturday, and Shealagh has already taken Damon to the hospital several times this week, I drive him in.

"I'm sorry you guys have to shuttle me back and forth all the time," Damon says.

"Come on, D-man, this is normal during the first year and we're prepared for it. It's why Mom's home full-time and I'm happy to do it when I'm here . . . The only thing you need to worry about is getting better!" I smile at my son, who looks frail and bowed.

When we reach the hospital, I ask Damon if he wants to wait by the entrance while I park. It's chilly outside and there's a steep hill down to the parking lot, which he'd have to climb. Damon nods, and I drop him by a bench out front before driving down to the lot.

When I return, I see Damon on a far corner of the bench, sitting in a narrow patch of bright sunlight. He's found the *one* blessed spot, and his red-crested head peeps out of his bulky anorak, craning upward to extract maximum warmth, light, and air before he must enter the hospital confines.

I sit on the bench by Damon and steal an extra few minutes in the slanting sun beside him, seizing the same glorious moment and briefly contemplating the same subversive thought.

What if we just stayed here and *refused* to go inside?

I recall Damon reading Melville's *Bartleby the Scrivener* on the plane back from L.A. and its famous words now echo for me in front of the hospital: "I would prefer not."

But then Damon starts to cough, and I know we have no choice. I make him put on his face mask before we walk inside, pass security, and run the gauntlet of chronically and acutely ailing patients that fills the emergency room. I raise my voice at the desk, explaining Damon is an immune-compromised patient and I need to get him out of this pathogen-teeming area. I get a few jaded, gimme-a-break scowls, but someone heeds me because we are soon ushered out of the waiting area and into a small cubicle inside.

To my dismay, Dr. Sanford, who promised she'd meet us, is nowhere to be found. I soon learn there are only two doctors for the whole ER, and they're both besieged. We have a long wait until one finally shows.

Our ER doctor is harried but sharp. She quickly grasps our case and leads us to a small private area where Damon can lie down. I tell her we need a regular room, away from the ER, and she nods. "Yes, but it would be easier if your son's cardiologist was here. I'll do what I can but I must run to my next patient now."

I get Damon comfortable, then go buy us food. We eat by his bed, then Damon tries to nap. But he's too restless, so he asks me about the paper I'm reading and we have a discussion about current events.

At some point, Damon falls asleep. He looks peaceful and settled, and I start to feel better about his condition.

The doctor comes by with Damon's blood results, circling two items. "Your son's liver enzymes are abnormal and his platelet count is very low. His team must deal with this." Then she runs off again. Since none of Damon's cardiologists is present, and I don't know exactly what these values mean—are they abnormal for a transplant patient or just for an average patient?—I focus on Damon's comfort and getting us onto the main floor.

A cardiologist drops by. She examines Damon but tells us nothing. She leaves.

By four P.M.—we arrived at noon—I begin to grow anxious about Damon. The ER is a dangerous place for my immune-compromised son, and I'm eager to get him out of here. But there's clearly a holdup with our room. After many calls and persistent pagings, by five P.M. I learn that the patient currently occupying the room meant for Damon refuses to leave.

He's a low-priority case, he's been cleared for discharge, but he simply *won't go.*

I explain to the nurse how urgent it is to get my son out of the ER. "Yes," she says, nodding.

Nevertheless, for the next five hours, I tussle with a series of inept hospital administrators and bureaucrats to get Damon into his own room. Everyone agrees he needs the bed and should have it. But no one knows how to get the other patient *out.*

I'm amazed the hospital cannot enforce its own rules due to the whim of one patient. But instead of ejecting *him,* they start pressuring *me* to accept an overnight bed in the ER for Damon. "It's out of the question!" I tell them. When they tell me the ER has its advantages, I demand to speak to the supervisor. I leave several messages until he finally calls me back. But to my astonishment, he *too* tries to get us to stay in the ER!

"I'm sorry, but we can't get the other patient to leave," the supervisor says.

"Are you serious? You expect me to endanger my son's life because you can't do your job? Get us a room or I'll file a complaint against you and your whole team!"

"The ER is not so bad and I'll make sure he gets a nice bed," he wheedles.

"My son is a *transplant* patient and he's *sick!*" I cry.

By nine P.M., after several hours more of this, I finally lose my patience and head for the ward. If they can't do it, I'll get the other patient out myself.

It's bad enough none of his cardiologists has seen Damon all day, knowing we had an *emergency*, but I won't let my son spend the night in the ER, a known incubator for infection. I'm furious and it's noted.

I storm up in the elevator, but there's a new supervisor who meets me as I step off. He apologizes hat in hand, admits the error, and promises to have the patient out forthwith.

It's eleven P.M. before Damon finally gets his own room on a regular ward. But perhaps because we had to work so hard to get here, once we arrive, everything quickly normalizes.

Damon is feeling better and the hospital room setup is so familiar, we make ourselves right at home. I check the phone and TV, unpack clothes, open up the armchair.

Damon is chirpy and seems more like himself. Maybe he's already recovered from whatever little problem he had.

The only bummer is that tomorrow night is his *Deadwood* debut, and I suspect he won't be discharged in time to watch it. Even if everything looks fine, the doctors will likely want to keep him under observation for at least another day.

Chapter 53

So for those who are interested, I will be on "Deadwood" this Sunday the 20th at 9:00 on HBO (channel 32 for most I think). The show is an hour and I don't know when exactly I'll be on but probably some point in the middle.

Now a word or two on Deadwood; it's not for everyone. It's very coarse and very vulgar and very violent. It takes a little getting used 2. When I watched the first episode, I was quite daunted but after you watch a couple and get into it you start 2 realize what a great show it really is . . . but maybe I'm biased. Either way this is not me trying 2 convince you or any1 to become a regular watcher of the show (though you're more than welcome 2), this just me keeping you all informed and giving you a little warning. And no I wasn't traumatized nor abused in any way when I went up 2 the set. Just 4 the record. I must say it was pretty cool watching the 2nd season and knowing all the people and seeing the scenes that I watched them shoot, it makes it a totally different experience.

—*From Damon's blog, March 14, 2005*

Damon has a decent night in the hospital and the next day, a Sunday, all seems to calm down. During morning rounds, the consensus is he has some kind of a cold and this is not a serious matter. Shealagh comes in the afternoon to relieve me and says Damon looks pretty good.

I'm scheduled to fly to Japan on Tuesday and have a talk to prepare, but with Damon in the hospital, I'm not sure I should bother. Shealagh suggests I draft my presentation. She's glad I'm ready to cancel, but for now she feels the situation is under control. "And you should definitely go if we don't need you here."

That night after I get home, Damon makes his national TV debut on *Deadwood*. Sadly, he can't watch it at a party with his friends, because he's in the hospital, and he can't watch it in the hospital because the place doesn't have HBO. I watch the show alone; it's too X-rated for Sam and Miranda. Happily, Damon's little scene is a gem and I get many compliments for him. I call Damon on his cell—even in the hospital, he answers reliably—and relay the tributes. Paula Malcomson calls to congratulate Damon, validating his professional bona fides. Gary Leffew also calls, but Gary only gets through to me. "Tell him we gonna ride to the mountaintop again, soon as he come outta there!"

The next day, a Monday, I head straight to the hospital after work. Damon sits up in bed, looking sharp and alert, while Dr. Mason, back on the case, beavers about. She has various people from infectious disease coming in to see Damon and trying to pinpoint what's causing his cold-like symptoms. By this stage, none of us has too many illusions about Dr. Mason—I even catch Damon frowning at one of her explanations—but we've gotten this far with her, and she's the only game in town, so we make the best of it.

I tell Dr. Mason that I'm scheduled to fly to Japan the following day, but I can easily cancel the trip if she thinks there's any reason, *any reason at all,* I should stay.

"No, make your trip—go, go!" Dr. Mason waves her arm breezily. "There's nothing to worry about here. We wouldn't even keep Damon in the hospital if he wasn't so close to his transplant. We're just being extra-cautious."

Dr. Mason tugs on her stethoscope, which she wears like a gym teacher's whistle. "It's always like this for the first year. We'll have Damon in whenever we suspect anything, and you can't put your entire lives on hold. Mostly it doesn't concern you, anyway . . . So go give your talk in Japan, and don't mind any of this. Everything's *fine* here."

"Yeah, Dad, I want you to go!" Damon pipes up.

"We *all* want you to go!" Shealagh chimes in, smiling.

"Can you bring me back some sushi?" Damon asks, fingering bland applesauce.

"You got it," I say. When Damon gets a call, I take Dr. Mason aside.

"What do you think is really going on?" I ask.

"He has something like a mild cold," Dr. Mason tells me, "and we think it's from a viral agent. We're just keeping him until we can determine exactly what it is, to be on the safe side. But it's a routine thing, and we have it totally under control. No worries."

I stay with Damon and Shealagh until the evening. As I gather my overnight bag and see Shealagh's bag in its place, I realize the hospital has turned into our second home.

Sensing the slightest sniffle, I refrain from hugging Damon good-bye because we're still scrupulous about his immune-compromised status. Instead, I just wave warmly to my son and blow him a kiss. "See you, D-man!"

"Bye, Dad," Damon says, waving back.

Shealagh steps out and walks me to the elevator. She gives me a big hug. "It's important for all of us—for Sam and Miranda and for me, as well as for Damon—that you keep plowing forward and not let our lives grind to a complete halt. We need you out there."

The next day, as we're sitting on the runway, I call the hospital for a final Damon check, half-expecting I'll never get off the ground because some impediment may yet crop up at the last minute. But when I reach Shealagh, she reports Damon is sleeping comfortably. "Everything is fine here," she informs me.

I smile and remind myself that we have entered a new, more positive phase.

We take off without incident but somewhere above the Bering Sea, our plane runs into serious turbulence, and we go into a sudden nosedive. It's more than the usual air bump, and we drop with alarming speed. In the brief, jolting seconds when we seem to be plunging to certain death, two thoughts flash before me: first, that I really would prefer to live; and second, if I am about to die, it means Damon, that durable son of mine, has survived me after all.

While the first thought induces terror and regret, the second is profoundly soothing and consoling, and actually brings a small smile to my lips.

I sacrifice an entire day and then some on the flight over, and by the time I get to my hotel, meet one of my hosts for a drink, and do e-mail, it's bedtime. I get up early the next morning and speak to Shealagh and Damon for over an hour. Damon had a rough night, spiking a fever, but now he feels better, as if the fever actually improved things.

I sign off and head to the National Institute of Science and Technology Policy to give my talk, "The Image of Scientists and Engineers." Later I meet with a member of the Japanese parliament and have dinner near Tokyo University.

On my way back to the hotel, I begin to fret about Damon. Although I'm not aware of any new problems, worrying about him is my default, and since we haven't spoken all day, I start to troubleshoot in my head, recalling that when I noted it sounded like he was improving, Damon said he wasn't improving, he was deteriorating. I pressed him to explain but he played it down, admitting he felt better today and was just letting off steam. But his remark returns to me now since Damon doesn't usually indulge in that kind of self-pity.

Alas, when I reach Shealagh on the phone, she is in a near-panic and informs me things have gotten very bad, very fast. "The doctors now believe Damon's *liver* may be infected. His liver enzyme levels are elevated, and he's broken out in these red spots everywhere. His platelet count is extremely low, and his body keeps chewing up the new platelets they're giving him. He's feverish, he looks shaky, and he seems *very* weak!"

Shealagh says the doctors have offered to move Damon to the ICU because he can get better care there, and she agreed, because she's worried. "They believe it could be a viral or bacterial infection, but they're still not sure what's going on!"

This news makes my heart shudder and turns everything around me to dust.

It's clear I have to return immediately. I don't know exactly what's going on, but I know I need to be there. I have little doubt we can fix this—isn't the worst behind us now?—but it's going to demand a full-court press.

"I hate to break up your trip but Damon always does better when you're around," Shealagh says. "He draws strength from you . . . And I need you too," she adds.

"Don't worry, it's only a question of how fast I can find a flight at this hour!" I check my watch. "It's now eleven P.M., so I probably won't get out until morning. But please let me have a word with Damon before I start calling around."

Shealagh puts Damon on, and at first he groggily objects to my cutting my trip short for him. "No, you don't need to!" It's an admission things are really bad if they need to call in the cavalry from Japan. But I can tell Damon is not himself and that he's in trouble.

"I'm on my way, D-man, and I will see you very shortly!" I tell him.

Shealagh starts to relax and even Damon quickly accepts the change in plans. By one thirty A.M., I book a seat on the first available flight out of Tokyo. My plane departs Japan on time and to my great relief, there are no delays. We land at JFK after fourteen hours, and I jump into a taxi and head straight to the hospital. I flash ID at the entrance, shoot up the elevator, and race down the hall and corridors, until I find Damon's room at the very end of the Cardiothoracic Unit ICU.

It's ten A.M. Friday morning, an hour *before* I left Japan on the same day.

I embrace Shealagh, who's amazed I made it so fast, and sling my suitcase in a corner before hurrying over to see my son.

Damon lies on the ICU bed with an IV in his arm, looking marginally bigger and older—he's been growing with his new heart. But he's pale, with a clipped, diminished look. A red pulsimeter on his fingertip indicates his oxygen saturation has dropped significantly, while his breathing is rapid and shallow. He's clearly in distress.

It hurts me to see my son looking so weak and beleaguered, especially after all the progress we've made. But Damon's face lights up when he spots me, and he flashes a beautiful smile, edged with embarrassment that he's in this state. "Hi, Dad."

I throw my arms around Damon, and we sit together on his bed. He is coherent, if slower and vaguer than usual. I show him the few trinkets I got him at the airport: a T-shirt stamped with sushi dishes, and a deck of royal Japanese playing cards. Damon, who's been asking for sushi, grins appreciatively at the T-shirt—nothing wrong with his sense of humor! I start unpacking the cards but he says, as if reminding me he still has homework to finish, "We can do that later, Dad, there's other stuff they want me to deal with right now."

"Sure." I step back and let the ICU team do its thing. There's a nurse with spiky brown hair, Hugh, who seems friendly and efficient, and an earnest young cardiology fellow, Dr. October. The ICU attending is a correct, compact Ghanaian, Dr. Ofuri.

I'm told Dr. Mason has not shown up at all and that Dr. Sanford, who's on the premises, is busy in the cath lab—she's supposed to arrive any minute.

We're in the hands of the ICU staff, generalists who have no history with Damon. They seem diligent enough but operate perforce on an assembly-line system, with interchangeable patients.

Right now, the ICU team is focused on Damon's low oxygen level. After an oxygen hose fails to help him, the doctors try an oxygen mask over Damon's face. But Damon *hates* the claustrophobic mask. "No!" he kicks against it. It's a delicate matter because we respect his feelings, but he *must* get more oxygen. We try to work out a compromise where Damon holds the mask over his own face. But it's a half measure, and Damon's saturation remains problematic.

Damon also struggles with his cyclosporine, the immune suppressant that comes in a big horse pill. Cardiology is still prescribing it, but Damon, who's having trouble swallowing, gags and resists. Shealagh finally gets him to take it, but it's a trial, and Damon looks ready to vomit, or cry, or both.

By eleven A.M., Dr. Sanford has still not shown up, which starts to rankle.

"I can't understand why cardiology has not yet taken charge of Damon's case, even after it's turned *critical!*" I protest to my wife. "What are they waiting for?"

Only last night, Shealagh was told Damon *urgently* needed to have a central line put in to receive the support he required, but it's eleven A.M. the next day and they still haven't taken him to the cath lab to do it. They're waiting for Dr. Sanford, who is in the cath lab doing a *routine biopsy.*

When I demand to see someone in charge, I get into an altercation with the cardiology fellow Dr. October. She's taking a blood sample from Damon, who squirms and asks me to please hold off.

"Sorry, D-man!" I apologize, mortified I might have *added* to his distress. But once Dr. October leaves, Damon tells me to go ahead and push the hospital.

"I just didn't want you to upset her when she had a needle in my vein!"

I hang back and stay with Damon, torn between my growing anger at the hospital and my tender feelings for him. Shealagh and I surround Damon and try to cordon him off. For a time, it's just the three of us again.

But then I notice that even safely ensconced between us, Damon looks increasingly stressed. His voice is shaky and quavering, and he doesn't seem like himself. He appears to be wandering mentally, and once or twice he completely loses his train of thought. He starts hallucinating, spying his sister on the staircase. Shealagh had warned me Damon was experiencing bouts of mental confusion, but seeing it for myself is devastating. Damon has always been an exemplar of lucidity. Now he begins muttering like a demented old man and speaking gibberish. Then, aware he's not making sense, Damon gets very frustrated and struggles to correct himself. Which is almost *more* painful to behold, because now he keeps cutting in, determined to set things straight, but then he forgets what he wanted to say and starts wandering again.

When the nurse comes by, I slip out with Shealagh and share my dismay at what I've just witnessed. "How could Mason let this occur? Everything was fine when I left on Tuesday! What the hell happened?"

Meanwhile, it's almost *noon* and Dr. Sanford has still not shown up.

"I can fly across two continents and an ocean, and race through two major cities, but she can't come up to see my son *from the fourth floor!*" I tell my wife. "And where-oh-where is Dr. Mason?" I cry, beseeching the heavens as much as Shealagh. "How can Damon's doctor in chief *not* come in to see her patient after such a setback? How much *sicker* does she need him to get?"

We're told it's Dr. Mason's day off.

I'm astonished because no physician assigned to us at Columbia in over sixteen years has ever acted like this. Desperate, I step forward and announce to the ICU staff that this situation is *totally unacceptable*.

"Where is Dr. Mason? Where is Dr. Sanford? Who is in charge, and what the hell is going on with my son?"

Dr. October snaps that she's already answered all my questions, and we must wait for Dr. Sanford before proceeding. I tell her my son can't afford to wait—he's going into a free fall while they're all standing around wringing their hands. "It's obscene!" I say sharply.

"Don't speak to me like that!" Dr. October says.

"My son is not getting adequate care and until he does, I'll speak to you any way that's necessary!" I retort.

Dr. October goes to complain about me to the ICU attending. Dr. Ofuri approaches and tries to be diplomatic but he just repeats the protocol, as if it is all out of his hands. I reject his do-nothing approach and clash with Dr. Ofuri as I did with Dr. October.

The nurse manager overhears the ruckus and comes over to try to resolve it. "Why don't you tell me what the problem is?" she says.

I review everything that's happened and explain my frustration and alarm.

"I've rushed back from Japan after learning my son had taken a sudden turn for the worse, yet there's still no one to explain how he could have deteriorated so fast, or what they're going to do about it! *Where is his doctor?* No one is taking responsibility for Damon's care! They still haven't put in a central access line, after telling us it was *urgent,* and they still don't have a treatment plan. Everyone is waiting for the cardiology transplant team to arrive, while my son is getting *sicker*! And they call this the ICU!" I exclaim.

The manager, who seemed interested in my views, tells me, "Don't raise your voice." I stare at her, realizing she has not heard a word I've said. I tell her I'll raise my voice until someone takes responsibility for this case and my son gets the care he needs.

Now the manager, nakedly harsh, says, "And don't point your finger!"

"What?" I cry. "My son is going into a spiral as we speak, his doctor *still* hasn't shown up and no one knows what to do, and you're concerned that I'm *pointing my finger*? You're lucky I'm staying this calm and collected!" I declare.

"You have no right to raise your voice *or* point your finger and if you don't stop *instantly,* I'll call security and have you removed from the premises!" the manager snarls.

I'm astonished she's turned herself into the injured party while my son lies in the ICU deteriorating. "Don't you feel any obligation for *the patient's* well-being?" I frown.

By now we have a crowd around us and we're in a nasty face-off. "I've called security and I'll have you *arrested* if you don't behave!" the manager says.

"You can call anyone you want," I reply, furious and pumped with adrenaline. "But Damon is not getting appropriate treatment and until he does, you'll have to deal with me!"

"Are you *threatening* me?" the manager asks with a glint in her eye.

"You're the only one making threats, I'm making a *promise,*" I shoot back.

"You better watch yourself!" she warns as the crowd looks on.

A pale, wild figure suddenly appears in the doorway, standing buck naked except for a tangle of lines and wires. He looks like an escaped marionette on a mission.

"I have to help Dad get rid of the bad people!" Damon announces in a half-crazed but defiant way, small fists clenched in angry solidarity. His red hair blazes, his face is fiery with indignation, and his arterial line looks in danger of popping out. "These people are saying bad things about you, Dad!"

I can't believe my eyes. My young lion has leapt from his sick bed and charged out of the room to defend *me*!

He stands there, the fiercest warrior-ally I've ever had, with a catheter threaded through his penis and big incision scar running down his chest. His mind flickers in and out, but his sense of justice, and his courage, burns pure.

I walk over and put my arms around Damon, patting his shoulders and reassuring him that everything is okay. *My amazing son.* I lead him back to the room, briefly checking his development—his big new heart has improved his circulation everywhere—before I help him back into bed.

Meanwhile, security has arrived in the form of two oversized, slouching cops. I step out and quickly determine what I must do if they try to put a hand on me. Fortunately, Shealagh intervenes with her mother's privileged position and her posh accent.

"My husband is just trying to get proper treatment for our son, who's very sick. Why don't you help find his doctor, if you want to be useful!" Shealagh says. "Doesn't anyone in this hospital care about *the patient*? What's the matter with everybody here!"

The cops look to the manager, who admits they're still waiting for the doctor. "But that's no reason to become *aggressive*," she says, albeit more sheepishly now.

One cop, who's been assessing the situation, turns to the nurse manager with a weary but dutiful sigh. "So whaddaya want us to do here?"

Hugh suddenly pops his head out of Damon's room. "His saturation is dropping!"

Shealagh and I rush inside.

A cop follows and peers in, as if we might escape through the window.

Damon's oxygen saturation has fallen to a dangerous level. Hugh tries holding a mask over Damon's face—it's better than strapping it on—but Damon pushes against it.

"If his numbers don't improve, we will have to intubate him," Dr. Ofuri states.

Shealagh and I try to soothe Damon, who's restive and uneasy. He mumbles.

By the time Damon is sufficiently stable so that I can step back into the hallway, the cops look very uncomfortable. They give me a pro forma warning and retreat.

"Well, I'm glad we straightened *that* out," the manager says before scurrying off.

I'm appalled but I don't know what to do. Time is running out and we're marooned here in the very last ICU room. I dig out my BlackBerry, check I have a signal, and go into overdrive, sending several SOSes. I've already contacted Dr. Chin but now I write Eric Rose, cc-ing Eric Kandel in the hopes of spurring Dr. Rose to respond, and plead for assistance, pulling out all the stops:

> Damon is deteriorating very rapidly and I am concerned that not enough is being done and people are dragging their feet in usual bureaucratic mode. His electrolytes are all over the place, platelets in single digits, oxygen so low they're about to intubate, shaking and gibbering like an old man with paranoid hallucinations—I left 3 days ago and he's not the same person! If there is anyone you can contact on our behalf to make sure they treat this with the urgency it deserves, I appeal to you now. Dr. Mason, the chief transplant cardiologist, is not here, and Dr. Sanford in my view is not doing all she can and should. I'm scared for my son and believe time is of the essence.

I also phone Dr. Hellenbrand, Damon's last doctor in this hospital before Dr. Mason. Dr. Hellenbrand has always been helpful, with a sense of moral, as well as medical, responsibility. He's also the head of the cath lab, where Damon needs to be.

Dr. Hellenbrand is in the OR, but his assistant promises to let him know about our situation ASAP.

"I'll get word to him the minute he finishes, I promise!" she says.

I go back to the ICU bed and stay with Damon. He is in visible distress and continues having trouble with his oxygen level and with his concentration. He mumbles something strange about a unicorn, until we realize he's drolly alluding to Hugh, the nurse whose loftily spiked hair could make him pass for a mythical horse with a single horn.

It's the last flash of Damon's whimsical, theatrical imagination before his breathing grows shallower and the ICU attending announces they must intubate him.

I feel like my son has just slipped one more step away from us but there's nothing we can do. He's in very bad shape.

By one thirty P.M., three and a half hours after my own fourteen-hour flight from Japan, Dr. Sanford shows up. She informs us that Damon has contracted an acute infection from the Epstein-Barr virus (EBV), and this infection has led to the dreaded "post-transplant lympho-proliferative disorder," or PTLD.

PTLD is a very serious condition in which the lymphocytes, white blood cells normally involved in the body's defense system, multiply rapidly and attack the vital organs. It's one of the three major threats for heart transplant patients, ranking just behind rejection and infection, and its consequences can be severe.

Damon's body is under attack, Dr. Sanford explains, and they will have to give him extensive support while trying to beat back this invasion. The doctors don't yet know whether Damon's lymphocytes have turned into cancerous cells that can reproduce by themselves or whether they're less advanced. But they have various tools in their arsenal, and now that they know what they're up against, they can take more careful, targeted aim.

"We're hopeful we can bring this under control, but we'll have to move *fast!*"

I try to ignore the brazen irony of the long-missing Dr. Sanford suddenly urging speed. Instead, I focus on her tone and body language. She seems to take a bookish satisfaction in imparting this information. Having just learned many of these facts herself, the results freshly arrived from a California lab, she's proud and flush with her new knowledge.

I don't ask Dr. Sanford why they couldn't figure this out *sooner*, since apparently it's a well-known complication. No one has mentioned the word "EBV" to us before, a term I know from previous research. Nor do I ask why they had to send out a standard PCR test from New York, a high-tech medical capital, all the way to California for an *urgent* result. And I don't even scream when Dr. Sanford tells us, as if she's just discovered the fact, that Damon must go to the cath lab *right away* so they can put in a central access line.

We must move forward, and Dr. Sanford is the only doctor we have right now. At least they know why Damon is sick. And we don't have another minute to lose.

Dr. Sanford says they're prepping Damon for the cath lab now, because they'll need full access for his supportive care. But they have good antivirals and other medications, as well as several experimental therapies to try. She also tells us we must *decrease* Damon's immune suppression because lowered immunity acts as *spur* for PTLD: "No more cyclosporine."

"But I just made him take his daily dose!" Shealagh cries. "You and Dr. Mason have been telling us to take it every day!"

"Look, some immune suppression is still necessary," Dr. Sanford backtracks. "We don't want Damon to have *rejection* amid these other issues, do we?"

My wife and I exchange sharp glances but we don't pursue this obvious screwup. "How do you think Damon contracted this infection?" we ask.

Dr. Sanford smiles like a well-rehearsed teacher. "EBV is very common. Damon probably picked it up from his siblings or his parents or even a friend . . . If anyone in the house had a slight cold or a cough, they could have infected him."

We go back to the ICU room, where Damon is being readied for the cath lab. There's a new sense of urgency now that we have the official diagnosis, and everyone is on full alert. I hear Dr. Hellenbrand will handle the procedure, which is a relief. But knowing that Damon has been harboring a secret, cancerlike infection is deeply unsettling.

Hugh asks me to help with the gurney. I grab one end when Glenda, Damon's first ICU nurse from infancy—she's a supervisor now—emerges from nowhere to give us a hand. So I know it's serious. Every second suddenly counts.

We swing Damon out of the ICU and run up the corridor. The gurney just fits into the elevator. We hop off and begin racing across the fourth floor with Damon balanced on the stretcher like a fragile package. We round several tight corners and sprint into the cath lab.

Someone hands me a consent form as Dr. Hellenbrand, a reassuring figure in his scrubs, shuffles over. Shealagh arrives, and we all briefly confer. But there's no time for lingering because Dr. Hellenbrand must perform what is by now an emergency procedure.

Shealagh and I vacate the premises and go into wait mode by a corridor bench.

It's a long, nerve-wracking wait. Damon's anatomy is tricky and his condition fragile. Yet they *must* find another access point into his bloodstream so they can deliver the requisite medication. Failure is not an option. As we sit in limbo, waiting to see if Dr. Hellenbrand can pull this off, I am amazed to find a live reply to my BlackBerry SOS! Only it's not from Dr. Rose, but from Eric Kandel, who's followed up on his own and, in just over an hour, tracked down the elusive, no-show Dr. Mason for me. Kandel writes:

> I just spoke to Dr. Mason, who would be pleased to take a call from you if you were to try and get a hold of her. She has the weekend off and will be in on Monday. However, she's been in touch with Damon and his condition and feels that even though he is very, very sick, she is hopeful they will get him through this successfully. As you probably know he has acute EBV which can be very serious. My prayers are with you.

I show the e-mail to Shealagh and we both shake our heads over Dr. Mason's behavior. Suddenly she's in the loop and pretending to be on top of things. Yet she's still taking *a three-day weekend* on the day her patient is rushed to the ICU, fighting for his life!

I feel my blood seethe. Only three days ago, Dr. Mason assured me Damon's symptoms were completely "routine" and all was "under control." Yet now that it clearly is *not* routine *nor* under control, she feels no sense of responsibility. Not only doesn't she come in to see her critically ill patient, she can't be bothered to call us and explain what went wrong. And for a final twist, she claims she'd "be pleased to take a call *from*" us—a call *we cannot make* because Dr. Mason has never given us any contact information!

Dr. Hellenbrand comes out of the cath lab and ambles toward us. At least we have one decent doctor on our side. Just seeing him restores my faith, even before he speaks.

The cath lab chief, still in scrubs, reports our son is fine. "I couldn't get in through Damon's neck but I managed to insert two access lines. They're both in Damon's groin area and though neither reaches the heart, both can deliver adequate doses of medication into the bloodstream. So we're okay on that score."

We thank Dr. Hellenbrand. He tips his head. It's what he does. But he tells us he thinks he's accomplished all he can for Damon. If we need him over the weekend, we have his number, but he's not sure what else he can offer.

"It's in other people's hands now," he says.

We nod grimly, wishing it were not so. Dr. Hellenbrand gives us a blunt, searching look. I watch him closely, because I know he cares about us but he won't bullshit.

"You're in for a very rough weekend. Call if you want. Good luck." He leaves.

Back on the ICU floor, there is open marveling at Dr. Hellenbrand's handiwork. Damon's groin now bristles like a bionic porcupine, boasting two erect clusters of quill-like IV tubes ready for medication delivery.

As the ICU team swings into action, I make a point of going over and apologizing to Dr. October and Dr. Ofuri for any earlier friction. "We really appreciate what you're doing. Thanks so much." They accept my apology, and we reengage in a congenial manner.

A technician rolls in a hemodialysis machine, "a kidney with a brain" geared for ICU patients. The contraption, known as a CVVH, consists of four pumps and filters that control all fluids into and out of Damon's body. We watch the rotary pumps whir quietly, like spools of film, and create a steady shushing sound as Damon's blood is filtered and waste matter removed into yellow bags. We take solace from the low, murmuring rhythm and the continuous nurturing action of the unit as we hover anxiously by Damon's bedside.

He dozes, flitting in and out of awareness.

Around seven P.M., there's a shift change and a new ICU attending replaces Dr. Ofuri, while Dr. October stays on. Dr. Sanford also departs but tries to reassure us, or perhaps to reassure herself, that they'll watch Damon all night and make every effort to stabilize him.

An hour later, Damon's blood pressure starts to drop and it becomes harder to keep it steady. The medical staff has been giving him intermittent infusions of red blood cells to maintain his pressure, but now he begins to seesaw and they have trouble stabilizing him.

"Up the epi one notch!" the doctor barks. Shealagh and I resign ourselves to a long, stomach-churning night as the ICU team battles back and forth.

We've been glued to the bedside for hours, talking to Damon and encouraging him even though we don't know how much he grasps. Shealagh has only left for the bathroom, and I haven't even done that in my fixation. But at one point, my jet lag, the raw fish I ate in Japan, and the unrelieved stress all get to me, and I make a beeline for the toilet.

As soon as I close the bathroom door, I become aware of a terrible pounding in my chest and a raw hammering in my skull, like the worked-over feeling when I sat in my corner between brutal rounds of my first boxing match against the Royal Military Academy Sandhurst. Only now it's worse, because I can't see my opponent and I don't know how to fight back. I shut my eyes and try to still the awful drilling pain, drifting to a calmer, more detached state, when a sharp knocking barges into my consciousness. At first, I think someone else wants to use the facilities, and I try to ignore them and regain quietude. But the banging persists, louder and fiercer, and then I realize it's Shealagh, and the banging is meant for me.

"Come quick! He's dying!" my wife shrieks through the closed door as I charge out in utter disbelief.

A long throng of medical personnel has crammed into the ICU room and crowded around Damon's bed. In the center, mounted above my son like the lightest, most acrobatic member of the team, squats the petite Dr. October, who's thumping Damon's chest and administering CPR with precise, vigorous strokes.

My son has gone into cardiac arrest!

The doctors are feverishly pushing in bagfuls of red blood while the cool ICU head instructs the nurse to administer doses of epinephrine. Everyone is watching the telltale monitor, which shows a long, flat, *totally inert* line.

I feel stunned and dazed but I refuse to believe this is the end. I approach the bed and grab Damon's leg, the closest I can get to him. All is happening in slow, crushing motion.

"Come on, D-man!" I push against heavy atmospheric resistance, like a diver at the bottom of the sea, and seek to reclaim my son, defiantly yanking him back from the underworld by his leg. "Come on, D-man, snap out of it, you're not going anywhere!"

I tug repeatedly at Damon's ankle, hearing the increasingly hollow, stubborn echo of my own small voice, when the line on the monitor suddenly *jumps*. The doctors all stare.

Shealagh yells at me to move closer to Damon; she's convinced he's responding to me. I edge nearer and continue urging Damon on, though I suspect it's the albumin or the extra shot of epinephrine that's galvanizing his body.

But whatever it is, Damon is reviving, and the terrible gloom starts to lift.

Damon's blood pressure rises, and all his vital signs perk up.

He's back on the big board, all lit up and posting solid numbers.

There's a deep, collective sigh in the ICU room. Everyone exhales, and then normal life returns almost as quickly as it was suspended.

The ICU reinforcements clear out and go back to their stations.

Damon's doctors quickly run an echocardiogram and determine that Damon's heart function still looks good. The ICU attending, a sinewy, unflappable type, estimates Damon arrested for one minute, ninety seconds tops.

"Since someone was pushing blood into his brain the whole time, I don't expect any lasting damage. But we won't know for sure until he regains consciousness. For now, we just need to keep him stable and let him rest."

Shealagh and I compose ourselves and try to assess the damage. Damon's face is very puffy, especially around the thick, goiter-like neck, while ventilator tubes snake out of his bloated lips and raw nostrils. A rash of tiny red pustules stipples his body. Most distressing, his vacant eyes swivel erratically in their sockets. We are told this is typical after an arrest, and it will subside once he snaps back, but it's still a worrisome sight.

We try not to lose heart and remind ourselves this is *Damon*. We've seen him come through so much—we've come through so much together—we'll get through this too.

"He's so naturally resilient. If we just let him get some rest and provide adequate support, his survival instincts will kick in," I tell Shealagh. "No one can stop Damon!"

"Yes, he's such a fighter, I'm sure he'll rally after a good night's sleep."

Hugh, our friendly nurse, overhears this and warns us not to underestimate what's happened. "He's had a sepsis, a life-threatening shock to the entire body where the blood cells spill out of the vessels. It's going to be a dicey few days, like walking on eggshells."

Near midnight, after Damon has stayed stable for a few hours, I call Dr. Bar-Or in Denver, two hours behind us. I tell my cousin about Damon's dramatic deterioration these past days, his sudden arrest, and all the support he's now on.

"It sounds like total organ failure—the leading cause of death in the ICU."

I wince. "What kind of numbers are we looking at?"

"About fifty percent of ICU deaths result from total organ failure," Dudu says.

I phone my parents, late-nighters, and explain we've had a setback. I don't go into details because they also need to be protected. My parents are due to fly the next day on a package vacation, a thank-you present from us for staying with our kids during Damon's transplant. They immediately offer to cancel their trip but I insist I still want them to go.

"There's nothing you can do for us here. Sam and Miranda are skiing in Vermont, and it will ease my mind and give me one *less* thing to worry about if you make the trip."

My parents are unhappy about leaving but reluctantly accede. I promise updates.

Shealagh and I spend the rest of the night in the ICU, sharing the single mattress on the window seat. We lie head to toe, twisting and writhing. Each of us rises often to check on Damon and to talk to the night nurse, who constantly struggles to adjust the machine and keep Damon stable.

I lie awake, exhausted but agonizing as I summon all the known data and review every detail and every twist and turn in my head. I conclude that Damon's current malaise actually began *three weeks earlier*, the night he told us of his shivery feeling. And I now see that this first crisis, when they insisted on treating him for rejection, never solved his problem but only *masked* it.

In retrospect, I grasp that as soon as he finished his course of immune-suppressant medication a week ago, Damon's underlying illness *returned*.

But instead of despairing, I take solace in this hypothesis. Because it means that Damon does not have a mysterious new illness, but only a continuation of his initial complaint. And so, as soon as we properly treat this original ailment, we should be able to bring everything back under control.

As I lie awake by the window, which I now notice for the first time offers a sweeping Renaissance-like vista of the city's rooftops and of the Hudson River, I realize this forty-hour day, which began for me in Tokyo and has been one of the longest and most shattering days of my life, has fallen on Good Friday.

If today was Damon's crucifixion, my hard-pressed imagination hazards, then shouldn't he soon rise up and return to us on Easter Sunday, or thereabouts?

I'm unsure of the exact resurrection sequence—do I recall a Bright Monday?—but I'm prepared to cut a lot of liturgical slack. I vow that if this miracle were to, in fact, materialize, I'd be perfectly willing to convert to Christianity by way of gratitude—or to Islam or Buddhism or to *any* religion or organized movement that could help Damon.

Anyone can have me, so long as they *give me back my son*.

Chapter 54

The next day, Saturday, is a busy day in the ICU, with many ups and downs, but grounds for hope.

Damon seems to stabilize, though he's still unconscious, and we all focus on the best treatment for his PTLD.

Dr. Mason finally appears in the late morning. Even *she* must respond to a cardiac arrest, not to mention a Nobel laureate's inquiries.

She bustles about Damon, listening to his chest and checking his bedside monitors. "It's very unusual to get an EBV infection and develop PTLD so *soon* post-transplant. I've never seen it this early and rarely even heard of it," Dr. Mason tells us with a show of confounded expertise. "The good news is that the early form of this illness is easiest to treat and has the best long-term prognosis. So you can take comfort from *that*."

An oncologist comes to discuss an experimental protocol involving a monoclonal antibody and a chemo agent. He gives me literature to read, but I've already discussed this approach with Dudu, and I know it's probably our best shot. I review it briefly with Shealagh before signing the consent.

"We've called in someone very special, one of the world's leading authorities on PTLD, to consult on Damon's case," the oncologist says with a touch of celebrity awe. And when the "famous" Dr. Manuela Orjuela arrives, she commands immediate attention with her striking appearance and dramatic manner. But she also displays a keen scientific mind and sharp diagnostic skills.

Dr. Orjuela believes Damon has an acute or "fulminant" case of PTLD, and she urges a very aggressive treatment. "I cannot fathom why Columbia waited *so long* to call me in!" she says. "But at this advanced stage, I recommend hitting your son with the combination therapy several times, so we really *zap* his lymphocytes."

But Dr. Mason, whose back may be up because a more high-powered woman doctor is in the room, takes issue with this approach. "I'm concerned Damon may not be strong enough to withstand a double dose of chemo in his current state. We need to find a balance between neutralizing the PTLD and keeping Damon stable."

Despite my growing disenchantment with her, I share Dr. Mason's concern. "What data do you have on comparable cases?" I ask Dr. Orjuela.

"The data pool for this illness is tiny, and one has to speak of individual cases," Dr. Orjuela replies. "But in my judgment and based on my experience, we need to go all-out to rescue Damon from this attack. All his organs, especially his liver and kidneys, suffered a big hit, and we must do everything to stem the assault. It's a risk, but I would take it."

"We can try one course of treatment and see how Damon responds," Dr. Mason says. "We could always bump it up after an interval if he does well. But I do not want to destabilize Damon, especially after what happened last night!"

Shealagh and I feel torn between these rival views, because like Dr. Mason, we also worry about Damon's fragile state. And it's possible Dr. Orjuela is too invested in this protocol. On the other hand, Dr. Orjuela specializes in PTLD and has seen more cases than Dr. Mason. She may be right that the risks of holding back outweigh the benefits.

In the end, the two women cannot agree and come to sharp words. But Dr. Mason, as the physician in charge of Damon's case, exercises the ultimate authority, and she makes the final call.

Dr. Orjuela storms off, insulted that her advice goes unheeded.

Damon gets one round of the combination therapy, and we await the results. He's having a marginally better day and shows small signs of improvement, though he remains asleep. But he seems to be stabilizing, and we derive a measure of relief from this.

While Dr. Mason checks Damon's lines and drips—like a fireman arriving one day late, she makes a big show of tidying up the after-blaze—I share my new theory with her. I'm determined to remain congenial and to extract any benefit I still can from her.

"I believe Damon may still be suffering from the original illness that brought him to the hospital three weeks earlier," I tell her. "And if it's really the same illness, this would be positive news, because it means Damon didn't just get hit with a sudden shock to the entire system from an EBV infection."

It's taken me painstaking work to solve this epidemiological puzzle in my head, and I'm pleased at how the pieces seem to fit together. But Dr. Mason is not impressed.

"Oh, of course, his donor was EBV positive!" she says with an insider's shrug, dismissing my entire reconstruction, not because it's wrong, but because it's so *obvious*.

His donor was EBV positive! These words, tossed out so casually, send me reeling. So she's known this all along? How could she not tell us? And why couldn't she *protect* Damon, if she knew? I want to scream but I suppress my anger so I can learn more while trying to process this shocking information.

If they gave Damon a donor heart with EBV, why didn't they look for an EBV infection *right away* when Damon first got sick, instead of waiting *three weeks* for his illness to rage unchecked? And don't they have standard precautions to take even earlier, from the first day of his transplant, if they knew he had such a ticking bomb? EBV is widespread in the population— I remember that from my own reading—but an immune-compromised, EBV-negative patient like Damon would have been especially susceptible and would merit extra protection if they knew they were giving him an EBV-positive heart!

And why didn't they ever breathe one word to us about the donor heart before now?

Only yesterday, Dr. Sanford said Damon probably got his EBV infection from one of us at home who had a cold. Is it possible Dr. Mason did not communicate such vital information to her colleague? Or that Dr. Sanford didn't see this on Damon's chart?

Unless Dr. Mason, despite her customary facade of all-knowingness, did not know this *herself* until today? Which would be just as unsettling, because she should have known it, and she should have acted on her knowledge.

These thoughts rush through my mind and leave me feeling even more sickened and angry. Could this entire crisis have been averted? What have they done to my son!

But it's all moot now. We're in this hole, and we must dig ourselves out.

Damon's cardiac arrest, however brief, is considered a signal event, and all day a parade of experts comes in to look at him. But it seems our best hope is still the experimental protocol. Shealagh and I spend the night on the same narrow window bed, entwined in the same uneasy state. We doze to the heaving rhythm of ICU machines while the nurses do impressive, night-long battle with the CVVH, juggling everything to keep Damon stable.

In the morning, I am buoyed because I think I detect an improvement in Damon's appearance. But it's Easter Sunday and I don't trust the possible influence of wishful thinking.

"What do you think?" I ask my wife, with her superior visual acuity.

"I also feel he definitely looks better today!" Shealagh replies. "I noticed it as soon as I woke up, but I didn't want to say anything and jinx it."

We stand quietly by Damon's bed and tick off the improvements we see.

Damon's facial swelling appears diminished. He no longer looks like a troll with an engorged neck, especially on the right side, where a big lump has subsided. Damon's arms don't look quite as puffy or swollen either. And the red pustules that had broken out all over Damon's body, while still visible, no longer look as vivid or virulent.

Damon remains unconscious, but even in slumber, his face looks more tranquil. He appears less under siege and more like his familiar, calmly contained and focused self.

Our hearts soar with reinvigorated hope.

"I keep inspecting him from different angles, to make sure it's real!" Shealagh says.

"The protocol must be taking effect. His body appears to have responded to the very first treatment," I say in grateful amazement.

We stay on this high all morning and throughout the early afternoon. But around two P.M., I notice that Damon's blood pressure is starting to slip again.

Maintaining his pressure is a constant juggling act: pushing in blood products and albumin as needed, with a bump in the epinephrine when there's no other recourse. Against this, one must balance the fact that he's retaining too much fluid and only essential items should be added to avoid overloading him.

Nonetheless, there are priorities, and the top one is to avoid another crisis and keep Damon stable. I've watched three ICU nurses in a row handle this ably, but now we get a new nurse who does not appear to know what she's doing.

As this nurse fumbles around, Damon's numbers continue heading south. It's like bad dream on replay, and there's nothing I can do to stop it.

Soon we have another full-blown crisis on our hands as the alarm goes off, and several doctors charge into the room. Gradually, they bring his pressure under control but the entire episode could have been avoided and sets him farther back.

We continue seesawing over the next twenty-four hours. By Monday, Damon's face looks more swollen, and I wonder if we should have listened to Dr. Orjuela's advocacy of a more aggressive course.

On the positive side, Damon finally regains consciousness. He presses our hands to show he understands what we're saying. We're immensely relieved that he's aware and functioning mentally. He's still very weak and groggy, and his eyes still wander at times, but he's clearly responding to our words, and we're overjoyed to have him back.

Dr. Lubritto, the liver specialist, comes by every day to visit. He is very concerned about Damon and mumbles that Damon's cardiologist, not he, should have caught this sooner.

"But as long as Damon stays stable," Dr. Lubritto says, "as long as he doesn't go *backward,* he's doing okay." The key is to keep him from further harm and to let his body recover. "There's nothing *irreversible* here!" Dr. Lubritto repeats in his high staccato.

By Tuesday, we seem to be in a good phase again. Damon had a peaceful night and seems stable. Sonja, a very devoted friend, has flown in to help with Sam and Miranda. In the morning, while the kids are in school, Sonja visits us in the ICU. She's had twenty years' experience as a hospital physician, and she says Damon does not look as bad as she feared. I don't know what she feared, but I take heart from this.

Sonja gives Shealagh a much-needed break and takes her out for a meal and a walk in the hospital garden. Shealagh gets some air and smells the trees and the river. We've been completely shut in for five days, and Shealagh stayed alone with Damon for three days before that.

By early afternoon, we're standing around Damon's bed and feeling more hopeful than we have since his cardiac arrest. The farther we get away from that precipitating event, and the more we can resume our lives and revert to a semblance of normalcy, the better our prospects seem.

Even the ICU head appears more sanguine than usual, telling us, "Damon is still poised on a very narrow beam. But as long as he doesn't tumble off, he's making progress, and the longer he manages to stay on, the better his chances. Every day that he doesn't fall off is a good day."

It seems like we're having a good day.

After Sonja leaves, Shealagh and I take turns going to the lounge and making calls. Once, we steal a break together and share coffee and a pastry.

"Our first child doesn't want to make it too easy on his parents!" Shealagh says dryly.

"No, he really likes to keep us on our toes," I reply. "But he's such a fighter and he's survived so much, he'll get through this."

"He has his special Damon powers!" Shealagh says, and I nod.

We stay in this cautiously optimistic groove till evening, when, just as the sun dips into the river, Damon's blood pressure falls. The nurse does not react but watches passively despite my urging, so I rush out to get the head nurse. But she's not there. Nor is anyone from our ICU team around. Frantic, I race up the hallway and spot a doctor sitting at a terminal. I plead for her help but she is apathetic. When I yell that it's *urgent* and shame her into responding, she goes to find a supervisor instead of coming herself, costing us more precious minutes.

By the time the ICU head and all the doctors have crowded around Damon, we have another crisis on our hands. They have to hit Damon with every weapon in their arsenal and overload him with more fluid—blood products, albumin, epinephrine—before they manage to bring his pressure back under control.

Deeply distressed and bristling at what I perceive to be another totally preventable setback, I demand a joint meeting with Dr. Mason and the ICU head Dr. Ofuri. They're both back on the case today. We go for privacy into the adjoining room, now empty.

I explain to the two supervising doctors what's happened *several times* now, and I ask if they can please instruct the nurses not to let the pressure drop so low before they bump up the dosage, because it creates a vicious cycle.

To my surprise, both physicians agree instantly with my analysis. Dr. Ofuri explains he's just come up with a new algorithm for intervention, and he will make sure everyone on Damon's ICU team understands the stricter standard we're advocating. Dr. Mason nods and concurs with everything. I've never had such a frictionless meeting with them, nor have they listened to me with such apparent deference. It's flattering but makes me wonder what I'm missing. Why would they treat me so nicely all of a sudden?

That night, per my request, the doctors establish a lower threshold for going up on the epi. But we never seem to fully recover from the previous setback.

We get a good nurse again, but even she can't get Damon back to sea level. The kidney machines are going at full tilt and being replaced regularly but Damon continues struggling. The staff is doing all the right things, but it's a terrible night, as we keep getting farther and farther away from the safety zone.

I can do all the calculations in my head—it's all I can do; my brain crunches nonstop—and I begin to despair when I realize we're near the point of no return.

Sleep is impossible. I get up and pace like an inmate on the eve of his own execution.

Daylight brings no relief. Damon now is so overloaded with fluid and so unstable that when the nurse tries to shift his *pillow,* his blood pressure plummets and we have a minicrisis to deal with. He seems to be hanging on by a thread.

Another parade of specialists troops in. But no one has a workable suggestion. They're just running down their checklist, and we're running out of time.

I scour my brain for any lead we might have overlooked. Our current problem is the kidneys, yet we haven't heard from anyone in that field. I know a renal expert at the University of Pennsylvania, and I've started composing an e-mail to him when the new ICU head, a crisp, self-assured brunette named Dr. Verani, asks me what I'm doing. I explain there might still be a kidney angle we haven't thought of, and I'm contacting a specialist

I know. Or maybe we could get a pulmonologist to weigh in on the respirator issue . . . But Dr. Verani just gives a quick, condescending shake of the head and tells me not to bother. "I know as much about the kidneys and the lungs as any specialist, and you won't learn anything new."

I feel deflated and sense the last, lingering breeze ebb from my sails.

"But if that's the case," I counter Dr. Verani, "then what's *your* plan?"

"Our plan is to continue what we're doing," she says. "We're providing every form of support we can, and there's nothing else we can do."

"With all due respect, that's just not good enough!" I tell Dr. Verani. "Because what you're doing *isn't working*, and Damon is *going downhill*." I shake my head. "If you don't have any new ideas, why not ask your colleagues at other hospitals? We're not just going to *give up* and resign ourselves to failure, or is that what you had in mind?"

Dr. Verani looks taken aback but I just roll on.

"I'm sure there's *one doctor* in *one ICU somewhere* who's been in a similar spot and who's found a solution for his patient. I know there's a way out of this, even if we can't think of it ourselves. We just need to find the right expert!"

Dr. Verani mulls my strong conviction. "That may not be a bad thing to try," she says. "I can send out an alert on my ICU Listserv, which links my colleagues across the country, and see if anyone responds. It's an excellent network, I check mine all the time."

I commend Dr. Verani for this suggestion, wondering why she hasn't thought of it before, and ask if she could please send out the alert ASAP, because I'm really worried.

"I'll get on it right away," Dr. Verani promises.

All day long, things continue to unravel. We're only moving in one direction now.

An air of unreality grips us. Time slows down, and people tiptoe around us. Everyone is solicitous and wary.

A psychologist appears and we send him flying. We're a little more polite to the pastor, but we have no time for him either. Someone offers me a cup of tea and though I understand what they're doing, I reluctantly accept because I can feel my strength ebbing.

By evening, the situation around Damon's bedside is turning grave. His numbers keep dipping and no one knows how to stop the slide. We have no more safety net—it lies in tatters—and the doctors are at a loss.

Damon's blood pressure continues to drop for the next hour, and all the machines and medicines and backup systems have been exhausted.

He's going down.

A hush has fallen over the room and there's a physical sense of emptiness and hopelessness. Of terminality.

All unnecessary staff have retreated. It's dark outside the window.

I don't believe this is happening.

Dr. Verani, who normally roves from room to room, comes in to supervise us. It's not a good sign. I ask her if she received any responses to her ICU alert regarding Damon. It's been eight hours. Dr. Verani says she's sorry, but she never got around to sending it.

Dr. Mason is summoned as a matter of protocol. She sweeps into the room and makes a show of putting her stethoscope to Damon's chest, even though his new heart is the one organ that's stayed strong throughout. We all stand by for several awkward minutes while she listens with exaggerated, detective-like concentration to Damon's heartbeat and his breathing, as if they could tell her anything useful at this stage.

Finally, Dr. Mason straightens up and remarks that Damon sounds a little "clearer" on the left side. Dr. Verani and the ICU nurses look away, clearly embarrassed. I get a sudden, queasy sensation—I've never seen Dr. Mason so transparent—and I wonder what else these past few days has been pure show.

But I quickly dismiss all such concerns. I have no more time for Dr. Mason or Dr. Verani. They're completely beside the point now.

Shealagh and I surround our son. He's regained consciousness and is aware of everything. Shealagh is reading to him from *The Picture of Dorian Gray*, the book he brought with him to the hospital. She's pouring all her tenderness into the reading, and Damon is absorbing every word, like a lullaby to the soul.

It's a brave, beautiful, loving act, braver than anything I can do. Mother and son share the deep, gorgeous consolation of art, which I, in a bitter irony of my misguided artisthood, cannot accept. I still want to save my son in the here and now, and I reject any move toward transcendence or sublimation as a form of surrender.

I'm focusing on vasopressin and dopamine and dobutamine. I'm still trying to figure out a way to raise Damon's blood pressure. I can't let him go, and I won't accept that it's over.

But he's fading, and everyone sees it. He lies there in a tangle of IV lines and tubes, his face grossly swollen with a crooked mouth jammed with a respirator and blubbery lips that fuse together at one end. His inert body, its organs ravaged by the untreated infection that has turned into a fulminant cancer, is puffed up from all the fluid he's retaining. And his eyes still swivel erratically.

Dr. Verani, feigning empathy, asks if we want to give Damon a sedative and let him drift away. Shealagh and I stare at one another in mutual horror. Damon is completely aware, and he's still with us! He keeps pressing our hands and responding to things we say.

There is no way in hell we're going to put our son to sleep and deprive our family of this time together!

I suddenly realize these ICU doctors are protecting *themselves*. They're afraid to look death in the face, even though it's their daily business, because they're fearful of confronting their own limitations.

And it's *not over*, as far as I'm concerned.

Damon is on a respirator and dialysis machine and every other form of critical life support, his body is grotesquely swollen and his face busted up, and his hold on existence is slipping away before our eyes. But he is still with us. Shealagh and I grab on to whatever part of him we can reach—anything untethered to tubes, lines, and machines, and not covered up with tape or other impediments.

Shealagh is on Damon's left, bent very low over her son and cooing into his ear as she trembles and tries not to fall apart. She holds on, a fierce, heartbroken lioness who won't stop tending her cub. I'm on Damon's right, my knees shaking, my throat constricting, and my eyes scalding. Even now, I don't want Damon to see me crying, and I keep turning away, ostensibly to reach for a glass of water on the cabinet, but really to try to blot my tears, which won't stop coursing. I fear if Damon sees me crying, he'll know the game is up. But my efforts are futile—it's like holding back my torrential love for him—and I resign myself to the stinging flow. We're beyond such pretense now.

We're all shedding our earthly roles and reverting to elemental cores.

I hold Damon's hand and look into his eyes. From some unknown place, I hear myself begin to tell him things I've never consciously formulated but now emerge with their own stamp of authority and their own momentum.

I tell Damon how much I love him and how proud I am of him. How proud he has always made me feel and what a privilege it is to have a son like him. That he is a magnificent, extraordinary human being, and that no parent could have wished for a more perfect child. That he is perfection itself, in every possible way, and that I cannot even imagine a finer young man or a more exquisite flower of humanity.

These words spill out in a hyperbolic-sounding gush, but there is not one ounce of embellishment in them. I am speaking plain truth, from a place where there is nothing but truth. The purity of love for a pure being, compounded by all the attachments and devotions of paternity and fatherhood. I need only reach into my inmost heart and show my son what's there, what's been there all along. And Damon, who can't speak because of the tube in his mouth and because of the illness raging in his blood, shows me he understands every word I'm saying. He nods with his tender eyes and flashes deep recognition. My praise meets with his profound approval because he knows it's all true, and that he's *earned* it.

There's no time left for false modesty. I'm only giving Damon his due.

Aware of the fleeting minutes, I'm desperate to let Damon know just how special he is and how much he means to me. To compress my boundless love into a nutshell. I tell Damon what a close and wonderful friend he has become. How I can talk to him about everything under the sun, including the most intimate and complex matters, and what a rare thing this is with anyone. To share such an affinity with one's own son is truly remarkable. I lean forward and whisper that if he promises not to tell my buddy David, I think he's turning into my best friend. Damon's eyes bat wildly, showing I've hit a sweet spot.

Meanwhile, Shealagh is cradling Damon's body and telling him what a brave boy he is, how proud she is of him. He's so full of courage. He is so strong and magnificent. She admires him and loves him with all her heart. He's her wonderful, amazing, fantastic boy.

Damon's courage never falters but his body is buckling.

We watch our son being dragged away from this world, his light slowly extinguishing.

The ICU staff presses in on us, encircling Damon. They're waiting to turn off his life support!

They've written him off already, and their impatience is palpable. And *shameless*.

I block them with my body, using my shoulder as both an impassive shield and a ready spear but unwilling to pay them any heed. They're too inconsequential to bother with. And they'd have to risk their own lives to get past me.

But Shealagh is *enraged* by their close, hovering presence and their unseemly eagerness to shut things down. She screams that they should back off and get away from our son.

It's a mother's piercing cry, and its irate fury carries unmistakable authority.

The forwardmost nurse retreats, and the entire ICU staff takes a step back. We focus back on our son.

Damon's cell phone suddenly goes off on the bedside table. It's an absurd intrusion, but it involuntarily stirs hope because of its mundane connection to Damon's world—a world that is still going on outside these walls.

No one answers, but we can see from the display screen the caller is Kyle.

Damon's dearest friend and soul mate somehow apprehends what's happening and reaches out to Damon at this precise moment. Kyle's name flashes several times across the screen as the cell phone groans and vibrates on the counter.

Briefly, Kyle is in the room with us, sharing her warmth and vitality and love.

Then the ringing stops, and the phone ceases its uncanny protest.

We lose the connection and are forced back to our grim scene.

Shealagh is still kneeling by Damon, wedged into a tight corner between his head, the IV pole, and various life support machines. It's hard for her to keep twisting and bending low to avoid the mass of equipment, so she tries to come out of her corner. But she quickly becomes enmeshed in a thicket of lines and wires, dropping to the ground to extricate herself and temporarily disappearing from sight. Almost immediately, Damon—as if to show the ICU staff he's not just alive but fully cognizant—notes his mother's absence, and he goes *ballistic*.

Damon thinks he's losing his mommy, and his face crumples. Invisible tears slash his eyes, and silent cries choke his respirator-clogged throat. His immobilized body writhes, and all his monitors go haywire.

You would not have thought Damon could look much worse, but he can. Because now he's not just suffering, he's *bereft*.

I alert Shealagh to what's happening and she rushes back, almost upending the IV pole and several monitors. She squeezes back into her corner and takes Damon's arm, placing her face directly alongside his. She whispers tenderly in her son's ear, until he's "calm" again.

Damon now has both his parents by his side, and there's a sense of completion. As if the outer ring of electrons has been filled, and he's stable again.

Except that Damon's *whole life* is decaying at an accelerated rate.

His blood pressure has dropped below 50, and he's crashing.

I start to kiss him over every available part of his face—his eyes, forehead, hair, cheek, nose—as I again tell him how perfect and beautiful he is. I'd been frustrated over the past week because I could not truly hug my son for fear of infecting him. But now all that has been mooted, if not mocked, and I just empty out my love and shower Damon with pent-up kisses.

I clasp as much of him as is claspable. His face is all busted up and taped over, but I can still see his beauty.

Shealagh is weeping as she sings softly into Damon's ear. She's had a terrible time these past years and been overwhelmed in so many ways, but in the end, she is strong for her son.

I've never felt weaker or more ineffectual. My son is dying before my eyes, and I don't know how to save him. There is no action in the entire universe I would not undertake on his behalf, but I have no action left to take.

I squeeze his hand and tell him how the two of us are going to go pick apples in Oregon. Damon's pupils flash wanly and he gives me a feeble squeeze back, or so I imagine.

Then he continues to fade.

His blood pressure has dropped below 40.

There's not a single life support system or drug that can help him any longer.

His body is completely inert, and his eyes are hollowing out.

Damon is collapsing, and the ICU vultures are buzzing again. They've stopped even pretending to sustain him and have turned off the CVVH machine.

They're just standing around, waiting for him to die.

It's effectively over, except that Damon is *still* with us. He's *still* hanging on, and I *still* can't accept the situation or give up on him.

"D-man, listen to me!" I lift my voice and appeal to him as if we're fellow soldiers fighting in the trenches and we could still win this war. "I want you to forget all these goddamn machines and this whole ridiculous setup here! Forget this silly hospital and all these silly doctors. Just go deep *inside*. I know you have the strength—it's time to use it. Okay?" I pump my fists, as I have so often for him, and urge Damon on with every fiber of my fraught being. "Come on, D-man, let's bust out of this joint and just go *home*!"

During Damon's first open-heart surgery, when he was six months old and weighed eleven pounds and things looked very bleak, I would shadow-box ferociously around his ICU bed—while his mobile played "Send in the Clowns"—and try to infuse my firstborn with the fighting spirit. So now I repeat my desperate exhortation, louder and fiercer each time—"Let's just blow this joint, D-man!"—while the impatient doctors smile and try to mask their disdain. They can't wait to shut everything off, including me, the ridiculous, pathetic father who's clearly in denial.

But my son hears me. From some region deep inside his stricken body— a place of love, and courage, and pride, and transcendent will—he starts responding.

The nurses and technicians stop in their tracks. Everyone looks stupefied. Damon's blood pressure has stopped dropping, and it begins to *rise*!

His numbers suddenly start to go up instead of down.

They climb out of their hole and keep climbing.

It's like a fantasy, a wish fulfillment, except it's measurably, verifiably real.

Damon's pressure reaches all the way to 90/70, which is viable. As if he's suddenly sprouted wings and lifted himself above certain disaster.

It has no physiological basis. It contradicts all the numbers and indicators. It's screwy. How can he reverse death?

I yell out my encouragement and applaud Damon's tour de force, a father overwhelmed by a command performance he asked for but never fully expected.

"Go, D-man, go! You're doing it, guy! Yes! We're almost home!"

Damon keeps it up, like a magician or a levitator confounding all the laws of gravity.

Who in the end can say what's possible?

The red digits on his blood pressure monitor stay in the safety zone, despite every sign to the contrary. There's absolutely *nothing* holding them up, save for pure will and determination. And maybe an act of grace.

"See, Dad, I can do it!" Damon tells me in the only language he has left. "I can do anything!"

"Yes, you can, that's my amazing boy!" I squeeze his hand and kiss him ardently.

My son is giving me a beautiful, awe-inspiring farewell gift.

Or possibly rewriting the future for us all.

We stand bolted to the floor and pray he can somehow find a way to sustain this.

He does.

Damon persists, despite all the forces against him. He maintains his pressure and keeps it above the danger line. He holds on.

But no one, not even Damon, can perform miracles forever.

Slowly, he starts to sink again.

Then he *plummets*.

And now there's nothing and no one to catch Damon, because he takes the whole world with him.

It's terrible.

Damon is dying.

My son is disintegrating before my eyes.

He is passing away.

The light in his eyes is receding but it's still there, and I hang on to it and keep talking to him. I again tell him how much I love him. The light gets dimmer and dimmer, like the faint glow from a star that died out billions of years ago. But the dimness remains visible, like a flickering shadow, even as it continues fading and receding. I track it to the most distant, infinitesimal lair in his pupil and I keep groping for single particles of him, like a man just struck blind, who still remembers the light and "sees" it as an afterimage even when it's gone.

Then there is true and total darkness.

Damon's indomitable spirit flies off, leaving only his body.

I hold my son, weeping, and kiss him all over his face.

The blood pressure monitor goes to zero, and they shut it off.

Dr. Mason puts on her condolence face, the shocked bystander, as Dr. Verani steps briskly forward and moves to separate me from my son, whom I'm still clasping. She takes possession of his body, wresting it away from me with cool efficiency, as if I no longer have the right to hold what's left of him and it belongs to her.

"I'm so sorry, Damon is *dead*."

Epilogue

Damon Daniel Weber died on March 30, 2005 — three days before my fiftieth birthday.

That's a misleading statement, since no one you love dies once.

Especially not a sixteen-year-old boy who was your first child.

They die for you repeatedly, over and over. You are condemned to relive their death, and to try to prevent it, and to fail, every time.

And how do you go on?

Your choices are despair, self-termination, numbness, violence, the law (socially sanctioned revenge), letting go (forgetting), starting over (razing the past), and the consolations of nature, society, philosophy, religion, fantasy, or art.

But nothing can change what happened, or bring back what's gone.

The hospital wanted us to leave the room right after Damon died, so they could make him look "like himself" again. We couldn't grasp what they meant — they seemed unnaturally excited, as if they could undo what we'd just witnessed.

We ignored them — they had zero credibility with us by this point — but eventually we had to leave the room for air, and when we came back, we were horrified at what they so proudly unveiled for our approval. They had removed all of Damon's tubes and IV lines and covered up his bloated, bruised arms. They had combed his hair and wiped his face and cleaned up his swollen features, even spreading shiny Vaseline across his cracked lips.

But this transparent makeover made him look far *less* like himself and more like a hollow, tidied-up corpse.

He was truly gone now.

The hospital wanted to know, delicately and without pushing us, but as soon as we could possibly tell them, because they couldn't hold it forever, what our plans were for *the body*.

I drew a total blank, since the thought that Damon might not walk out of that hospital alive had never crossed my mind. Shealagh suggested calling Rabbi Kloner, who was responsive and helpful, proving, if proof be needed, that religion still has a role to play in modern life.

Sonja came to pick us up from the hospital. We drove home in a state of shock but realized that despite the late hour and our desire to grant our two remaining children even one more night of peace, we had to wake them up and break the news immediately. The tragedy would alter their lives regardless of when we told them about it, but they'd never forgive us if we held back the information for even one hour. We could no longer pretend we had any control.

We woke Sam up in his room and told him, then we went upstairs into Miranda's room and told her, and then the four of us huddled together on the king-size mattress in our bedroom, sobbing and clinging to one another like shipwrecked survivors on a raft.

The following day we had to take care of funeral business and suffer through the unspeakable agony of picking out a casket for Damon.

I had to write an obituary for my son, an unnatural act. I ignored the steep per-word charge—the obituary wound up costing us as much as the funeral, but words matter to me, and I had many different kinds of debt to repay—and then I begged *The New York Times* to include a photograph, because I knew Damon's face would have a bigger impact than all my words.

Sitting around our kitchen table that first stunned morning, Shealagh, Sam, Miranda, and I decided that in lieu of flowers, we would ask that any contributions be sent to an award established in Damon's name. Since theater had been his first love and since Brooklyn Tech had been his final theater home, on the spot we created the Damon Weber Theater Prize at Brooklyn Technical High School. The annual award would recognize a promising student at Damon's school who excelled in acting, directing, or writing for the theater.

The New York Times obituary with Damon's photo was published on

April 4. There was also a prominent story in the *New York Post*, accompanied by the same photo, only bigger, and headlined "Tragic Teen Star." The *Post* article began:

> Grieving family members are working to boost a Brooklyn high school's theater program in memory of their son—a teen actor who died a little more than a week after making his breakthrough television debut.

The story quoted the heartbroken father, the Brooklyn Tech principal, and the television writer David Milch, whose comments were reported thus:

> David Milch, the creator and executive producer of *Deadwood*, who worked with Damon in Santa Clarita, Calif., for two weeks over the summer, said, "He was wonderful . . . In his moment, and in the work that he was doing with us, he was perfect."

The *New York Times* obituary and the *New York Post* article, as well as the wide nexus of people we knew, generated hundreds of condolence cards and e-mails. A surprising number of actors, many who did not know Damon, wrote out of solidarity with one of their own. Among the many affecting notes we received, Shealagh and I were struck by a letter from Andre Lawe, Damon's Jamaican-born home instructor who spent many hours with Damon during his last year—when not preparing for exams, the two were often up to their eyeballs in mischief:

> I never believed in an angel, that is until I met Damon. How could one continue to doubt when his presence spoke such kindness?
>
> We often talked about different things, movies, music, school and life. Yet he was never uncomfortable to speak about the battles he was facing. I often remarked about his strength and determination: added to that he never showed a sign of fear. Through his reflection, I saw myself and how much I fell short. For I could never become the kind of human being he was. But then no human could ever be like him because he was above us. It was clear that heaven had loaned us an angel.

We held the funeral service at Temple Beth Emeth in Brooklyn, the same synagogue where Damon had his Bar Mitzvah. The place was packed—Rabbi Kloner could not recall seeing it so full, except during the High Holy Days.

Perhaps the most unexpected and strangely gratifying sight was watching over a hundred students and teenagers filling the front pews. It turned out Damon was known by far more than his own circle of friends and was something of a local legend at Brooklyn Tech. The small, smiling redheaded boy who could, and did, talk to everyone, displaying easy confidence, natural empathy, and an engaging wit, had been dubbed by many, anomalously, as "the coolest kid in the school." And even those who did not subscribe to this view knew who Damon was. Most of these kids had never confronted death, certainly not of a peer, and they showed up in force, with shocked, uncomprehending, and grief-struck faces.

Their vital, teeming presence, with tender hearts on sleeves, helped us get through.

The worst moment for me came just before we started, when the funeral home director took me aside and explained that as a matter of procedure, someone had to identify Damon's body. We agreed to spare the rest of the family, so the two of us went to the front of the stage, where the wooden coffin rested on a stand. The director lifted the lid of the casket. I saw a wax dummy of Damon, a compact, bloated figure with a puffy face and a big, coarse coif of red hair that was the empty outline of my son. I nodded, and the director closed the lid.

I still haven't shaken that image.

Several people spoke about Damon. Keith came up with WWDD, for "What Would Damon Do?" describing Damon's wise judgment and resourcefulness as a guide for life. Max and Zak recalled Damon's utterly fearless, grinning stage dive into the crowd during a rock concert, and how they envied his sublime confidence that someone would catch him. Kyle's love and heartbreak over the loss of her lifelong friend and confidante shone through every word she uttered. Andre Lawe, who was so late I thought we'd need to scrub him, emerged at the last moment from the shadows like a spectral figure or a heavenly messenger himself and imparted his deep, mellow spirituality with rueful aplomb. Krista talked about Damon as a serious and selfless student of theater, and announced that a second prize honoring him, the Damon Weber Award for Artistry and Citizenship, was being established by the NYU Looking for Shakespeare program. And Paula Malcomson, in a gesture of pure loving kindness, flew in from Los Angeles to speak about working with Damon on the set of *Deadwood*. Paula's dazzling blondness added a touch of glamour and evoked Damon's own shining radiance.

Sonja gave a physician's perspective on Damon's illness and praised his heroism, as well as that of his parents in battling a flawed system. My mother, Helga, was terse and eloquent about the loss of her beloved grandson, and Sam, normally shy in public, was brave in standing up before the entire assembly, his voice shaking, and expressing his enormous love and admiration for his older brother and his undying gratitude for all Damon had taught him. "He didn't just tell me, he showed me!" It was Sam's twelfth birthday, and though he would stand in the same spot a year later for his own Bar Mitzvah, he had just stepped out in a big way for the first time.

Shealagh and Miranda stood with Sam and me but were too distraught to speak.

I provided a brief narrative of Damon's life and a context for his death, since many people had no idea what had happened beyond the brute fact of his demise. I also thanked all the people who helped us along the way. Among the myriad scenes from Damon's rich but truncated life, I recalled the day in Truro, Massachusetts, when Damon and I built a sand castle on Ballston Beach and then spent four frantic hours battling the incoming tide, furiously retreating, redigging, and rebuilding our original structure and refusing to let our drenched mud mound be swept away, until, exhausted and sweaty, with our muscles and fingernails aching and the light fading, we finally declared sweet victory as the tide peaked and our puny flag was still flying.

There were many other scenes and memories but what most concerned me as I spoke was hewing to the high road and not letting my carefully contained wrath spill out. I had a bitter, trembling sense of fury and outrage locked up in my heart along with my grief, and I knew with a certainty, just as the sun rises every morning, that as soon as this was over, I would have to strap on my armor and go to war in an all-out hunt for justice if it was the last thing I did.

But that was for later, and though it had to be done, I knew it wouldn't bring Damon back. Right now, I could not let any of those feelings mar the beauty that was Damon's life, nor detract from our obligation to mourn my extraordinary son with full rites and honors.

We drove from the synagogue in Brooklyn to the cemetery in the Bronx. David had flown in from Seattle and, along with Sonja, helped us manage the carpool logistics. My parents sat with us in the first limo.

We had been at Woodlawn Cemetery a decade earlier for the funeral of Peggy Day, Shealagh's maternal great-aunt, but this was an altogether different affair. The Days had been a prominent New York family—Ben Day, who gave his name to a form of engraving, owned the New York *Sun*, the main city paper in the nineteenth century, and his relations were prosperous bankers and inventors, while Peggy's celebrated husband, Clarence Day, authored *Life with Father*, the Broadway hit of its decade, which became a classic Hollywood film. Damon had spent many great summers with us at Peggy's house in Truro and enjoyed extended heart-to-hearts with the sharp, vivacious bluestocking who remained the life of any party into her nineties. Now Damon would be laid to rest beside Peggy, whose lifespan had exceeded his by a multiple of six.

We were directed to the tranquil, tree-shaded family plot with the successive generations laid out in simple granite markers. The site was dominated by a high stone sculpture depicting a handsome Victorian mother reading from an open book to her tousle-haired son, who sits on her lap in his plus fours and gazes up with adoration and wonder. The rough approximation of Shealagh and Damon, and of the scene I had just witnessed in the hospital, was almost unbearable.

We stood in a wide, forlorn circle around the open gravesite. Shealagh's cousin Rory spoke briefly about the Days and their openness to all comers, welcoming the Webers. My father, his voice quavering, read a melancholic poem from Sir Walter Scott, "Coronach," and I read a defiant dirge from Dylan Thomas, "And Death Shall Have No Dominion." (I had asked my friend John Farrell, a literature professor, for any relevant father-son passages from Shakespeare or the classics, and he had consulted several colleagues, but to our surprise there seemed to be very little.)

We sang two songs: "He's Got the Whole World in His Hands," which Damon had played on the piano when he first got home from his transplant—the songbook on our living room piano was still open to this page when we returned from the hospital for the last time—and "The World's Greatest" by R. Kelly, an R & B favorite of Damon's that Sam had astutely suggested. The mood was very grim and somber and when the singing started to falter, Kyle's musician father, Andre, stepped in with his strong, melodious voice and helped lift and carry us over the hump.

By the time Rabbi Kloner recited the Burial Kaddish and they started lowering the coffin into the ground, there was a hush, followed by quiet sobbing. A few teenagers broke down and wept openly. Shealagh had her arms around Sam and Miranda, all propping each other up and crying quietly, while I stood closest to the grave, almost on top of it, on my own. No one could come near me now because I was completely focused on Damon. I watched a wooden box bearing his remains knock against the sides of the freshly dug pit as it was hoisted down unevenly by creaky pulleys. I made Damon a last promise about setting things right, and I gave him a last kiss. I knew that what was being buried was not just the body of my sixteen-years-and-eight-months-old son, or a big part of me and of my family, but also a normal vision of life.

We sat shiva for the requisite seven days and kept an open house, thanks to very kind neighbors who pitched in. They formed shifts and took turns helping in the kitchen with food and drink and cleaning up at night. For "shiva furniture"—plain wooden benches—the funeral home dropped off two flimsy cardboard boxes, so absurd and useless they made Sam and Miranda giggle hysterically. Mostly we sat out on patio furniture in our backyard by the peach tree and the fig tree that Damon had only recently helped me prune.

For the first days we were surrounded by relatives and good friends from high school and college and beyond, and it was almost like a reunion. But then this group started to leave, and we felt raw and exposed again. Shealagh withdrew to her bed, and I had to greet the remaining visitors on behalf of the family. Many kind people, including professional colleagues and strangers who'd known Damon, or whose children had known Damon, continued to come and pay their respects. Sonja manned the phone and answered the door in the best English butler tradition, until she needed to return home. David, who gave me a personal outlet, had to go back to his family. And then, bereft of these two best friends and buffers, we felt the full chill again.

On the last day of shiva, I received a rejection letter from the writing program I'd applied to. I'd completely forgotten about my application and had been warned I was taking a step back by returning to school, but it was still a rejection in an area that mattered to me—or would have mattered to me if I could have felt anything. I was so numb by this point, I couldn't register any sensation, like a frozen man who must look down to grasp that he's been shot in the stomach. I knew the bullet holes couldn't be a good sign, even if I didn't feel any pain, and that they meant something else I cared deeply about had just been taken from me. I tried resigning myself with a fatalistic shrug—maybe it was for the best, since I was losing *everything* at the same time—when I heard a dim, defiant voice, like the guardian of my own soul, react angrily on my behalf to this attempted double burial. *Not only do you kill my boy, but now you want to kill the boy in me!*

We decided we needed a complete getaway, so after the shiva, Shealagh, Sam, Miranda, and I flew to Newfoundland, Canada, where we'd never been before, nor did we know a soul. It had the advantage of being stark and beautiful and situated on the very edge of the continent.

We stayed in a modest hotel overlooking the harbor in St. John's, ate in family restaurants, and hiked and explored the area, involuntarily reconstituting ourselves as a family of four. Everywhere we went, we saw and felt Damon's presence—in the close, smiling face of the chalky moon on Signal Hill and in the wild, wind-whipped promontory of Cape Spear. We kept active during the day, and at night we all bedded down in the same room and cried ourselves quietly to sleep.

We returned to New York. I went back to work and Sam and Miranda went back to school. Shealagh stayed home.

My wife and I repeatedly discussed the unsettling events leading to our son's death. He'd had a successful heart transplant and was doing well, and we were both convinced he need not have died if the hospital had only followed the standard treatment protocol. But we needed to be sure we hadn't missed something or overreacted emotionally.

We did a cold chronology and ran it backward and forward. We searched for alternative explanations. Shealagh became obsessed with researching everything known about the infection that had killed Damon. She spent hundreds of hours online, staying up all night to track down arcane studies and references. I conducted less research, though I read Shealagh's material, because I had done the deepest dive possible in the hospital the night before Damon died, and I knew what had happened. But part of me still wanted to discover we were wrong and it was all inevitable, so we could absolve ourselves, as well as the hospital, of responsibility and not have to deal with dredging it all up, reliving the horror, and accusing such a formidable, renowned institution.

In the end, the evidence was even more overwhelming than we'd understood. EBV infection was not some rare event but appeared in all the literature, underlined and in bold, as one of the most common and dangerous—if not *the* most common and dangerous—of all threats for patients like Damon. It was routinely described as "the bugaboo of heart transplants." Yet Dr. Mason and her team of four, who provided little continuity of care but instead rotated shifts so no one was ever fully responsible—"the person responsible is the person on call," Mason would state at her deposition, denying that even as *medical director* she had any ongoing responsibility—never treated Damon for EBV-driven PTLD until the battle was already lost.

Why hadn't the hospital treated Damon for EBV infection at the time he first presented as a high-risk patient with every symptom of this notorious, well-documented killer, and with no sign of rejection? Dr. Mason would later admit under oath that once the hospital knew Damon's donor was positive for EBV, they should have been on the lookout for any indications of EBV infection, and that infection was as common a complication as rejection. Yet she and her team persistently ignored every symptom of EBV infection and kept treating Damon for rejection—the opposite treatment!

But Dr. Mason knew what treatment she *should* have administered because, as we soon learned, in 2004, over a year *before* Damon's death, she coauthored, with Dr. Sanford, a chapter on pediatric heart transplantation in a Columbia textbook. Writing as an acknowledged expert, Dr. Mason advised practitioners that when a patient develops PTLD from an EBV infection, as Damon had, "treatment for the disease includes reduction or temporary cessation of immunosuppression. This approach is effective in the majority of cases."

Yet she never followed her own advice and gave Damon a chance.

Why had Dr. Mason *increased* Damon's immune suppression instead of *decreasing* it and letting his body use its normal defenses to fight off this infection in its earlier stages, as she told fellow professionals was the standard of care?

Damon was the toughest fighter I ever knew but it turned out the hospital not only didn't help him, they actually *prevented* him from fighting back with his own strength. When they upped his immune suppression, they disabled his natural defense system and left him exposed to EBV and then PTLD, choking off his ability to defend himself and rendering him effectively powerless.

Outraged and sickened, Shealagh and I agreed we had no choice but to try to initiate legal action against Dr. Mason, her fellow physicians, and Columbia for Damon's death. We didn't have the resources to hire a team of lawyers to take on the powerful hospital and the well-heeled doctors, so we sought representation on a contingency basis. We knew it would be costly for any attorneys to challenge this hospital and these doctors, so it wasn't easy. But Shealagh and I felt we owed it to Damon to demand accountability for what had happened and to fight for him even after he was gone. We also owed it to our children, Samuel and Miranda, and to ourselves. And we owed it to other children and other parents we did not know because we believed we might prevent future disasters by exposing the responsible parties and their misguided practices.

On Father's Day weekend, I drove Sam to northern Vermont to begin a summer session of circus camp. He'd seen a performance of Circus Smirkus in Oak Bluffs, Massachusetts, and decided it would be cool to join a youth circus. We took a leisurely two days for the drive and wallowed in the motel pool, played basketball, and went to the movies on the way up. It was gratifying to just hang out and be together.

But by Sunday afternoon, our first Father's Day without Damon, Sam and I were both relieved when I dropped him off with his new peers at the camp. In the car driving back on my own, a cascade of emotions suddenly poured out, and I found myself crying and screaming at the top of my lungs, during which time I flew past every vehicle on the road, including a Dodge Charger driven by a Vermont state trooper, who was not too pleased about being overtaken. After the angry trooper warned me to keep my hands on the steering wheel, and after he ran my license and registration through his computer, he seemed to ease up, as if he knew I was not a threat and could smell the tang of sadness and tears suffusing the interior of my car.

"Lots on your mind, huh?" the trooper said. He was a tall, rangy young man.

"Buried my son a little while ago."

He'd heard a lot of lines but he knew this wasn't one. The trooper shook his head. "I couldn't imagine that . . . But you don't want to hurt your family any more, do you? You need to drive more carefully." He handed back my license and let me go.

Miranda insisted on celebrating Father's Day the next day, a Monday, so as soon I got home from the office, she blindfolded me and led me downstairs to the kitchen, where she had strung a big HAPPY FATHER'S DAY! banner and wrapped lots of tiny presents in pretty paper. There was a handsome table and wineglasses with flower petals on the rims. Miranda gave me a bronze quill pen with a long feather, a tub of ink, and a bound leather notebook.

"Everyone buys you books to read, Dad, but I want you to write one!" She gave me a sweet kiss, then lingered near my face to discover my various imperfections.

Miranda didn't want to go to sleepaway camp like Sam but she took horseback riding lessons daily. She did well, training hard and advancing in dressage and cross-country and jumping. She also mucked out the stables and took younger kids on rides.

Shealagh donated a ton of psychology textbooks to the Salvation Army and washed her hands of her former profession. A gifted craftsperson, she decided to take up furniture restoration, a longtime interest—Damon, among others, had encouraged her to pursue this—and the following year, she decamped to Wales for a renowned summer course in furniture making, specializing in chairs. We converted our garage into a state-of-the-art workshop for her.

In August of that first summer, we settled for several weeks in our country place in the Catskill Park. Sam and Miranda didn't want to sleep alone in the low upstairs bedroom where all three children had stayed for so many years, playing games and listening to Damon's bedtime stories, so their devoted mother became an honorary sibling and slept beside them in Damon's bed.

On Monday, August 8, I was sitting in the one-room writing shack, where Damon would bring me a mug of morning coffee from the main house and signal brunch was imminent—I could hear his high rubber boots scraping across the grass and then the slow creak of the screen door as he knocked politely before he pushed into my lair and his golden smile lit up the whole place as he handed me the steaming coffee, his bright eyes settling on my computer screen or a book on my shelf that he'd ask me about with his warm, inquisitive bird's gaze. On that day, which would've been Damon's seventeenth birthday, I found myself starting to write this memoir about Damon.

It was the one gift I could still give him, and give to the rest of my family. And it was the only place I had left to go for myself, since I could not abide living in a Damon-less world.

I entered my first Olympic triathlon a month later. I knew I was ill prepared but the race had become linked for me with Damon, so there was no backing down. And I had the advantage of knowing I could suffer through anything. The man in the transition area beside me was an Israeli who'd lost his leg in the Lebanon war and competed with a prosthetic limb, which he took off for the swim and strapped back on for the bike and the run.

Our family attended weekly sessions at the Healing Center, a modest Brooklyn facility focused on helping children cope with loss. Sam and Miranda enjoyed going to the Volcano Room to whale away at padded objects. They kept diaries and read from them. Shealagh and I also found solace in our tiny parents' group, no more than four people at one time. We met another woman who'd lost her child after a heart transplant at Columbia under

Dr. Mason's care. We did not know the details of her case, but even the Healing Center staff commented on this remarkable coincidence.

In the fall, we found a law firm who felt our case had merit, and in the spring of 2006, a week before the first anniversary of Damon's death—and a month before the first Damon Weber Theater Prize was awarded at Brooklyn Tech in an emotional ceremony attended by a hundred and fifty people—we filed suit against Dr. Mason and New York-Presbyterian Hospital/Columbia University Medical Center, alleging carelessness, negligence, and malpractice in Damon's death. We also registered a complaint against Dr. Mason with the New York State Department of Health Office of Professional Medical Conduct. I felt, along with the memoir I had started writing about Damon, that I was keeping my promise to my son.

On the first anniversary of Damon's death, we visited his gravesite in Woodlawn Cemetery. My parents, my sister, and several of Damon's friends had paid their respects earlier and left poems and other mementos. Shealagh, Sam, Miranda, and I spent a few heartbreaking hours at the site, planting bright yellow daffodils and arranging colorful marbles on top of his grave, then going off separately to be alone, until none of us could take it anymore, and we left.

We did the same thing the next year, and the year after.

In August 2009, five days before Damon would have turned twenty-one, Amelia Mason, after failing for three years to produce Damon's medical records, testified at her deposition that all of Damon's preoperative and postoperative clinical records had been shipped to an off-site storage facility and "could not be located despite multiple best efforts." New York-Presbyterian Hospital/Columbia University Medical Center, one of the foremost medical centers in the country, if not in the world, had apparently lost all the most critical medical information pertaining to Damon's heart transplant and the post-transplant infection that killed him.

On Damon's twenty-first birthday, we all visited the cemetery once again.

What do people mean when they talk about a mourning period, or any fixed limit on sorrow and loss, as if it had an expiration date, after which it is no longer valid?

Damon Daniel Weber officially died on March 30, 2005, except no one that you love dies once or ever stops not being alive, and nothing you do can change what happened or bring back what's gone.

Nevertheless, you can still fight—for truth, justice, beauty, memory, love, and the fiercely evolving human future . . .

Damon, three years old and smiling on a wintry January evening, is buttoned up in a snug navy blue and bottle green anorak and a Thomas the Tank Engine wool hat to match. We're strolling along the southwest perimeter of Prospect Park when a light snow starts to fall. The redheaded child glances up at the sky with his bright blue eyes and puts out his hands to touch the twinkling white confetti. The crystalline particles dissolve in his palms, delicate and wet and vaporous. Delighted, he yanks off his cap so he can feel the glistening snow drops on his hair and his face, raising his beaming gaze skyward. He lets the vanilla fractals tickle his nose.

We're about to tell him to put the cap back on so he won't catch cold, but he's having too much fun, running in circles and chasing the scurrying flakes like elusive white butterflies in a rain forest. Besides, the air is pleasant, almost balmy. And Damon's excitement is contagious. Shealagh and I feel inspired by this sudden burst of animation from our exuberant only child.

Damon is beguiled and transfixed by the miracle of snow. He marvels as the clustering, diamond-shaped flakes settle over the ground and the trees, transforming all around him into an enchanted white playground. He pumps his arms in the air and stamps his feet and begins to dash through the carpeted streets in an ecstatic rampage. He runs and yelps and cavorts, shaking his fists at the sky in a blizzard of joy, a madcap snow dance before the gods of the upper air.

Shealagh and I chase after our son, sprinting to catch up with this dervish, who's whooping and hollering as if there is no tomorrow.

The heavenly firmament is raining down its glittering alabaster treasure, and Damon can't believe this bounty. He wants to touch it and smell it and taste it, but most of all, to celebrate it. He keeps dashing through the streets with giddy, outstretched arms, pounding the snowy asphalt with his little legs and reaching for the fertile sky, as if he could grasp and salute all nature's glory in one great, grinning embrace.

He's the happiest little boy in the world, and his face is filled with wonder at the unfolding and eternal splendor of life.

Grahamsville, NY 8/8/05—Windsor Terrace, Brooklyn—Isle of Skye, Scotland—The Writers Room, New York City—Truro, Massachusetts—Vegas Diner, Bay Ridge—Delta Airlines—Oak Bluffs, Martha's Vineyard—F train, IRT Line—*Grahamsville, NY 8/8/09*

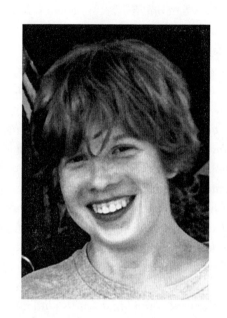

Author's Note

On more than one occasion, Damon—who knew me as well as anyone ever has, and who was rarely off point—would walk up and say, "You should write a children's book, Dad." I always felt vaguely flattered but also a little guilty as, unlike many writers, I'd never even *considered* writing a children's book. Even within our family, my father Robert was the real storyteller and my wife Shealagh the most engaging story reader. So I wasn't sure what to make of my son's idea, which he seemed to repeat with increasing conviction over the years, going so far as to wag his finger and smile at me with his bright-eyed, preternatural wisdom.

"*You*—you should write a children's book, Dad!"

Baffled but intrigued, I resolved that if ever I *did* write a children's book, it would be about Damon in some way.

So now, as I approach my acknowledgments, it strikes me that perhaps *Immortal Bird* is the book Damon meant. It is not a children's book in the traditional sense, but it is about a child and his growth to the verge of young adulthood. It is a book about Damon's life, tragically cut short, and although I labored over it for several years, in one sense it is the most involuntary thing I've ever written. While the material was dauntingly painful and I found myself taking frequent emotional breaks—literally lying down to catch my breath as I waited for the paralyzing anguish to pass—I never experienced a whiff of writer's block or the hesitation or uncertainty that comes from creative impasse. This book *always* had momentum and a sure sense of purpose, and it *always* had Damon's bright spirit and his palpable presence behind it. I knew what I had to do from the start and my son guided and kept me company while I did it, staying with me to the very end.

The son is father to the man, and in this instance, perhaps the real author of the book.

Acknowledgments

As I stumbled in the darkness following Damon's death, two friends encouraged me to write a book about him. As obvious as that may now seem, then it came to me as a revelation and a lifeline. I wish to thank David Milch, the writer and television producer, and Nancy Milford, the biographer and teacher, for their personal advice during that difficult period.

My first reader was the journalist and author Katherine Eban and she played a key role in steering me to a first-person account. Katherine was an excellent sounding board throughout and revealed herself to be a first-rate editor as well as a kind friend.

Kathy Robbins, the first and only agent I approached with this manuscript, agreed to represent me after reading sixty pages, which changed the whole course of this book. I've never had a literary agent in my corner before—I've published three books and written several others—and it really makes a difference. And no one does it better than Kathy, a dedicated, morally centered professional with an incisive grasp of the creative process and the marketplace. Kathy and two of her agency associates, Rachelle Bergstein and Michael Gillespie, gave me excellent notes and feedback throughout. I thank Rachelle and Mike and predict a great future for them both, and I salute Kathy for her generous spirit, sharp acumen, and tenacious, tough-minded engagement. She is a great agent and a good friend to have.

Among readers of the first draft, I wish to thank my wife Shealagh, my partner in all things Damon, for whom getting through these intensely personal pages took enormous courage; my parents Robert and Helga, who suffered their own deep loss but persevered; my longtime friend David Brumer, always there in every way; Arthur Singer Jr., the Joe DiMaggio of philanthropy, a barometer of intelligence, wise judgment, and good taste; the writer Richard Rhodes, a unique talent, and the psychologist Ginger Rhodes, his sympathetic wife; and Jason Epstein, an early champion, preparer of great feasts, and a legend, who seems either to have been involved in or present at the birth of virtually every important book and publishing development of the last half century.

I also sent the early ms to a dear college friend, the critic and editor Robert Tashman, who was dying at the time from pancreatic cancer. I didn't expect Bob to read it—I'm not sure I wanted him to, it was more a gesture of love—but he took time in his final months to peruse the first section. Bob was unusually positive and complimentary and then added, in that inimitable way dreaded by many well-known writers from his days at *Granta* and *The New York Review of Books*: "But I have some issues." Bob died before he could enumerate them but I know he's up in heaven, waiting to tell me, and I look forward, if I ever get there, to hashing them out with him.

Dr. Paul Marantz and Dr. Joseph Feldschuh, two outstanding physicians with broad knowledge and experience, reviewed the manuscript from a medical perspective. I thank them for their close and careful reading.

Michael Rudell, my literary lawyer, is one of the best-kept secrets around—those of us fortunate enough to work with him all know this—so I'm ambivalent about outing him. In the field of entertainment law, he is, truly, supreme. Michael was an early believer in me, long before this book, and he has provided wise counsel on multiple fronts over many years. I'm grateful to him and pleased to count him among my friends. Neil Rosini, a top attorney who works with Michael, reviewed my manuscript with impressive thoroughness and care.

Jonathan Karp, executive vice president and publisher at Simon & Schuster, responded swiftly to the draft manuscript with an immediate offer, always heartening to an author. A truly gifted and sensitive editor as well as a smart, savvy publisher, he oversees every aspect of production and marketing with a deft hand. Jon still has the look of a boy wonder, but he is a wise and accomplished man with real depth of feeling, and I am grateful for his unstinting support and consideration.

Among Jon's talented and committed team at Simon & Schuster, I'd also like to thank Nicholas Greene, editorial assistant; Loretta Denner, production editor; George Turianski, production manager; Christopher Lin, jacket designer; Jackie Seow, art director; Ruth Lee-Mui, interior designer; Alexis Welby, associate director of publicity; Jessica Abell, marketing coordinator; Marie Florio, rights manager: and Elisa Rivlin, general counsel.

My thanks also to Louise Quayle, foreign rights director for The Robbins Office.

I wish to salute and thank Judith Donnel, Joseph Miklos and Joseph Awad of Silberstein, Awad and Miklos for representing us in our lawsuit against New York Presbyterian/Columbia University Medical Center. For those who question the value of trial lawyers, they give ordinary people without a voice a chance to seek justice and accountability from powerful institutions that might otherwise commit harm with impunity.

I must also acknowledge The Writers Room in New York City, the nation's oldest and largest urban writer's colony, where I've been a member since Damon's birth. I wrote my first books in The Writers Room and although I only managed to slip in for short stints on this manuscript, The Writers Room is a gift to all writers and my spiritual home. Its existence sustains me even when I'm not there, and its light burns 24/7, thanks in no small measure to its dedicated Board and its exceptional executive director, Donna Brodie.

Most of all, I could never have undertaken such a project without the explicit encouragement and support of my family. Shealagh, Sam and Miranda each agreed they wanted me to tell Damon's story and all generously shared their recollections as best they could. I especially wish to thank Shealagh, for whom reliving these events was unspeakably painful. I incorporated every memory or scene she shared, and I changed anything she asked. Nevertheless, this is a father's memoir, constrained by my experience and perspective, and as such it cannot possibly do justice to Shealagh's extraordinary love for Damon or her unique and amazingly close bond with her son. Rarely has a mother poured so much of herself and so much love into a child, or met with such reciprocal love and adoration. Nor can this memoir fully honor Sam and Miranda's love for their brother and their remarkably deep connection with him. It can only hint at what they all had, and lost.

My wife and children honored the long hours of work and seclusion this book demanded and stood with me in wanting to resurrect Damon for the world. Each, in his or her own way, made sacrifices to help bring this book into being. For all that and more, I am deeply and eternally grateful to my immortal family.

About the Author

Doron Weber was born in Israel, grew up in New York, and was educated at Brown University, the Sorbonne, and Oxford, where he was a Rhodes Scholar. He has worked as a newspaper boy, busboy, waiter, and taxi driver and is the coauthor of three published nonfiction books and various articles. For fifteen years he has directed programs at the Alfred P. Sloan Foundation, a nonprofit institution that supports science, education, and the arts.